Benign Prostatic Hyperplasia and Lower Urinary Tract Symptoms

Guest Editors

JERRY G. BLAIVAS, MD
JEFFREY P. WEISS, MD

UROLOGIC CLINICS
OF NORTH AMERICA

www.urologic.theclinics.com

November 2009 • Volume 36 • Number 4

SAUNDERS an imprint of ELSEVIER, Inc.

W.B. SAUNDERS COMPANY
A Division of Elsevier Inc.

1600 John F. Kennedy Blvd. ● Suite 1800 ● Philadelphia, PA 19103-2899

http://www.theclinics.com

UROLOGIC CLINICS OF NORTH AMERICA Volume 36, Number 4
November 2009 ISSN 0094-0143, ISBN-13: 978-1-4377-1279-7, ISBN-10: 1-4377-1279-7

Editor: Kerry Holland

Urologic Clinics of North America (ISSN 0094-0143) is published quarterly by Elsevier Inc., 360 Park Avenue South, New York, NY 10010-1710. Months of issue are February, May, August, and November. Business and Editorial Offices: 1600 John F. Kennedy Blvd., Suite 1800, Philadelphia, PA 19103-2899. Periodicals postage paid at New York, NY and additional mailing offices. Subscription prices are $291.00 per year (US individuals), $463.00 per year (US institutions), $333.00 per year (Canadian individuals), $568.00 per year (Canadian institutions), $414.00 per year (foreign individuals), and $568.00 per year (foreign institutions). Foreign air speed delivery is included in all *Clinics* subscription prices. All prices are subject to change without notice. **POSTMASTER:** Send address changes to *Urologic Clinics of North America*, Elsevier Health Sciences Division, Subscription Customer Service, 3251 Riverport Lane, Maryland Heights, MO 63043. Customer Service: 1-800-654-2452 (US). From outside the United States, call 1-314-447-8871. Fax: 1-314-447-8029. E-mail: JournalsCustomerServiceusa@elsevier.com (for print support) and JournalsOnlineSupport-usa@elsevier.com (for online support).

Reprints. For copies of 100 or more, of articles in this publication, please contact the Commercial Reprints Department, Elsevier Inc., 360 Park Avenue South, New York, New York 10010-1710. Tel.: 212-633-3813; Fax: 212-462-1935; E-mail: reprints@elsevier.com.

Urologic Clinics of North America is covered in MEDLINE/PubMed (*Index Medicus*), *Excerpta Medica, Current Contents/ Clinical Medicine, Science Citation Index,* and *ISI/BIOMED.*

Printed and bound by CPI Group (UK) Ltd, Croydon, CR0 4YY

Transferred to Digital Print 2011

Contributors

GUEST EDITORS

JERRY G. BLAIVAS, MD
Clinical Professor of Urology, Weill Cornell
Medical College, Department of Urology,
New York; Adjunct Professor
of Urology, Department of Urology,
SUNY Downstate Medical School,
Brooklyn, New York

JEFFREY P. WEISS, MD, FACS
Professor of Urology, SUNY Downstate
Medical School, Brooklyn; The James
Buchanan Brady Foundation, Department of
Urology, Weill Medical College of Cornell
University, New York, New York

AUTHORS

GREGORY B. AUFFENBERG, MD
Department of Urology, Feinberg School
of Medicine, Northwestern University,
Chicago, Illinois

JERRY G. BLAIVAS, MD
Clinical Professor of Urology, Weill Cornell
Medical College, Department of Urology,
New York; Adjunct Professor of Urology, SUNY
Downstate Medical School, Department of
Urology, Brooklyn,
New York

WADE BUSHMAN, MD, PhD
Robert and Delores Schnoes Professor
of Urology, Department of Urology, University
of Wisconsin Medical School, Clinical Science
Center, Madison, Wisconsin

ROBERT F. DONNELL, MD, FACS
The Department of Urology, The Medical
College of Wisconsin, Milwaukee,
Wisconsin

BRIAN T. HELFAND, MD, PhD
Department of Urology, Feinberg School
of Medicine, Northwestern University,
Chicago, Illinois

KARL J. KREDER, MD
Professor and Vice Chair, Department
of Urology, University of Iowa, Iowa City, Iowa

BRIAN V. LE, MD, MA
Resident, Department of Urology
Northwestern University, Feinberg
School of Medicine, Chicago, Illinois

GARY E. LEACH, MD
Director, Institute for Continence,
Tower Urology, Los Angeles, California

LORI B. LERNER, MD
Assistant Professor of Urology, Section
of Urology, VA Boston Healthcare System;
Boston University School of Medicine, Boston,
Massachusetts

KEVIN T. McVARY, MD, FACS
Department of Urology, Feinberg School
of Medicine, Northwestern University,
Chicago, Illinois

JENNIFER L. MEHDIZADEH, MD
Fellow, Tower Urology, Los Angeles,
California

STEVEN P. PETROU, MD
Professor of Urology, Consultant,
Department of Urology, Mayo Medical
School, Mayo Clinic Florida, Jacksonville,
Florida

CHARLES R. POWELL, MD
Assistant Professor, Department of Urology,
Indiana University School of Medicine,
Indianapolis, Indiana

MATTHEW P. RUTMAN, MD
Assistant Professor, Department of Urology,
Columbia University College of Physicians
and Surgeons, New York, New York

ANTHONY J. SCHAEFFER, MD
Chair, Department of Urology Northwestern
University, Feinberg School of Medicine,
Chicago, Illinois

DAVID D. THIEL, MD
Assistant Professor of Urology, Senior
Associate Consultant, Department of Urology,
Mayo Medical School, Mayo Clinic Florida,
Jacksonville, Florida

DANIEL A. THORNER, DO
Department of Urology, SUNY Downstate
Medical School, Brooklyn, New York

MARK D. TYSON, BS
Dartmouth Medical School, Hanover, Hanover,
New Hampshire

JEFFREY P. WEISS, MD, FACS
Professor of Urology, SUNY Downstate
Medical School, Brooklyn; The James
Buchanan Brady Foundation, Department of
Urology, Weill Medical College of Cornell
University, New York, New York

MATTHEW S. WOSNITZER, MD
Department of Urology, Columbia University
College of Physicians and Surgeons, New
York, New York

Contents

Historically, benign prostatic hyperplasia (BPH) has been a major focus of urologic practice and surgery. But a simplistic causal relationship among prostatic enlargement, progressive obstruction, lower urinary tract symptoms, retention, and complications of retention has been challenged by recognition of the incomplete overlap of prostatic enlargement with symptoms and obstruction. The result has been a greater focus on symptoms than prostatic enlargement and a shift from surgery to medical treatment. Therefore, the question can be asked whether BPH per se, the glandular enlargement as it contributes to bladder dysfunction, or hyperplastic enlargement as a biomarker for generalized lower urinary tract dysfunction are concerns. This article addresses these issues.

The approach to a patient with benign prostatic hyperplasia and lower urinary tract symptoms (LUTS) begins with a detailed history. The goal is to clearly identify the patient's urinary complaints, including frequency of micturition, urgency, urge incontinence, weak stream, the need to push or strain, hesitancy, intermittency, dysuria, and hematuria. Bladder diaries and symptom questionnaires are useful as adjuncts to information that is acquired in the history. The voiding diary is an essential part of the workup. The voiding diary differs from a simple frequency-volume chart in that it incorporates not only the frequency, voided volume, urge episodes, pad usage, and fluid intake but also the data related to patient activities. It allows patients to have a more thorough self-evaluation of their LUTS.

The role of urodynamics in the evaluation of lower urinary tract symptoms in men with benign prostatic hyperplasia is controversial despite the additional information regarding bladder function and outlet obstruction it provides. This controversy is primarily based on outcome studies that suggest men without proved bladder outlet obstruction may benefit from outlet reduction with medication or surgical resection. The aim of this article is to describe the role of urodynamic studies in the evaluation of benign prostatic hyperplasia, including illustration of existing urodynamic techniques, reviewing best practice guidelines and current literature, and providing recommendations for use of urodynamics in clinical practice.

Benign prostatic hyperplasia is characterized by smooth muscle and epithelial proliferation primarily within the prostatic transition zone that can cause a variety of problems for a patient, the most frequent being bothersome lower urinary tract symptoms. In most cases, medical therapy has become the first-line treatment modality of choice, with a variety of pharmacologic mechanisms proving to be beneficial. Several large trials have shown the efficacy of alpha-receptor blocking and 5-alpha reductase inhibiting medications when used alone and in combination. Newer data has shown the benefit of anti-muscarinic medications in specific populations who suffer from bladder outlet obstruction causing storage urinary symptoms. Phytotherapeutic supplements are numerous and used frequently; however, data supporting safety and efficacy is limited, making treatment recommendations difficult. The available clinical trial data for all of these types of therapy is discussed in this article.

Transurethral resection of the prostate (TURP) is the historical gold standard therapy for lower urinary tract symptoms secondary to obstruction from benign prostatic hyperplasia (BPH). Over the last 15 years, medical therapy (alpha blockers and 5-alpha-reductase inhibitors) and the advent of office-based prostatic ablation for BPH have altered the treatment landscape of men suffering from lower urinary tract symptoms. Efficacy and morbidity of newer minimally invasive surgical therapies are often compared with traditional TURP data from the 1960s and 1970s. Technologic improvements in lighting, resectoscope design, lens crafting, anesthetic care, and surgical technique have dramatically improved the efficacy, morbidity, and mortality of the modern TURP. This review outlines the indications, technique, and outcome data of the modern TURP and its variant, the saline bipolar TURP. Current indications and outcomes of simple prostatectomy (open, laparoscopic, and robotic) are also reviewed.

Laser-based treatments have emerged in the past 15 years as an alternative to transurethral resection of the prostate (TURP) for treatment of symptomatic benign prostatic hyperplasia. Increasing demand for a minimally invasive procedure to alleviate lower urinary tract symptoms with greater efficacy and fewer side effects has led to the introduction of various lasers. The excellent clinical outcomes, low morbidity, technical simplicity, and cost-effectiveness of GreenLight laser photoselective vaporization have made this technology a valid and efficacious clinical alternative to TURP.

The high-powered holmium laser is an excellent tool for the surgical treatment of benign prostatic hyperplasia. This article discusses the background of holmium use in the prostate and describes the surgical techniques of holmium laser ablation of the prostate and holmium laser enucleation of the prostate. Operative challenges are reviewed with suggestions as to how to avoid these problems or deal with them when they arise. Surgical outcomes and a thorough literature review are both presented.

The establishment of guidelines, pharmacologic therapies, improved understanding of lower urinary tract symptoms (LUTS) versus benign prostate hyperplasia (BPH), respect for patient-centered goals, and improved discrimination of the patient with occult prostate cancer have empowered change in the management of LUTS. These developments have allowed urologists to recognize the limitations of transurethral prostatectomy as the gold standard and search for "ideal therapies" to provide treatments with an improved relief of symptoms, decreased complication rate and cost, to correct BPH-associated morbidities and prevent future morbidities. Prognostic parameters and their ability to predict progression may be important in the future of LUTS management and selection of therapy.

Bladder diverticula are common enough to be encountered by most urologists in practice but are reported less frequently in the literature than they were 50 years ago. Some patients can be managed nonoperatively, whereas others will need surgical intervention consisting of bladder outlet reduction and possibly removal of the diverticulum itself. In addition to the decision to operate, the timing of each intervention deserves careful consideration. Cystoscopy, computed tomography with contrast, urodynamic studies, cytology, and voiding cystourethrography play important roles in informing the clinician. Many new techniques for treatment of the bladder outlet and the diverticulum are available, such as laparoscopy and robotic surgery.

The overlap of pain and urinary voiding symptoms is common for urologic patients. The etiology of these syndromes is frequently multifactorial and due to disorders of the bladder and/or prostate. The evaluation and treatment of these syndromes continues to evolve. Here we summarize the general approach to evaluation and treatment of these pain syndromes.

This article examines real-life case histories of men with routine and not so routine conditions underlying lower urinary tract symptoms (LUTS), and demonstrates the utility of what has become our standard evaluation: repeated bladder diaries, urinary flow rate postvoid residual urine flow, cystoscopy, and videourodynamics, as well as the routinely used LUTS questionnaire. Each case history was sent to each of the other authors of this monograph who, on a case by case basis, answered queries and made relevant comments. The patient evaluations and case histories are discussed by top experts who have authored articles in this issue.

GOAL STATEMENT

The goal of *Urologic Clinics of North America* is to keep practicing urologists and urology residents up to date with current clinical practice in urology by providing timely articles reviewing the state of the art in patient care.

ACCREDITATION

The *Urologic Clinics of North America* is planned and implemented in accordance with the Essential Areas and Policies of the Accreditation Council for Continuing Medical Education (ACCME) through the joint sponsorship of the University of Virginia School of Medicine and Elsevier. The University of Virginia School of Medicine is accredited by the ACCME to provide continuing medical education for physicians.

The University of Virginia School of Medicine designates this educational activity for a maximum of 15 *AMA PRA Category 1 Credits*™ for each issue, 60 credits per year. Physicians should only claim credit commensurate with the extent of their participation in the activity.

The American Medical Association has determined that physicians not licensed in the US who participate in this CME activity are eligible for a maximum of 15 *AMA PRA Category 1 Credits*™ for each issue, 60 credits per year.

Credit can be earned by reading the text material, taking the CME examination online at http://www.theclinics.com/home/cme, and completing the evaluation. After taking the test, you will be required to review any and all incorrect answers. Following completion of the test and evaluation, your credit will be awarded and you may print your certificate.

FACULTY DISCLOSURE/CONFLICT OF INTEREST

The University of Virginia School of Medicine, as an ACCME accredited provider, endorses and strives to comply with the Accreditation Council for Continuing Medical Education (ACCME) Standards of Commercial Support, Commonwealth of Virginia statutes, University of Virginia policies and procedures, and associated federal and private regulations and guidelines on the need for disclosure and monitoring of proprietary and financial interests that may affect the scientific integrity and balance of content delivered in continuing medical education activities under our auspices.

The University of Virginia School of Medicine requires that all CME activities accredited through this institution be developed independently and be scientifically rigorous, balanced and objective in the presentation/discussion of its content, theories and practices.

All authors/editors participating in an accredited CME activity are expected to disclose to the readers relevant financial relationships with commercial entities occurring within the past 12 months (such as grants or research support, employee, consultant, stock holder, member of speakers bureau, etc.). The University of Virginia School of Medicine will employ appropriate mechanisms to resolve potential conflicts of interest to maintain the standards of fair and balanced education to the reader. Questions about specific strategies can be directed to the Office of Continuing Medical Education, University of Virginia School of Medicine, Charlottesville, Virginia.

The faculty and staff of the University of Virginia Office of Continuing Medical Education have no financial affiliations to disclose.

The authors/editors listed below have identified no professional or financial affiliations for themselves or their spouse/partner:

Gregory B. Auffenberg, MD; Wade Bushman, MD, PhD; Brian T. Helfand, MD, PhD; Kerry K. Holland (Acquisitions Editor); Karl J. Kreder, MD; Brian V. Le, MD, MA; Gary E. Leach, MD; Jennifer L. Mehdizadeh, MD; Steven P. Petrou, MD; Charles R. Powell, MD; William Steers, MD (Test Author); David D. Thiel, MD; Daniel A.Thorner, DO; Mark D. Tyson, BS; and Matthew S.Wosnitzer, MD.

The authors/editors listed below identified the following professional or financial affiliations for themselves or their spouse/partner:

Jerry G. Blaivas, MD (Guest Editor) owns stock/ownership in Engogun, HDH; is a consultant for Pfizer and for Bayer; and is an industry funded researcher/investigator for AMS.
Robert F. Donnell, MD serves on the Advisory Committee/Board for NIH and AUA (Guidelines committee), and is an industry funded research/investigator for EDAP.
Lori B. Lerner, MD serves as a preceptor for Lumenis, Inc.
Kevin T. McVary, MD, FACS is an industry funded research/investigator for GSK, Lilly/ICOS, and Allergan; is a consultant for Pfizer, Lilly/ICOS, and Allergan; and is on the Speakers' Bureau for GSK, Lilly/ICOS, and Sanofi-Aventis.
Matthew P. Rutman, MD is a consultant for American Medical Systems, and is on the Speakers' Bureau for Pfizer and Laborie Medical Technologies.
Anthony J. Schaeffer, MD is on the Speakers Bureau and Advisory Committee/Board for American Urological Association, is an author for Haymarket Media, Inc., and is a consultant for Alita Pharmaceuticals, Inc., NovaBay Pharmaceuticals, Inc., American Medical Systems, J. Reckner Associates, Inc., and Pfizer Inc.
Jeffrey P. Weiss, MD (Guest Editor) is a consultant for Pfizer, Ferring, Allergan, and Vantia.

Disclosure of Discussion of Non-FDA Approved Uses for Pharmaceutical Products and/or Medical Devices.
The University of Virginia School of Medicine, as an ACCME provider, requires that all faculty presenters identify and disclose any off-label uses for pharmaceutical and medical device products. The University of Virginia School of Medicine recommends that each physician fully review all the available data on new products or procedures prior to clinical use.

TO ENROLL

To enroll in the Urologic Clinics of North America Continuing Medical Education program, call customer service at 1-800-654-2452 or visit us online at www.theclinics.com/home/cme. The CME program is available to subscribers for an additional fee of $195.00.

Urologic Clinics of North America

THE CLINICS ARE NOW AVAILABLE ONLINE!

Access your subscription at:
www.theclinics.com

Urologic Clinics of North America

FORTHCOMING ISSUES

February 2010

Advances and Controversies in Prostate Cancer
William K. Oh, MD and Jim C. Hu, MD, MPH,
Guest Editors

RECENT ISSUES

August 2009

Vasectomy and Vasectomy Re...
Guest Editors
Jay I. Sandlow, MD,
Guest Editor

May 2009

Preface

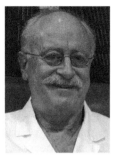 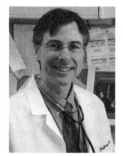

Jerry G. Blaivas, MD   Jeffrey P. Weiss, MD
Guest Editors

You read publications like the *Urologic Clinics of North America* to learn more about a subject; we write to learn more about the same subjects. Writing forces the author to think about things differently. Writing has a permanency to it; with that permanency comes a responsibility to be sure that everything written down is the truth and that it can be backed up by scientific scrutiny or the author's own experience. Either way, the author must stand by what he or she writes. When one edits the same principles apply, and the wisdom and experience of the editor amplify the learning experience for the reader. The editor asks questions of the author, asks him to clarify certain points, document others, and express his own opinions. So what did we learn from authoring and editing this edition of *Urologic Clinics of North America*? The first thing we learned is how little we really know about the long-term consequences of the things we do. In the article on case studies (which was selected, in part, because of the long follow-up), no patient was followed for even a decade. Most follow-ups ranged from 6 months to a few years, and that is in the life of men who are now expected to live into their eighth, ninth, or tenth decade. With the exception of TURP and open prostatectomy (which few urologists do as primary treatment), none of the recommended ablative prostate surgeries have been done for very long. Even for these treatments, there are woefully few long-term studies. Nevertheless, based on those few studies and our own experience, TURP and open prostatectomy have an excellent short- and long-term outcome with respect to efficacy. That excellent outcome comes at a price measured in short- and long-term morbidity, which is well documented in many of

the articles in this issue. It is such morbidity that fueled the search for less morbid procedures, leading to minimally invasive surgeries, and to KTP and holmium laser surgeries, which in the short term seem to be as efficacious as the gold standards.

Another thing we learned is that, as a profession, we have lowered the bar of expectations for successful treatment of LUTS. Many patients, it is believed, are treated and "satisfied" with conservative therapies whose efficacy is much less than can be obtained by surgery. Further, some patients are treated with conservative therapies affording good symptomatic relief, yet the underlying condition insidiously progresses and may lead to hydronephrosis, renal failure, and bladder decompensation. Patients exhibiting both of these phenomena are presented in the article on case studies.

In Dr Bushman's article, he describes factors associated with the progression of BPH, the relationship to aging, PSA levels, and prostate growth and their interaction with symptom progression and the development of urinary retention. He also discusses mechanism for LUTS improvement through surgical outlet reduction. From Dr Bushman, we learned about the presence of "chronic inflammation" in the prostates of men with BPH and the possible relationship between this and the subsequent development of prostate cancer. Where does this inflammation come from and what does it mean? He cites evidence for urinary reflux into the prostatic ducts and suggests that this may lead to bacterial colonization or infection and, by implication, inflammation. We wonder, does BPH cause symptoms in the absence of prostatic obstruction and is inflammation the cause?

Urol Clin N Am 36 (2009) xi–xiii
doi:10.1016/j.ucl.2009.09.001

urologic.theclinics.com

We also learned about the relationship between obesity, fasting plasma glucose, diabetes with prostatic enlargement, and the association of obesity with inflammation and oxidative stress, factors that have been associated with BPH. Further, Dr. Bushman notes that the prevalence of LUTS increases with age in both men (even in the absence of BPE) and women and suggests that ischemia may be a contributing factor.

Dr Bushman asks a most provocative question "If the pathophysiology of LUTS is multifactorial, and prostatic enlargement and obstruction is a major contributor in only some patients, why does surgery work so well in most patients?" He offers a tantalizing answer: "The effects of aging and outlet resistance synergize to increase exposure and susceptibility to free radical damage to the detrusor, and LUTS are a symptomatic manifestation of these degenerative changes in the same way that symptoms of CHF are for the heart. Recalling the central role of afterload reduction in the treatment of CHF, is it possible that TURP works in the case of LUTS not by 'relieving obstruction' per se but by reducing afterload?"

Drs Thorner and Weiss summarize the major available questionnaires, patient-reported (subjective), and objective outcome instruments useful in characterizing symptoms, bother, and treatment of patients with BPH.

The role of urodynamics in the evaluation of BPH is reviewed by Drs Mehdizadeh and Leach. They describe and illustrate existing urodynamic techniques, review best practice guidelines, and provide recommendations for the use of urodynamics in clinical practice.

The article by Drs Auffenberg, Helfand, and McVary provides a definitive compendium of the current status of medical therapy of BPH including alpha antagonists, 5 alpha-reductase inhibitors, anticholinergics, nutraceuticals, and combination therapies. They state that "combination therapy (with alpha blockers and 5 ARI's) is rapidly emerging as a mainstay of therapy, especially for patients with bothersome LUTS and an enlarged prostate...not only (does it) provide symptom relief, it is the only therapy shown to alter disease progression." They review studies refuting the commonly held belief that anticholinergics are contraindicated in the presence of BOO and cite short-term studies documenting its safety and some efficacy; however, they also correctly note that "nearly every study pertaining to anti-muscarinics...excluded those with higher-grade obstructions as evidenced by an elevated PVR or low Qmax. As a result, the risk of AUR in those with higher grade BOO is unknown. No study has shown significant improvement in symptoms from the use of antimuscarinic agents alone." As patient AT shows in the article on case studies, some patients do derive significant benefit by anticholinergics alone. Nevertheless, the combination of anticholinergics and alpha blockers makes the most sense at the present time and this too is "combination therapy."

We were disappointed to learn how little progress has been made in the field of phytotherapeutics. According to the authors there are simply insufficient quality studies (or clinical experience) to provide enough information to offer a firm opinion as to their safety and efficacy. They do offer a glimmer of hope that future research, under the guidance of the National Institute for Diabetes and Digestive and Kidney Diseases, will provide some insights.

In their article, Drs Thiel and Petrou masterfully review the gold standards of prostatectomy performed through electroresection in its current state of development and open techniques, including laparoscopic and robotic modifications of the latter.

In the article by Drs Wosnitzer and Rutman, the authors review the evolution of KTP photoselective laser ablation for treatment of prostatic obstruction and compare this newer procedure with the gold standard TURP.

In their article, Drs Lerner and Tyson review holmium laser applications of the prostate and propose HoLEP as a surgical alternative to TURP and open prostatectomy with potentially greater safety and efficacy at the expense of a more difficult learning curve.

Dr Robert Donnell presents an exhaustive and informative review of MIST procedures, including TUMT, TUNA, alcohol injection therapy, Botox, and urethral stenting. In clear and concise language, he discusses the past, present, and a glimpse at the future of these techniques. Presently, it seems that none of these techniques has lived up to their promises. The most promising of the MIST techniques are those that result in thermoablation; so far, this is best accomplished with TUMT techniques. Dr Donnell points out that thermoablation is reliably accomplished by heating the prostate to temperatures greater than 70°C. Techniques heating to less than 45°C (hyperthermia) and 45°C to 70°C (thermotherapy) are far less efficacious. The utility of MIST techniques lies in the future (if at all).

Drs Powell and Kreder provide an insightful look at causes, diagnosis, and management of bladder diverticula and related topics of impaired detrusor contractility and low bladder compliance, potential complications of intervention versus nonintervention, and technical variations of available surgical therapies.

In their article, Drs Le and Schaeffer offer a detailed analysis of the main genitourinary pain syndromes (prostatitis including CPPS, interstitial cystitis, and pelvic floor pain) and suggest a highly useful approach to patients presenting with LUTS and pelvic pain.

Finally, Dr Blaivas hosts a spirited roundtable panel discussion of evaluation and management of a number of conventional and not-so conventional cases of clinical problems associated with BPH.

So, are clinicians better off from a practical standpoint than 40 years ago? At that time there was no standard of care other than surgical outlet reduction through open or transurethral prostatectomy. Bladder diverticulectomy was and remains an uncommonly performed operation useful in a small number of well-selected patients. Over the past four decades urologists have seen added to their armamentarium a variety of medicines, such as uroselective alpha blockers and antimuscarinics and 5 alpha-reductase inhibitors that proved to both benefit symptoms of BPH and reduce the risk of urinary retention. Diagnostic aids, such as voiding diaries, LUTS questionnaires, noninvasive and invasive urodynamic studies, prostate ultrasound, and PSA, allow clinicians to prescribe such medications alone or in combination on a rational basis to maximize their efficacy. Minimally invasive, office-based procedures using thermoablative techniques are potentially efficacious substitutes for formal outlet reducing operations, which in turn have been made safer through application of lasers and advanced electronic circuitry to vaporize and resect the prostate with less chance of hemorrhage, hyponatremia, or hemolysis than was the case previously. We do not yet have a clear picture of the cost-effectiveness and relative outcomes of such manifold competing therapies, although TURP and open prostatectomy remain standards for comparison of all newer modalities treating prostatic obstruction and its consequences in the bladder. In this age of concern for efficient medical expenditure, it is incumbent on members of our specialty to determine which of these treatments work well enough and are affordable enough and safe enough to persist in the evolving era of rationed health care.

Finally, despite the fact that clinicians have come a long way since the introduction of urodynamics nearly 40 years ago, there are still some basic questions to be addressed: (1) What is the relationship between BPH, BPE, prostatic obstruction, prostatitis, impaired detrusor contractility, detrusor overactivity, and sensory urgency? (2) Are the current methods of diagnosing urethral obstruction accurate (Schafer, Abrams-Griffiths, and ICS nomograms)? (3) What is the best way to diagnose obstruction in the face of impaired detrusor contractility? (4) In men with obstruction, is relief of obstruction necessary for a successful treatment outcome? (5) Is prostatic ablative surgery or prostatectomy indicated only in patients with proved outlet obstruction or is there a nonspecific effect of prostatectomy, which ameliorates symptoms regardless of the underlying condition? (5) Should treatment be selected on the basis of symptoms or the underlying pathophysiology? (6) Are there specific therapies that can be directed at one particular condition, such as detrusor overactivity or impaired detrusor contractility?

With the advent of reliable instruments to document symptoms (questionnaires and diaries) and the ability to define and quantitate the underlying pathophysiology (multichannel videourodynamic studies), clinicians now have the technical ability to answer these questions. Treatment should be tailored to the specific underlying pathophysiology, but well done clinical trials are necessary to determine if this is true.

Jerry G. Blaivas, MD
Department of Urology
Weill Cornell Medical College
New York, NY, USA
SUNY Downstate Medical School
Brooklyn, NY, USA

Jeffrey P. Weiss, MD
Department of Urology
SUNY Downstate Medical School
Brooklyn, NY, USA

E-mail addresses:
jblvs@aol.com (J.G. Blaivas)
jeffrey.weiss@downstate.edu (J.P. Weiss)

Etiology, Epidemiology, and Natural History

Wade Bushman, MD, PhD

KEYWORDS

- Prostatic enlargement • Metabolic risk factors
- Lower urinary tract symptoms

Historically, benign prostatic hyperplasia (BPH) has been a major focus of urologic practice and surgery. However, a simplistic causal relationship among prostatic enlargement, progressive obstruction, lower urinary tract symptoms, retention, and complications of retention has been challenged by recognition of the incomplete overlap of prostatic enlargement with symptoms and obstruction. The result has been a greater focus on symptoms than prostatic enlargement, and a shift from surgery to medical treatment. Therefore, the question can be asked whether BPH per se, the glandular enlargement as it contributes to bladder dysfunction, or hyperplastic enlargement as a biomarker for generalized lower urinary tract dysfunction (LUTD) are concerns. This article addresses these issues.

Recent observational studies have uncovered a remarkable association of BPH with various manifestations of LUTD, including lower urinary tract symptoms (LUTS), erectile dysfunction (ED), and chronic pelvic pain syndrome (CPPS). How does one make sense of this? Should BPH be considered the primary mechanism for LUTD? Or should BPH be considered just one facet of a generalized pathophysiologic process affecting aging men? An unbiased approach would entertain both possibilities: acknowledging the long-recognized role for BPH in the development and progression of LUTS while recognizing that etiologic factors for development of BPH likely have collateral impacts on other facets of lower urinary tract function.

Traditionally, the definition of BPH has been stratified to include histologic BPH, macroscopic glandular enlargement, BPH-related symptoms, and BPH-related complications (retention, renal failure, stones). Although this stratification is appealing in its simplicity, the potentially intertwined nature of prostatic hyperplasia, LUTS, and other symptoms of LUTD suggest that this stratification may not be particularly helpful in sorting out the development and natural history of BPH and associated symptoms.

ETIOLOGY
The Etiology of Prostatic Enlargement

BPH is characterized histologically as a progressive enlargement of the prostate gland resulting from a nonmalignant proliferative process that includes both epithelial and stromal elements. Growth results from proliferation of fibroblasts/myofibroblasts and epithelial glandular elements near the urethra in the transition zone of the prostate gland.[1–4] The hyperplastic process is multifocal and exhibits a variegated histology with variable proportions of stromal nodules and glandular hyperplasia. The histology of BPH was carefully described by McNeal.[5,6] During the initial phase of BPH small hyperplastic nodules appear in the periurethral area and gradually increase in number. A second phase of BPH, generally occurring in men older than 60 years, involves a dramatic and simultaneous increase in size of glandular nodules McNeal[5] noted that the histologic appearance of stromal tissue in BPH nodules resembled the histologic appearance of developmental mesenchyme and hypothesized that BPH is caused by "embryonic processes reawakened in a distorted form in adult life."

Endocrine influences have been postulated to play an important role in BPH. Androgen

Department of Urology, University of Wisconsin Medical School, K6–562 Clinical Science Center, 600 Highland Avenue, Madison, WI 53792, USA
E-mail address: bushman@surgery.wisc.edu

Urol Clin N Am 36 (2009) 403–415
doi:10.1016/j.ucl.2009.07.003
0094-0143/09/$ – see front matter © 2009 Elsevier Inc. All rights reserved.

urologic.theclinics.com

stimulation is required for fetal prostate growth and development[7] but are considered to play only a permissive role in the pathogenesis of BPH. Androgen levels in the prostate are not significantly different in BPH and normal tissues, and currently no evidence shows an increase in BPH incidence for men undergoing androgen supplementation therapy.[8–14] However, estrogens or a changing ratio of androgens to estrogens in aging men has been speculated to play an important role in the pathogenesis of BPH. This hypothesis is based on two main observations.

First, the ratio of testosterone to estradiol steadily declines in aging men.[15] Second, experimental manipulation of estradiol levels in animal models can cause benign prostatic enlargement. Dogs and humans are believed to be the only mammals with a significant incidence of spontaneous BPH, and treatment of young dogs with androgen plus estrogen hormones leads to an earlier onset and greater extent of benign prostatic enlargement.[16,17] Similarly, treatment of mice with androgen plus estrogen hormones leads to benign prostatic enlargement[18–21] (Talo and colleagues 2005; Ishii and colleagues 2006; McPherson and colleagues 2008). Recent studies implicating obesity and BPH could reflect an increased estrogen/testosterone ratio in obese men resulting from increased aromatization of testosterone in peripheral tissues.

Prostatic inflammation is a common feature of the adult prostate and is associated with the development and progression of BPH. Acute and chronic inflammation are extremely common histologic findings in the adult human.[22–27] McNeal[28] found inflammation in 44% of prostate tissue samples in an autopsy series in men without evidence of other prostate disease, whereas Bennett and colleagues[29] reported inflammation in 73% of prostates examined. The origin of inflammation in the prostate remains a subject of debate and is likely multifactorial. Evidence exists for urinary reflux into the prostatic ducts,[10] and bacterial colonization/infection in surgical specimens of BPH seems to be common. Among patients who underwent transurethral resection of the prostate (TURP) and had preoperatively sterile urine, 38% of specimens grew bacteria when the tissues were morcellated and cultured.[30] Other possible causes of inflammation include noxious dietary constituents, autoimmune mechanisms, oxidative stress associated with androgen action, and systemic inflammation associated with the metabolic syndrome.[31]

A retrospective study of 3942 prostatic biopsies identified as consistent with BPH showed inflammation in 1700 (43.1%; 25). A study of specimens obtained from 80 men who had no symptoms of prostatitis but underwent TURP for treatment of BPH found inflammation to be uniformly present.[32] In another study that evaluated tissue removed with radical prostatectomy, inflammation was found in tissue samples of 35 of 40 patients who had BPH, and prostatic inflammation was associated with significantly greater prostate weight than that observed in patients who had no prostatic inflammation.[33]

In a prospective study of autopsy specimens obtained from 93 men who had histologic evidence of BPH, chronic inflammation was found (primarily in the transitional zone) in 75% of prostates examined compared with 55% of prostates not affected by BPH.[22] Prostate biopsy of 8224 men enrolled in the Reduction by Dutasteride of Prostate Cancer Events (REDUCE) trial showed inflammation in more than three quarters of the biopsies. Chronic inflammation was more common than acute inflammation (78% vs 15%, respectively).

Inflammation also correlates with prostatic enlargement and symptomatic progression. Evidence of inflammation on baseline biopsy in the Medical Therapy of Prostatic Symptoms (MTOPS) trial correlated with prostate volume (41 versus 37 mL; $P = .0002$), suggesting a significant role in prostatic enlargement.[34] Inflammation also correlated with symptomatic progression, risk for urinary retention, and need for surgery.[35] In a recent analysis of the data from the REDUCE trial, Nickel and colleagues[36,37] reported a weak but statistically significant association between chronic inflammation and symptom severity.

Several studies have identified associations suggesting metabolic risk factors for the development or progression of BPH. The Baltimore Longitudinal Study of Aging examined whether obesity, fasting plasma glucose, and diabetes were associated with prostatic enlargement.[38,39] This analysis, authored by a collaborator in this proposal, showed a positive correlation of body mass index with prostate volume. The risk was increased for very obese men. The association of obesity with BPH has been supported by other studies. Hammersten and Hogstedt, 1999 observed that prostatic growth correlated with BMI, and Giaovannucci and colleagues 1994 found that obesity was associated with an increased risk for BPH surgery.

One mechanism through which obesity has been postulated to promote hyperplasia is increased peripheral aromatization of testosterone with a resulting increase in the estrogen/testosterone ratio. Another postulated mechanism involves the association of obesity with inflammation and oxidative stress; factors that have been associated with BPH. Other studies have shown that men diagnosed with BPH have a higher incidence of diabetes than the general population, and that diabetes is associated with more severe symptoms[40] (Michel and colleagues 2000; Hammerstein and colleagues 2001). Part of the explanation may be that diabetes can be a primary cause of lower urinary tract symptoms, but the studies cited earlier suggest that metabolic factors may influence the development and progression of LUTS indirectly by increasing the rate of prostatic enlargement.

Association of Benign Prostatic Hyperplasia and Prostate Cancer

BPH and prostate cancer are dysregulations of prostate growth control that share an increasing prevalence with advancing age. This association was recently reviewed by Alcaraz and colleagues 2009. Furthermore, 83% of prostate cancers develop in prostates where BPH is also present.[41] The zonal location of BPH and cancer is generally distinct, but approximately one quarter of prostate cancers arise in the transition zone.[42] Some reports show that the rate of growth of BPH is correlated with the risk for prostate cancer.[43–46]

Recent histopathologic studies of human prostatectomy specimens identified lesions characterized by proliferating epithelial cells and activated inflammatory cells (proliferative inflammatory atrophy [PIA]) in juxtaposition to areas of prostate intraepithelial neoplasia (PIN) and prostate carcinoma (CaP).[47] Based on this and subsequent studies, chronic inflammation is now widely considered a critical element in the genesis of CaP, and PIA is now widely considered a likely precursor of PIN and CaP[48–50] (Palapattu and colleagues 2004). The metabolic syndrome has also been implicated as a risk factor for prostate cancer (reviewed in Alcaraz and colleagues 2009).

In summary, epidemiologic evidence of an association between BPH and prostate cancer is being complemented by discovery of shared etiologic influences that may explain the association.

Etiologic factors for lower urinary tract dysfunction

Recent studies have indentified a tantalizing general coincidence regarding the presence of LUTD, including LUTS, ED, and CPPS, in patients who have BPH. Certainly, LUTS have been historically associated with benign prostatic enlargement. More recently noted is the strong association between ED and LUTS and the finding that both conditions may be improved by medical treatment of either LUTS or ED[51–54] (Kaplan and colleagues 2006).

The coincidence of pelvic pain in men who have BPH also has been noted recently. Although pain has not classically been considered a feature of BPH, a recent study by Clemens and colleagues[55] suggested considerable overlap of voiding symptoms and pain, with as many of 34% of men who had LUTS reporting pain symptoms. The mechanistic basis for these associations is a subject of considerable interest.

Aging is associated with increasing lower urinary tract symptoms independent of prostatic enlargement. The prevalence of LUTS increases with aging in both men and women (**Fig. 1**).[56–62] Comparisons of storage and voiding symptoms show comparable trends of increasing symptoms with age, although the overall prevalence is higher in men. The simplest and probably best explanation for this is that most voiding symptoms are a consequence of nonprostatic factors that operate similarly in both sexes. The higher prevalence in men might be explained by the superimposed effect of prostatic enlargement and obstruction.

The reasons for the aging-associated increase in LUTS are not well understood. Aging is associated

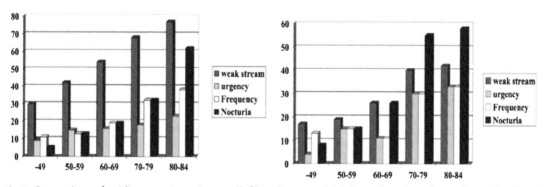

Fig. 1. Comparison of voiding symptoms in men (*left*) and women (*right*) as a function of age. (*From* Nordling J. The aging bladder—a significant but underestimated role in the development of lower urinary tract symptoms. Exp Gerontol 2002;37(8–9):991–9; with permission.)

with changes in detrusor morphology, detrusor innervation, and bladder metabolism that may affect bladder function. Partial denervation has been linked to increased excitability of the detrusor, leading to detrusor instability. Aging is associated with decreases in detrusor contractility that result in diminished urinary flow and variable degrees of incomplete emptying. Indirect effects of aging on bladder function may also accrue from degenerative changes in bladder innervation and vascular supply. Coronary artery disease, ischemic heart disease, and vascular risk factors have been found to be associated with BPH symptoms, leading to speculation that pelvic ischemia may be a contributing factor in the development of LUTS.[63]

The recognized association between BPH and ED may reflect a shared etiologic connection with cardiovascular disease. The importance of cardiovascular risk factors in the development of ED is well recognized. Recent evidence suggests that the autonomic and cardiovascular systems may also be involved in the development and progression of BPH and LUTS. Studies have shown a higher prevalence of hypertension in men who have BPH, a positive correlation between the duration of hypertension and prostate size, and a greater risk among men who have hypertension to develop urinary retention and require BPH surgery.[64,65] These correlations have fueled speculation that hypertension and BPH symptoms are linked by the metabolic syndrome and overactivity of the sympathetic nervous system.[53,66]

Prostatic inflammation may be a primary cause of lower urinary tract symptoms through influencing bladder sensation and function.[67,68] Development of prostatic inflammation may trigger and be exaggerated by neurogenic inflammation. Multiple studies support the occurrence of neurogenic inflammation in the bladder, and neurogenic inflammation of the bladder results in many of the symptoms associated with LUTS.[69–72]

The concept that chronic inflammation accompanying BPH may sensitize afferent nerve fibers of the bladder, resulting in development of LUTS, is supported by the fact that the bladder and prostate share innervation and also the observation that inflammation of one pelvic organ can result in cross-sensitization of other pelvic viscera.[73–76] Although BPH has not been traditionally considered to be a painful condition and a patient complaint of pain has often been used to distinguish BPH from prostatic inflammation,[77] a far greater number of men diagnosed with BPH describe the presence of pain than was previously recognized.[55,78] Pain associated with ejaculation has been reported by a substantial number of patients diagnosed with LUTS caused by BPH.[79–81] In one study of 3700 men who had BPH-related LUTS, 688 (18.6%) reported pain on ejaculation.[82]

The role of prostatic inflammation and afferent sensitization in development of pelvic of pelvic pain is unknown but a promising area of further study.

EPIDEMIOLOGY
The Epidemiology of Prostatic Enlargement

BPH is an age-related process with a histologic prevalence of approximately 10% for men in their 30s, 20% for men in their 40s, 50% to 60% for men in their 60s, and 80% to 90% for men in their 70s and 80s. Androgens and aging are necessary for the development of BPH, but the etiology of prostatic hyperplasia is poorly understood.[34,47]

Prostate volume increases with age. In the Olmstead study, median prostate volumes were 21, 27, 32 and 34 mL in the 5th, 6th, 7th, and 8th decades, respectively. This study calculated a 1.6% average annual increase in prostatic volume.[83] The rate of enlargement varied considerably at the individual level, but patients who had larger baseline volumes tended to experience more rapid enlargement (**Fig. 2**). Strong suggestions have been found of geographic variations in prostate size, with several studies showing significantly lower size in Japanese, Chinese, and Indian men compared with American and Australian men[84] (Tsukamotyo and colleagues 1996; Jin and colleagues 1999).

The Incidence of Lower Urinary Tract Symptoms and Urinary Retention in Aging Men

LUTS are prevalent among aging men (see **Fig. 1**). Surveys of an unselected population of men aged 40 to 79 years in Olmstead county, Minnesota, showed moderate to severe symptoms in 13% of the men aged 40 to 49 years and 28% of men older than 70 years. Symptoms of urgency, nocturia, weak stream, intermittency, and sensation of incomplete emptying were most strongly correlated with age (Chute, 1993). Bosch and colleagues[85] surveyed 502 men aged 55 to 74 years in the Netherlands using the International Prostate Symptom Score (IPSS) and identified a prevalence of severe and moderate symptoms in 6% and 24%, respectively.

In a comprehensive review of the epidemiology of acute urinary retention that combined data from various epidemiologic studies, Roehrborn[86] found that the estimated incidence of acute urinary retention is 0.5% to 2.5% per year.

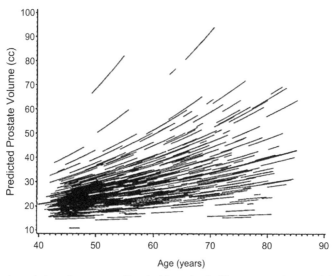

Fig. 2. Plot of predicted prostate volumes as estimated by mixed effects regression model. Each line represents individual subject and thick line represents population average. (*From* Rhodes T, Girman CJ, Jacobsen SJ, et al. Longitudinal prostate growth rates during 5 years in randomly selected community men 40 to 79 years old. J Urol 1999;161(4):1174–9; with permission.)

What is the Relationship Between Benign Prostatic Hyperplasia and Lower Urinary Tract Symptoms?

Recent studies have highlighted the comparable incidence of LUTS in men and women, and implicated various potentially contributing factors, including the effect of aging on the bladder and nervous system, and the effects of metabolic derangements, autonomic overactivity, diabetes, neurologic disease, and age- and cardiac-related changes in the pattern of body-water regulation. What does this signify regarding the role of BPH and prostatic enlargement in the development of LUTS?

The Olmstead County Study of Urinary Symptoms and Health Status[87] showed that prostatic enlargement, peak flow rate, and LUTS were all age-dependent. Analysis of the data adjusting for age showed that men who had significant prostatic enlargement (>50 cm³) were 3.5 times more likely to have moderate-to-severe LUTS (**Fig. 3**). This finding suggests that significant prostatic enlargement is a significant driver in development of LUTS. However, the overall contribution of prostatic enlargement to LUTS in this unselected group of men was calculated to be small. Similarly, Bosch and colleagues[88] observed only a weak correlation of prostate volume with IPSS, peak flow, and post-void residual urine volumes.

The explanation for this is simply that most men, even those who have significant symptoms, have prostate volumes less than 50 mL. In an analysis of 354 symptomatic men, Vesely and colleagues[89] reported a mean prostatic volume of 40.1 ± 23.9 cm³. Ezz and colleagues[90] reported a mean prostate volume of 43 ± 20 cm³ among 803 patients who had mild to severe LUTS. One might infer from these data that prostate volume is an important determinant of symptoms in men who have significant prostatic enlargement but not in those who have only modest degrees of enlargement.

An interesting study examining the correlation of specific parameters of prostate enlargement to symptoms found that length of the transition zone was the dimension most strongly correlated with symptom severity.[91] This study suggests that prostatic enlargement alone does not determine symptom severity, but also the elongation of the transition zone and, presumably, its effect on outlet resistance.

What is the Relationship Between Obstruction and Lower Urinary Tract Symptoms?

Several different studies have shown a significant correlation between diminished urinary flow rate and LUTS (see **Fig. 3**).[85,89,90,92,93] However, maximum flow rate is a function of both detrusor function and outlet resistance. The correlation of maximum flow rate therefore may reflect a contribution of impaired detrusor function, increased outlet resistance, or both. Nitti and colleagues[94] performed urodynamic studies on 83 patients (mean age, 67 years) who had symptoms of BPH. Of these, 34% were considered obstructed, 20% deemed unobstructed, and 46% believed to be equivocal according to the Abrams-Griffiths

A   **B**

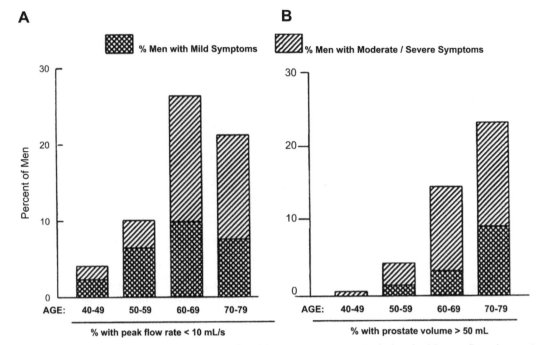

Fig. 3. Cross-hatched bars represent subjects with mild or no symptoms. Single hatched bars reflect those with moderate to severe symptoms, so that total height of stacked bars represents total percentage within that age decade meeting criteria. (A) Percentage of men randomly selected from community with peak urinary flow rate of less than 10 mL/s by age decade. (B) Percentage of men randomly selected from community with prostate volume of more than 50 mL. (*From* Girman CJ, Jacobsen SJ, Guess HA, et al. Natural history of prostatism: relationship among symptoms, prostate volume and peak urinary flow rate. J Urol 1995;153(5):1510–5; with permission.)

nomogram. No significant differences were seen in total, obstructive, or irritative scores among the three groups. In fact, the urodynamic parameter that exhibited a significant correlation was detrusor instability, present in 54% of patients who had irritative symptoms.

Netto and colleagues[95] performed urodynamic studies on 217 patients who had moderate or severe symptoms and identified obstruction in 53% and 83%, respectively. Yalla and colleagues[96,97] performed urodynamic studies on 125 men (mean age, 67.7 years) who had micturitional urethral pressure profilometry (MUPP) and observed a prevalence of obstruction in 76% and 78% of men who had moderate or severe symptoms, respectively. No correlation was observed between the severity of obstruction and the severity of symptoms. In another urodynamic study of 222 patients who had a clinical diagnosis of BPH and a maximum flow rate of less than 15 mL/s, 80% were obstructed.[98]

Finally, the ICS-"BPH" study evaluated 933 patients who had LUTS. Of this group 57% were obstructed. The presence of obstruction was significantly correlated with urgency and urge incontinence but not with any other symptom. Although these studies show that urodynamic

evidence of outlet obstruction is prevalent in men who have moderate to severe LUTS, with an incidence ranging from 34% to 80%, the presence or absence of obstruction does not reliably correlate with either specific symptoms or their overall severity.

Given the similar incidence of LUTS in men and women and the incomplete association of urodynamic evidence of obstruction with symptoms in men, it is tempting to deemphasize the role of outlet obstruction. However, aohHoqwlthough other etiologic factors are important, perhaps even more so than outlet obstruction, the preponderance of evidence indicates that outlet obstruction is present in most men who have moderate to severe LUTS. Furthermore, surgical treatment of outlet obstruction remains a highly effective therapy for LUTS, with symptomatic success rates that clearly outshine any other medical therapy.

If the pathophysiology of LUTS is multifactorial and prostatic enlargement and obstruction is a major contributor in only some patients, why does surgery work so well in most patients?

In an editorial comment on the paper by Yalla and colleagues[96] John McConnell pointed out that urodynamic evidence of obstruction is not a prerequisite for surgery. He noted that the success rate for surgery is higher for patients who have obstruction, but pointed out that most patients who do not have obstruction who undergo transurethral resection of the prostate also experience successful symptomatic outcomes. Nothing in the field of BPH-related research has been as perplexing as this simple fact: that surgical interventions for outlet obstruction improve symptoms remarkably well, even in patients for whom urodynamic testing does not show obstruction. One potential explanation for this paradox is that nomograms for diagnosing obstruction are unreliable, particularly in those who have impaired detrusor contractility. These patients may well be obstructed and would benefit from surgical reduction of urethral resistance. Thus, there is room for healthy debate about the mechanism through which surgery produces symptomatic improvement and whether it depends on reducing outlet resistance.

An intriguing and instructive parallel may be found in the use of afterload reduction in treatment of congestive heart failure (CHF). The heart experiences several age-related changes.[99] These include myocyte apoptosis and myocyte hypertrophy, impaired mitochondrial respiratory enzyme function, a shift in myosin isoform from rapid to slow ATP hydrolyzing forms, increased extracellular collagen and elastin, diminished compliance, prolonged ventricular contraction and slower left ventricular filling, decline in the number of sinoatrial pacemaker cells, increased atrioventricular delay, and increased ectopy.[99–102] Aging has been termed *blunted hypertension*, and hypertension has been considered *accelerated aging*.[103] This symmetry reflects a common mechanism in the effects of aging and hypertension on the heart: both result in increased energy use, increased glycolysis and reactive oxygen species generation, decreased antioxidant defenses, and increased free-radical damage. Oxidative stress is considered the major mechanism for aging and stress-related damage and seems to be a final common pathway for the synergistic effects of aging and hypertension on the heart.[102,104,105]

When of sufficient severity, damage to the heart produces the condition of heart failure. Afterload reduction is a central therapeutic intervention for CHF. Reduction of the heart's workload globally improves cardiac function and ameliorates the symptoms of heart failure.[106,107] What is noteworthy and particularly important is that afterload reduction is an effective treatment of CHF, even when increased afterload (ie, hypertension) is not a contributing factor. In other words, reducing the afterload globally improves heart function even when the afterload is not significantly increased.

The aging bladder has many similarities with the aging heart. Clinically, diminished bladder capacity, diminished compliance, detrusor overactivity, decreased contractility, decreased Q_{max} and incomplete emptying are seen. The physiologic and cellular changes associated with aging include myocyte hypertrophy, increased electrical coupling, increased ectopic activity, impaired mechanical coupling, impaired mitochondrial enzyme function, decreased contractility, increased extracellular collagen/elastin deposition, and diminished compliance[59,108–114] (Elbadawi and colleagues 1998). Remarkably, animal models of bladder outlet obstruction produce many of the same changes, including myocyte hypertrophy, impaired mitochondrial enzyme function, decreased contractility, increased extracellular collagen/elastin deposition, diminished compliance, increased work demand, and increased energy use.[115–122]

As in the heart, the deleterious effects of aging and increased afterload on the bladder share a common mechanism, including increased glycolysis and free radical generation, decreased (mitochondrial) antioxidant defenses, and increased oxidative stress and free-radical damage. This comparison suggests that the effects of aging and outlet resistance synergize to increase exposure and susceptibility to free radical damage to the detrusor, and that LUTS are a symptomatic manifestation of these degenerative changes in the same way that symptoms of CHF are for the heart. Recalling the central role of afterload reduction in the treatment of CHF, TURP may work in the case of LUTS not by relieving obstruction, per se, but by reducing afterload. This conceptualization coincides with the empiric observation that TURP is highly effective in treating LUTS even when obstruction cannot be shown through urodynamic criteria. As long as the peak flow rate is less than 15 mL/s, wherein some combination of increased outlet resistance or detrusor contractile dysfunction may be inferred, surgery to reduce outlet resistance is highly successful.

This analysis accounts for the multifactorial origin of LUTS in aging men and women, recognizing a special role for prostatic enlargement in some men, and identifies TURP as an intervention that is uniquely effective in men because surgical reduction of afterload is usually only applied in men. Anecdotal success has been observed in treating women who have bladder neck obstruction and LUTS with TURP.[123,124]

With respect to the understanding of BPH/LUTS and the role of surgery, this suggests that past attempts to understand and predict the efficacy of surgery for LUTS based on obstruction have failed not only because the definition of obstruction is relative and arbitrary but also because the efficacy of surgery lies in reducing outlet resistance and decreasing afterload rather than remedying a pathologic condition of abnormally increased outlet resistance.

NATURAL HISTORY
The Natural History of Lower Urinary Tract Symptoms

Lee and colleagues[125] reported the natural history of LUTS in a large cohort of symptomatic men followed for 5 years without treatment. This observation showed a significant worsening of storage and voiding symptoms in general. Some patients experienced a spontaneous improvement in symptoms, but the general trend was strongly and significantly negative. Obstructive symptoms (hesitancy, weak stream, and incomplete emptying) and nocturia showed the greatest mean increases in symptoms.

The Risk for Acute Urinary Retention

The overall risk for AUR has been estimated to be 0.5% to 2.5% per year. However, the risk is cumulative and increases with age and symptom severity (**Fig. 4**). Several studies, including Proscar Long-term Efficacy and Safety Study (PLESS) and MTOPS, have shown a strong correlation of AUR risk with prostatic enlargement. In the PLESS study, the incidence of AUR was increased three-fold in patients who had a prostate volume greater than 40 mL (1.6% vs 4.2%). An even greater (eight-fold) increased risk was seen in patients who had a prostate-specific antigen (PSA) level greater than 1.4 ng/mL (0.4% vs 3.9%). Symptom severity is also correlated with risk for retention (see **Fig. 3**), as is a maximum flow rate less than 12 L/s. Using the data from the Olmstead Study, Jacobsen[126] estimated that the risk for AUR for a 60-year-old man who has moderate to severe symptoms over 10 years is 13.7%.

Effect of Unrelieved Outlet Obstruction on Detrusor Function

Several recent studies have examined the natural history of subcategories of men who have LUTS. In a 10-year follow-up of symptomatic men who had urodynamically showed bladder outlet obstruction, Thomas and colleagues[127] observed a significant increase in detrusor overactivity and decreased peak flow rate. Given the absence of a control group of unobstructed men, how the presence of outlet obstruction influences the rates of increase in detrusor overactivity and decrease in peak flow rate that occur with aging is unclear. Although the effect of unrelieved obstruction on detrusor function has been of concern, no compelling data supports the notion that unrelieved bladder outlet obstruction increases the risk for detrusor decompensation and chronic retention.[128–130]

Summary

Despite the apparently modest role of prostatic enlargement in the generation of LUTS, prostatic enlargement has been shown to be significantly associated with symptomatic progression and development of urinary retention. Other factors are also important. Longitudinal population-based studies have provided significant data on the risk for BPH symptoms and symptomatic progression. The Olmsted County study implicated age, severe

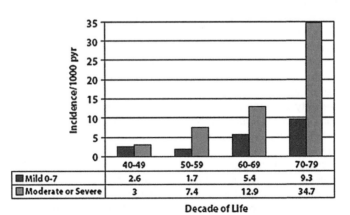

	40-49	50-59	60-69	70-79
■ Mild 0-7	2.6	1.7	5.4	9.3
▦ Moderate or Severe	3	7.4	12.9	34.7

Decade of Life

Fig. 4. Cumulative incidence of urinary retention. (*From* Roehrborn CG. The epidemiology of acute urinary retention in benign prostatic hyperplasia. Rev Urol 2001;3(4):187–92; with permission.)

symptoms, prostatic enlargement, high serum PSA, low peak flow rate, and increased post-void residual urine volume as risk factors for AUR and surgery. Many of these findings have been corroborated by MTOPS or Alfuzosin Long-term Efficacy and Safety Study (ALTESS).

Among the different studies, prostate volume and elevated PSA are most consistently associated with symptomatic progression. A higher risk for AUR and symptomatic progression is seen in patients whose symptoms fail to respond to medical therapy (Roehrborn, 2008). Significant issues remain. The role of PSA testing as a marker of BPH, for example, remains a topic of discussion.

Although PSA may be a useful index of prostatic volume and an indicator of relative risk for symptomatic progression, the risk for progression is multifactorial and the specific contribution of PSA testing to improving patient management and outcomes remains to be shown. Similarly, one might ask what is the significance of an enlarged prostate without symptoms? An array of cross-sectional and observational studies suggesting a general correlation of prostatic enlargement with increased risk for symptomatic progression suggest that men who have enlarged prostates have a higher risk for developing LUTS and AUR. However, in the present state of knowledge, the latter does not justify early pharmacologic intervention to reduce the risk for development of symptoms.

THE FUTURE

If the current understanding of BPH has one critical weakness, it is that clinical studies have tended to regard patients who have BPH as having one condition characterized by LUTS. This approach has not accounted for the uniqueness of individual patients. One patient may be relatively young, have severe obstructive symptoms (hesitancy, intermittency, diminished stream, and need to strain) with little in the way of irritative symptoms (frequency, urgency, nocturia) and a relatively small prostate. Another patient may be elderly, have little in the way of obstructive symptoms but severe irritative symptoms and a very large prostate. Although both of these patients would be considered to have LUTS, they really couldn't be more different.

A major need is to understand the pathophysiology of LUTS in individual patients; to elucidate contributions of prostatic enlargement, aging of the bladder muscle, associated medical conditions, metabolic factors, prostatic inflammation, or other as-yet-to-be-identified factors; and to understand how these individual contributing factors influence the response to treatment and risk for clinical progression. These are the challenges that lie ahead.

REFERENCES

1. Bierhoff E, Vogel J, Benz M, et al. Stromal nodules in benign prostatic hyperplasia. Eur Urol 1996;29: 345–54.
2. Meigs JB, Mohr B, Barry MJ, et al. Risk factors for clinical benign prostatic enlargement in a community-based population of healthy aging men. J Clin Epidemiol 2001;54:935–44.
3. Michel MC, Mehlburger L, Schumacher H, et al. Hyperinsulinaemia as a risk factor for developing benign prostatic hyperplasia. J Urol 2001;163(6): 1725–9.
4. Verhamme K, Dieleman J, Bleumink G, et al. Incidence and prevalence of lower urinary tract symptoms suggestive of benign prostatic enlargement in primary care-the Triumph project. Eur Urol 2002;42:323–8.
5. McNeal J. Pathology of benign prostatic hyperplasia. Insight into etiology. Urol Clin North Am 1990;17(3):477–86.
6. McNeal JE. Origin and evolution of benign prostatic enlargement. Invest Urol 1978;15(4):340–5.
7. Thomson AA, Marker PC. Branching morphogenesis in the prostate gland and seminal vesicles. Differentiation 2006;74(7):382–92.
8. Gooren L. Androgen deficiency in the aging male: benefits and risks of androgen supplementation. J Steroid Biochem Mol Biol 2003;85(2–5):349–55.
9. Green JS, Holden ST, Bose P, et al. An investigation into the relationship between prostate size, peak urinary flow rate and male erectile dysfunction. Int J Impot Res 2001;13(6):322–5.
10. Kaufman JM. The effect of androgen supplementation therapy on the prostate. Aging Male 2003;6(3): 166–74.
11. Kirby RS, Lowe D, Bultitude MI. Intra-prostatic urinary reflux: an aetiological factor in abacterial prostatitis. Br J Urol 1982;54(6):729–31.
12. Marks LS, Mostaghel EA, Nelson PS. Prostate tissue androgens: history and current clinical relevance. Urology 2008;72(2):247–54.
13. Masumori N, Tsukamoto T, Kumamoto Y, et al. Japanese men have smaller prostate volumes but comparable urinary flow rates relative to American men: results of community based studies in 2 countries. J Urol 1996;155(4):1324–7.
14. Mostaghel EA, Nelson PS. Intracrine androgen metabolism in prostate cancer progression: mechanisms of castration resistance and therapeutic implications. Best Pract Res Clin Endocrinol Metab 2008;22(2):243–58.

15. Belanger A, Candas B, Dupont A, et al. Changes in serum concentrations of conjugated and unconjugated steroids in 40- to 80-year-old men. J Clin Endocrinol Metab 1994;79(4):1086–90.

16. Coffey DS, Walsh PC. Clinical and experimental studies of benign prostatic hyperplasia. Urol Clin North Am 1990;17(3):461–75.

17. Collins GN, Lee RJ, Russell EB, et al. Ultrasonically determined patterns of enlargement in benign prostatic hyperplasia. Br J Urol 1993;71(4):451–6.

18. Fingerhut B, Veenema RJ. Histology and radioautography of induced benign enlargement of the mouse prostate. Invest Urol 1966;4(2):112–24.

19. Ricke WA, McPherson SJ, Bianco JJ, et al. Prostatic hormonal carcinogenesis is mediated by in situ estrogen production and estrogen receptor alpha signaling. FASEB J 2008;22(5):1512–20.

20. Ricke WA, Ishii K, Ricke EA, et al. Steroid hormones stimulate human prostate cancer progression and metastasis. Int J Cancer 2006;118(9):2123–31.

21. Streng TK, Talo A, Andersson KE, et al. A dose-dependent dual effect of oestrogen on voiding in the male mouse? BJU Int 2005;96(7):1126–30.

22. Delongchamps NB, de la Roza G, Chandan V, et al. Evaluation of prostatitis in autopsied prostates—is chronic inflammation more associated with benign prostatic hyperplasia or cancer? J Urol 2008;179: 1736–40.

23. de la Rosette JJ, Witjes WP, Schäfer W, et al. Relationships between lower urinary tract symptoms and bladder outlet obstruction: results from the ICS-"BPH" study. Neurourol Urodyn 1998;17(2): 99–108.

24. Kohnen PW, Drach GW. Patterns of inflammation in prostatic hyperplasia: a histologic and bacterial study. J Urol 1979;121:755–60.

25. Kramer G, Marberger M. Could inflammation be a key component in the progression of benign prostatic hyperplasia? Curr Opin Urol 2006;16:25–9.

26. Steiner G, Gessl A, Kramer G, et al. Phenotype and function of peripheral and prostatic lymphocytes in patients with benign prostatic hyperplasia. J Urol 1994;151:480–4.

27. Theyer G, Kramer G, Assmann I. Phenotypic characterization of infiltrating leukocytes in benign prostatic hyperplasia. Lab Invest 1992;66:96–107.

28. McNeal JE. Regional morphology and pathology of the prostate. Am J Clin Pathol 1968;49(3):347–57.

29. Bennett BD, Culberson DE, Petty CS. Histopathology of prostatitis [abstract]. J Urol 1990;143: 265.

30. Weiss JP, Wein A, Jacobs J, et al. Use of nitrofurantoin macro-crystals after transurethral prostatectomy. J Urol 1983;130:479.

31. De Marzo AM, Platz EA, Sutcliffe S, et al. Inflammation in prostate carcinogenesis. Nat Rev Cancer 2007;7:256–69.

32. Nickel JC, Downey J, Young I, et al. Asymptomatic inflammation and/or infection in benign prostatic hyperplasia. BJU Int 1999;84:976–81.

33. Gerstenbluth RE, Seftel AD, MacLennan GT, et al. Distribution of chronic prostatitis in radical prostatectomy specimens with up-regulation of bcl-2 in areas of inflammation. J Urol 2002;167: 2267–70.

34. Roehrborn CG. Benign prostatic hyperplasia: an overview. Rev Urol 2005;7(9):S3–14.

35. Roehrborn CG. Definition of at-risk patients: baseline variables. BJU Int 2006;97(Suppl 2):7–11 [discussion: 21–2].

36. Nickel JC, Roehrborn CG, O'Leary MP, et al. The relationship between prostate inflammation and lower urinary tract symptoms: examination of baseline data from the REDUCE trial. Eur Urol 2008;54: 1379–84.

37. Nickel JC. Inflammation and benign prostatic hyperplasia. Urol Clin North Am 2007;35:109–15.

38. Parsons JK, Carter HB, Partin AW, et al. Metabolic factors associated with benign prostatic hyperplasia. J Clin Endocrinol Metab 2006;91(7):2562–8.

39. Popp KA. Assignment of patients into the classification of cardiomyopathies. Circulation 1992; 86(5):1622–33.

40. Boon TA, Van Venrooij GE, Eckhardt MD. Effect of diabetes mellitus on lower urinary tract symptoms and dysfunction in patients with benign prostatic hyperplasia. Curr Urol Rep 2001;2(4):297–301.

41. Bostwick DG, Cooner WH, Denis L, et al. The association of benign prostatic hyperplasia and cancer of the prostate. Cancer 1992;70(Suppl 1):291–301.

42. Carson C, Rittmaster R. The role of dihydrotestosterone in benign prostatic hyperplasia. Urology 2003;61(4 Suppl 1):2–7.

43. Hammarsten J, Högstedt B. Calculated fast-growing benign prostatic hyperplasia–a risk factor for developing clinical prostate cancer. Scand J Urol Nephrol 2002;36(5):330–8.

44. Hammarsten J, Högstedt B. Hyperinsulinaemia as a risk factor for developing benign prostatic hyperplasia. Eur Urol 2001;39(2):151–8.

45. Hammarsten J, Högstedt B. Clinical, anthropometric, metabolic and insulin profile of men with fast annual growth rates of benign prostatic hyperplasia. Blood Press 1999;8(1):29–36.

46. Hedelin H, Johansson N, Ströberg P. Relationship between benign prostatic hyperplasia and lower urinary tract symptoms and correlation between prostate volume and serum prostate-specific antigen in clinical routine. Scand J Urol Nephrol 2005;39(2):154–9.

47. De Marzo AM, Marchi VL, Epstein JI, et al. Proliferative inflammatory atrophy of the prostate: implications for prostatic carcinogenesis. Am J Pathol 1999;155:1985–92.

48. Nelson WG, De Marzo AM, DeWeese TL, et al. The role of inflammation in the pathogenesis of prostate cancer. J Urol 2004;172(5 Pt 2):S6–11.

49. Nelson WG, De Marzo AM, Isaacs WB. Prostate cancer. N Engl J Med 2003;349(4):366–81.

50. Nelson WG, De Marzo AM, DeWeese TL. The molecular pathogenesis of prostate cancer: Implications for prostate cancer prevention. Urology 2001;57:39–45.

51. Köhler TS, McVary KT. The relationship between erectile dysfunction and lower urinary tract symptoms and the role of phosphodiesterase type 5 inhibitors. Eur Urol 2008.

52. McVary K. Lower urinary tract symptoms and sexual dysfunction: epidemiology and pathophysiology. BJU Int 2006;97(Suppl 2):23–8 [discussion: 44–5].

53. McVary KT, Rademaker A, Lloyd GL, et al. Autonomic nervous system overactivity in men with lower urinary tract symptoms secondary to benign prostatic hyperplasia. J Urol 2005;174(4 Pt 1):1327–433.

54. Rosen RC, Wei JT, Althof SE, et al. Association of sexual dysfunction with lower urinary tract symptoms of BPH and BPH medical therapies: results from the BPH Registry. Urology 2009; 73(3):562–6.

55. Clemens JQ, Markossian TW, Meenan RT, et al. Overlap of voiding symptoms, storage symptoms and pain in men and women. J Urol 2007;178(4 Pt 1):1345–8.

56. Dubeau CE. The aging lower urinary tract. J Urol 2006;175(3 Pt 2):S11–5.

57. Dutkiewicz S, Witeska A, Stepień K. Relationship between prostate-specific antigen, prostate volume, retention volume and age in benign prostatic hypertrophy (BPH). Int Urol Nephrol 1995; 27(6):763–8.

58. Elbadasi A, Diokno AC, Millard RJ. The aging bladder: morphology and urodynamics. World J Urol 1998;16(Suppl 1):S10–34.

59. Nordling J. The aging bladder—a significant but underestimated role in the development of lower urinary tract symptoms. Exp Gerontol 2002; 37(8–9):991–9.

60. Ozayar A, Zumrutbas AE, Yaman O. The relationship between lower urinary tract symptoms (LUTS), diagnostic indicators of benign prostatic hyperplasia (BPH), and erectile dysfunction in patients with moderate to severely symptomatic BPH. Int Urol Nephrol 2008;40(4):933–9.

61. Ozden C, Ozdal OL, Urgancioglu G, et al. The correlation between metabolic syndrome and prostatic growth in patients with benign prostatic hyperplasia. Eur Urol 2007;51(1):199–203, discussion 204–6.

62. Palapattu GS, Sutcliffe S, Bastian PJ, et al. Prostate carcinogenesis and inflammation: emerging insights. Carcinogenesis 2005;26(7):1170–81.

63. Nandeesha H. Benign prostatic hyperplasia: dietary and metabolic risk factors. Int Urol Nephrol 2008;40:649–56.

64. Guo LJ, Zhang XH, Li PJ, et al. Association study between benign prostatic hyperplasia and primary hypertension. Zhonghua Wai Ke Za Zhi 2005;43(2): 108–11.

65. Steers WD, Clemow DB, Persson K, et al. Tuttle the spontaneously hypertensive rat: insight into the pathogenesis of irritative symptoms in benign prostatic hyperplasia and young anxious males. Exp Physiol 1999;84(1):137–47.

66. Kasturi S, Russell S, McVary KT. Metabolic syndrome and lower urinary tract symptoms secondary to benign prostatic hyperplasia. Curr Urol Rep 2006;7(4):288–92.

67. Geppetti P, Nassini R, Materazzi S, et al. The concept of neurogenic inflammation. BJU Int 2008;101(Suppl 3):2–6.

68. Giovannucci E, Rimm EB, Chute CG, et al. Am Obesity and benign prostatic hyperplasia. J Epidemiol 1994;140(11):989–1002.

69. Compérat E, Reitz A, Delcourt A, et al. Histologic features in the urinary bladder wall affected from neurogenic overactivity–a comparison of inflammation, oedema and fibrosis with and without injection of botulinum toxin type A. Eur Urol 2006; 50:1058–64.

70. Marchand JE, Sant GR, Kream RM. Increased expression of substance P receptor– encoding mRNA in bladder biopsies from patients with interstitial cystitis. Br J Urol 1998;81:224–8.

71. Nazif O, Teichman JM, Gebhart GF. Neural upregulation in interstitial cystitis. Urology 2007;69(Suppl): 24–33.

72. Pang X, Marchand J, Sant GR, et al. Increased number of substance P positive nerve fibres in interstitial cystitis. Br J Urol 1995;75:744–50.

73. Qin C, Malykhina AP, Akbarali HI, et al. Cross-organ sensitization of lumbosacral spinal neurons receiving urinary bladder input in rats with inflamed colon. Gastroenterology 2005;129:1967–78.

74. Rudick CN, Chen MC, Mongiu AK, et al. Organ cross talk modulates pelvic pain. Am J Physiol Regul Integr Comp Physiol 2007;293:R1191–8.

75. Ustinova EE, Gutkin DW, Pezzone MA. Sensitization of pelvic nerve afferents and mast cell infiltration in the urinary bladder following chronic colonic irritation is mediated by neuropeptides. Am J Physiol Renal Physiol 2007;292:F123–30.

76. Ustinova EE, Fraser MO, Pezzone MA. Colonic irritation in the rat sensitizes urinary bladder afferents to mechanical and chemical stimuli: an afferent origin of pelvic organ cross-sensitization. Am J Physiol Renal Physiol 2006;290:F1478–87.

77. Nickel JC, Saad F. The American Urological Association 2003 guideline on management of benign

prostatic hyperplasia: a Canadian opinion. Can J Urol 2004;11(2):2186–93.

78. Nickel JC. The overlapping lower urinary tract symptoms of benign prostatic hyperplasiz and prostatitis. Curr Opin Urol 2006;16:5–10.

79. Brookes ST, Donovan JL, Peters TJ, et al. Sexual dysfunction in men after treatment for lower urinary tract symptoms: evidence from randomized control trial. Br Med J 2002;324:1059–61.

80. Frankel SJ, Donovan JL, Peters TI, et al. Sexual dysfunction in men with lower urinary tract symptoms. J Clin Epidemiol 1998;51:677–85.

81. Rosen R, Altwein J, Boyle P, et al. Lower urinary tract symptoms and male sexual dysfunction: the multinational survey of the aging male (MSAM-7). Eur Urol 2003;44:637–49.

82. Nickel JC, Elhilali M, Vallancien G, ALF-ONE Study Group. Benign prostatic hyperplasia (BPH) and prostatitis: prevalence of painful ejaculation in men with clinical BPH. BJU Int 2005;95: 571–4.

83. Rhodes T, Girman CJ, Jacobsen SJ, et al. Longitudinal prostate growth rates during 5 years in randomly selected community men 40 to 79 years old. J Urol 1999;161(4):1174–9.

84. Ganpule AP, Desai MR, Desai MM, et al. Natural history of lower urinary tract symptoms: preliminary report from a community-based Indian study. BJU Int 2004;94(3):332–4.

85. Bosch JL, Kranse R, van Mastrigt R, et al. Reasons for the weak correlation between prostate volume and urethral resistance parameters in patients with prostatism. J Urol 1995;153(3 Pt 1):689–93.

86. Roehrborn CG. The epidemiology of acute urinary retention in benign prostatic hyperplasia. Rev Urol 2001;3(4):187–92.

87. Girman CJ, Jacobsen SJ, Guess HA, et al. Natural history of prostatism: relationship among symptoms, prostate volume and peak urinary flow rate. J Urol 1995;153(5):1510–5.

88. Bosch JL, Hop WC, Kirkels WJ, et al. The International Prostate Symptom Score in a community-based sample of men between 55 and 74 years of age: prevalence and correlation of symptoms with age, prostate volume, flow rate and residual urine volume. Br J Urol 1995;75(5):622–30.

89. Vesely S, Knutson T, Damber JE, et al. Relationship between age, prostate volume, prostate-specific antigen, symptom score and uroflowmetry in men with lower urinary tract symptoms. Scand J Urol Nephrol 2003;37(4):322–8.

90. Ezz el Din K, Kiemeney LA, de Wildt MJ, et al. Correlation between uroflowmetry, prostate volume, postvoid residue, and lower urinary tract symptoms as measured by the International Prostate Symptom Score. Urology 1996;48(3):393–7.

91. Lee T, Seong DH, Yoon SM, et al. Prostate shape and symptom score in benign prostatic hyperplasia. Yonsei Med J 2001;42(5):532–8.

92. Girman CJ, Panser LA, Chute CG, et al. Natural history of prostatism: urinary flow rates in a community-based study. J Urol 1993;150(3):887–92.

93. Vulchanova A, Wang L, Li X, et al. Immunocytochemical localization of the vanilloid receptor 1 (VR1): relationship to neuropeptides, the P2X3 purinoceptor and IB4 binding sites. Eur J Neurosci 1999;11:946–58.

94. Nitti VW, Kim Y, Combs AJ. Correlation of the AUA symptom index with urodynamics in patients with suspected benign prostatic hyperplasia. Neurourol Urodyn 1994;13(5):521–7 [discussion: 527–9].

95. Netto Júnior NR, D'Ancona CA, de Lima ML. Correlation between the International Prostatic Symptom Score and a pressure-flow study in the evaluation of symptomatic benign prostatic hyperplasia. J Urol 1996;155(1):200–2.

96. Yalla SV, Sullivan MP, Lecamwasam HS, et al. Correlation of American Urological Association symptom index with obstructive and nonobstructive prostatism. J Urol 1995;153(3 Pt 1):674–9 [discussion: 679–80].

97. Zlotta AR, Teillac P, Raynaud JP, et al. Evaluation of male sexual function in patients with Lower Urinary Tract Symptoms (LUTS) associated with Benign Prostatic Hyperplasia (BPH) treated with a phytotherapeutic agent (permixon), tamsulosin or finasteride. Eur Urol 2005;48(2):269–76.

98. Madersbacher S, Klingler HC, Schatzl G, et al. Age related urodynamic changes in patients with benign prostatic hyperplasia. J Urol 1996;156(5): 1662–7.

99. Svanborg A. Age-related changes in cardiac physiology. Drugs Aging 1997;10(6):463–72.

100. Lakatta EG, Levy D. Arterial and cardiac aging: major shareholders in cardiovascular disease enterprises: part II: the aging heart in health: links to heart disease. Circulation 2003;107(2):346–54.

101. Lewis JF, Maron BJ. Cardiovascular consequences of the aging process. Cardiovasc Clin 1992;22(2): 25–34.

102. Roffe C. Aging of the heart. Br J Biomed Sci 1998; 55(2):136–48.

103. Lakatta EG. Similar myocardial effects of aging and hypertension. Eur Heart J 1990;11(Suppl G):29–38.

104. Susic D, Frohlich ED. Hypertension and the heart. Curr Hypertens Rep 2000;2(6):565–9.

105. Varagic J, Susic D, Frohlish E. Heart, aging, and hypertension. Curr Opin Cardiol 2001;16(6): 336–41.

106. Carson P. Pharmacologic treatment of congestive heart failure. Clin Cardiol 1996;19(4):271–7.

107. Hollenberg SM. Vasodilators in acute heart failure. Heart Fail Rev 2007;12(2):143–7.

108. Elbadawi A, Hailemariam S, Yalla SV, et al. Structural basis of geriatric voiding dysfunction. VI. Validation and update of diagnostic criteria in 71 detrusor biopsies. J Urol 1997;157(5):1802–13.

109. Jensen KM, Bruskewitz RC, Madsen PO. Urodynamic findings in elderly males without prostatic complaints. Urology 1984;24(2):211–3.

110. Saito M, Ohmura M, Kondo A. Effect of ageing on blood flow to the bladder and bladder function. Urol Int 1999;62(2):93–8.

111. Schäfer W. Urodynamics in benign prostatic hyperplasia (BPH). Arch Ital Urol Androl 1993;65(6):599–613.

112. Tse V, Wills E, Szonyi G, et al. The application of ultrastructural studies in the diagnosis of bladder dysfunction in a clinical setting. J Urol 2000;163(2):535–9.

113. Tsukamoto T, Masumori N, Rahman M, et al. Change in International Prostate Symptom Score, prostrate-specific antigen and prostate volume in patients with benign prostatic hyperplasia followed longitudinally. Int J Urol 2007;14(4):321–4 [discussion: 325].

114. Van Mastrigt R. Age dependence of urinary bladder contractility. Neurourol Urodyn 1992;11:315–7.

115. DiSanto M, Stein R, Chang S, et al. Alteration in expression of myosin isoforms in detrusor smooth muscle following bladder outlet obstruction. Am J Physiol Cell Physiol 2003;285:C1397–410.

116. Di Silverio F, Gentile V, De Matteis A, et al. Distribution of inflammation, pre-malignant lesions, incidental carcinoma in histologically confirmed benign prostatic hyperplasia: a retrospective analysis. Eur Urol 2003;43:164–75.

117. Greenland JE, Brading AF. The effect of bladder outflow obstruction on detrusor blood flow changes during the voiding cycle in conscious pigs. J Urol 2001;165(1):245–8.

118. Greenland JE, Hvistendahl JJ, Andersen H, et al. The effect of bladder outlet obstruction on tissue oxygen tension and blood flow in the pig bladder. Br J Urol 2000;85(9):1109–14.

119. Lu SH, Chang LS, Yang AH, et al. Mitochondrial DNA deletion of the human detrusor after partia bladder outlet obstruction-correlation withurodynamic analysis. Urology 2000;55(4):603–7.

120. Lu SH, Wei YH, Chang LS, et al. Morphological and morphometric analysis of human detrusor mitochondria with urodynamic correlation after partial bladder outlet obstruction. J Urol 2000;163(1):225–9.

121. Luo J, Dunn T, Ewing C, et al. Gene expression signature of benign prostatic hyperplasia revealed by cDNA microarray analysis. Prostate 2002;51(3):189–200.

122. Nevel-McGarvey CA, Levin RM, Haugaard N, et al. Mitochondrial involvement in bladder function and dysfunction. Mol Cell Biochem 1999;194:1–15.

123. Blaivas JG, Flisser AJ, Tash JA. Treatment of primary bladder neck obstruction in women with transurethral resection of the bladder neck. J Urol 2004;171(3):1172–5.

124. Boluyt MO. Matrix gene expression and decompensated heart failure: the aged SHR model. Cardiovasc Res 2000;46(2):239–49.

125. Lee AJ, Garraway WM, Simpson RJ, et al. The natural history of untreated lower urinary tract symptoms in middle-aged and elderly men over a period of five years. Eur Urol 1998;34(4):325–32.

126. Jacobsen SJ, Girman CJ, Lieber MM. Natural history of benign prostatic hyperplasia. Urology 2001;58(6 Suppl 1):5–16 [discussion: 16].

127. Thomas AW, Cannon A, Bartlett E, et al. The natural history of lower urinary tract dysfunction in men: minimum 10-year urodynamic follow-up of untreated bladder outlet obstruction. BJU Int 2005;96(9):1301–6.

128. Al-Hayek S, Thomas A, Abrams P. Natural history of detrusor contractility–minimum ten-year urodynamic follow-up in men with bladder outlet obstruction and those with detrusor. Scand J Urol Nephrol Suppl 2004;215:101–8.

129. Andersson KE. Storage and voiding symptoms: pathophysiologic aspects. Urology 2003;62(5 Suppl 2):3–10.

130. Antunes AA, Srougi M, Dall'oglio MF, et al. The role of BPH, lower urinary tract symptoms, and PSA levels on erectile function of Brazilian men who undergo prostate cancer screening. J Sex Med 2008;5(7):1702–7.

Benign Prostatic Hyperplasia: Symptoms, Symptom Scores, and Outcome Measures

Daniel A. Thorner, DO[a], Jeffrey P. Weiss, MD[a,b,*]

KEYWORDS
- BPH • Questionnaires • LUTS • Outcomes
- Voiding dysfunction

The approach to a patient with benign prostatic hyperplasia (BPH) and lower urinary tract symptoms (LUTS) begins with a detailed history. The goal is to clearly identify the patient's urinary complaints, including frequency of micturition, urgency, urge incontinence, weak stream, the need to push or strain, hesitancy, intermittency, dysuria, and hematuria. Causes of these symptoms gleaned from the history include urinary tract infection, prostatic obstruction, BPH, bladder cancer, prostate cancer, urolithiasis, urethral stricture disease, and neurologic causes (eg, Parkinson disease, cerebrovascular accident). In patients experiencing urinary frequency or polyuria, the symptoms may be caused by nonurologic conditions, such as polydipsia, diabetes mellitus, and diabetes insipidus. Similarly, nocturia may be associated with factors other than prostatic obstruction or BPH, including detrusor overactivity, sensory urgency, abnormal drinking patterns, congestive heart failure, venous insufficiency, or polydipsia. The use of prescription drugs and over-the-counter medications should be discussed because some medications affect detrusor contractility (eg, anticholinergics) or increase bladder outflow resistance (eg, alpha agonists). Bladder diaries and symptom questionnaires are useful as adjuncts to information acquired in the history.

Questionnaires are especially useful in evaluating patients in that they afford the patient and physician an opportunity to efficiently record the nature, frequency of occurrence, severity, and degree of bother of the patient's LUTS. However, questionnaires are not an end unto themselves; rather, they serve as a useful adjunct to history taking. Merely reading the questionnaire makes the patients think more intently about their symptoms, but not all patients are compliant. Some do not answer the questions at all; others answer them without even thinking; and some do not understand the questions and answer them incorrectly. It is important, therefore, that the patients be specifically queried for the accuracy of their answers. The purpose, function, and characteristics of each of the more common LUTS questionnaires can be seen in **Table 1**. The International Prostate Symptom Score (IPSS), also known as the American Urological Association Symptom Index, has been recommended for the assessment of severity of patients' LUTS.[1] However, the IPSS cannot differentiate between patients with BPH and those with other causes of voiding dysfunction; therefore, its utility is mostly as a general guide to symptom severity. The Overactive Bladder Symptom Score,[2] the Urgency Perception Score,[3] and the Urgency Perception Scale[4] are the 3 questionnaires that focus on urgency-associated symptoms, and these are useful in determining patient response to treatment. In addition, the Patient Global Impression of Improvement[5] questionnaire is a simplistic

[a] Department of Urology, SUNY Downstate Medical School, 445 Lenox Road, Box 79, Brooklyn, NY 11203, USA
[b] The James Buchanan Brady Department of Urology, Weill Medical College of Cornell University, New York, NY, USA
* Corresponding author. The James Buchanan Brady Department of Urology, Weill Medical College of Cornell University, New York, NY.
E-mail address: urojock@aol.com (J.P. Weiss).

Urol Clin N Am 36 (2009) 417–429
doi:10.1016/j.ucl.2009.07.001
0094-0143/09/$ – see front matter. Published by Elsevier Inc.

Table 1
Instruments used in the evaluation of men with BPH and LUTS

Instrument	Origination	Function	Number of Questions	Other Features or Disadvantages
International Prostate Symptom Score[1]	1992	Primarily used in the clinical management of men with LUTS. Also used in research studies investigating the medical/surgical management of patients with voiding dysfunction in treatment response	7	Instrument is nonspecific in that it is not able to differentiate between patients with BPH and those with other forms of voiding dysfunction. It is weighted toward voiding as opposed to storage symptoms
Overactive Bladder Symptom Score[2]	8/2007	Quantitates all aspects of overactive bladder symptoms (OAB) Total possible score is 28	7	Questions are in graded response format Contains urgency subscale Assigns severity score (28 being the worst) May be useful as an OAB outcome instrument
Urgency Perception Score[3]	1/2007	Objectively quantifies severity/degree of OAB/urgency	1	When used as outcome instrument, improvement based on decrease in grade of usual reason for voiding or decrease in number of urgency voids. Sometimes used in combination with urgency severity score
Patient Global Impression of Improvement (PGII)[5]		Used to evaluate patient condition pre- and postsurgery.	Single item-graded response	Treatment failure based on PGII ≥ 4
King's Health Questionnaire Assessment[6,7]		Quality of life assessment Used for evaluation of clinical response in BPH patients	7 domains	Most useful when used in patients with OAB Also used as an assessment tool for urinary incontinence
The Pittsburgh Sleep Quality Index[8]	5/1998	Assesses sleep quality and disturbances over a 1-mo period Quantitates patient's level of sleep disturbance associated with nocturia	19 items (7 component scores)	Standardized version of areas routinely assessed in patients with sleep disturbance Used in patients with sleep/wake complaints
LUTS Outcome Score[9]	2004	Outcome instrument used in patients receiving treatment for LUTS	8 items (assigned score of 0–2)	Unlike the International Prostate Symptom Score, it combines subjective, semisubjective, and objective parameters
Urgency Perception Scale[4]	2005	Used to assess perceived urinary urgency; specifically used to evaluate patient response to antimuscarinic treatment	1	Used as outcome instrument In comparison to Urgency Perception Score, similar function when evaluating patient response to treatment; however, fewer response options make it less specific

assessment of how the patient feels after treatment, and it does not evaluate LUTS specifically. The King's Health Questionnaire,[6,7] which is not a symptom score, focuses on the bother owing to LUTS and incontinence and on overall quality of life, including personal, social, and emotional perspectives. The Pittsburgh Sleep Quality Index[8] is an instrument used to assess patient sleep patterns and interruptions that can be associated with LUTS, but it does not evaluate specific voiding symptoms in patients. Some questionnaires double as outcome instruments in assessing response to treatment. For example, the LUTS Outcome Score is used in patients receiving treatment for LUTS, and it combines subjective and objective parameters.[9] This score may easily be ciphered with the data derived from the IPSS, uroflow, postvoid residual volume, voiding diary, and a single question regarding whether treatment administered resulted in cure, improvement, or same or worse status. Subanalysis of components of these questionnaires allows for the determination of what drives patients to seek treatment and what in fact gets better (or not) in response to such therapy. The International Consultation on Incontinence Modular Questionnaire contains several modules designed to evaluate LUTS (including subsets of incontinence, overactive bladder, nocturia, and neurogenic and pediatric conditions) and vaginal and bowel symptoms.[10]

The voiding diary (Appendix) is an essential part of the workup; the time and volume of each void and a description of associated LUTS should be noted. The voiding diary differs from a simple frequency-volume chart in that it not only incorporates frequency, voided volume, urge episodes, pad usage, and fluid intake but also includes data related to patient activities and allows patients to have a more thorough self-evaluation of their LUTS. Above all, the voiding diary allows the physician to assess a patient's voiding patterns (ie, frequency, nocturia, incontinent episodes) during his ordinary life activities. The maximum voided volume gleaned from the diary is useful as a guide for determining the optimal infusion rate during cystometry and for estimating the minimum volume that should be infused. Completing a voiding diary requires that the patient be self-motivated, as diligence is needed to record and accurately reflect voiding patterns. It is also important that the physician spends time providing the patient with detailed instructions for the voiding diary. Most important of all is that the physician and staff emphasize the diagnostic importance of the diary. In some research studies, voiding diaries are kept for up to a week, but for routine clinical practice, a 24-hour diary will suffice.[11] It has been shown that charts can be increasingly complex yet acceptable and practical for patients to complete, provided that appropriate instruction is given.[12] For assessment of nocturia, the patient should record the time he or she goes to bed with the intention of falling asleep and the time he or she awakens for the day. These data are essential to clearly define characteristics of nocturia, such as nocturnal polyuria and nocturnal bladder capacity. Pad weight testing allows for detection and quantification of urine loss during a defined period of time. It is diagnostic for incontinence but not for its cause. Pad weight gain during a 24-hour period (wet pad weight minus dry pad weight) is assessed and used to determine the level of incontinence. Ideally, 24-hour diary and pad-weight-testing period should be representative of a normal day; notation should be made as to whether the patient felt that the LUTS were better or worse than normal. These can be used as outcome instruments to record patient symptoms at baseline and after therapeutic intervention (ie, surgical or medical treatment). The Appendix provides an example of 1 type of voiding diary that incorporates patient symptoms (reasons for voiding) and incontinent episodes.

APPENDIX: SUPPLEMENTARY DATA

Supplementary data associated with this article can be found in the online version at doi:10.1016/j.ucl.2009.07.001.

REFERENCES

1. Barry MJ, Fowler FJ Jr, O'Leary MP, et al. The American Urological Association symptom index for benign prostatic hyperplasia. J Urol 1992;148:1549.
2. Blaivas JG, Panagopoulos G, Weiss JP, et al. Validation of the Overactive Bladder Symptom Score. J Urol 2007;178:543.
3. Blaivas JG, Panagopoulos G, Weiss JP, et al. The urgency perception score: validation and test-retest. J Urol 2007;177:199.
4. Cardozo L, Coyne KS, Versi E. Validation of the urgency perception scale. BJU Int 2005;95(4):591.
5. Yalcin I, Bump R. Validation of two global impression questionnaires for incontinence. Am J Obstet Gynecol 2003;189:98–101.
6. Espuña Pons M, Castro Diaz D, Carbonell C, et al. [Comparison between the "ICIQ-UI Short Form" Questionnaire and the "King's Health Questionnaire" as assessment tools of urinary incontinence among women]. Actas Urol Esp 2007;5:502 [In Spanish].
7. Awa Y, Suzuki H, Hamano S, et al. Clinical effect of alpha 1D/A adrenoreceptor inhibitor naftopidil on benign prostatic hyperplasia: an international prostate symptom score and King's Health Questionnaire assessment. Int J Urol 2008;8:709.

8. Buysse DJ, Reynolds CF 3rd, Monk TH, et al. The Pittsburgh Sleep Quality Index: a new instrument for psychiatric practice and research. Psychiatry Res 1989;2:193.

9. Weiss JP, Blaivas JG, Tash Anger JA, et al. Development and validation of a new treatment outcome score for men with LUTS. Neurourol Urodyn 2004;23(2):88.

10. Avery K, Donovan J, Peters TJ, et al. A brief and robust measure for evaluating the symptoms and impact of urinary incontinence. Neurourol Urodyn 2004;23(4):322–30.

11. Brown JS, McNaughton KS, Wyman JF, et al. Measurement characteristics of a bladder diary for use by men and women with overactive bladder. Urology 2003;61(4):802–9.

12. Abrams P, Klevmark B. Frequency volume charts: an indispensable part of lower urinary tract assessment. Scand J Urol Nephrol 1996;30(179):47–53.

APPENDIX: SUPPLEMENTARY DATA

International Prostate Symptom Score (IPSS)1

Please answer the following questions about your urinary symptoms.
Write your score for each question at the end of each row.

Over the past month, how often have you...	Not at all	Less than 1 time in 5	Less than half the time	About half the time	More than half the time	Almost always	Your Score
1. ...had a sensation of not emptying your bladder completely after you finished urinating?	0	1	2	3	4	5	
2. ...had to urinate again less than two hours after you finished urinating?	0	1	2	3	4	5	
3. ...stopped and started again several times when you urinated?	0	1	2	3	4	5	
4. ...found it difficult to postpone urination?	0	1	2	3	4	5	
5. ...had a weak urinary stream?	0	1	2	3	4	5	
6. ...had to push or strain to begin urination?	0	1	2	3	4	5	

And finally..	None	Once	Twice	3 times	4 times	5 times or more	
7. Over the past month, how many times did you most typically get up to urinate from the time you went to bed at night until the time you got up in the morning?	0	1	2	3	4	5	

Add up your total score and write it in the box.							Total

From Barry MJ, Fowler FJ Jr, O'Leary MP, et al. The American Urological Association symptom index for benign prostatic hyperplasia. J Urol 1992;148:1549; with permission.

OAB Symptom Score2

OAB Questionnaire

NAME: _____ DATE: _____

1. How often do you usually urinate during the day?
   - ☐ no more often than once in 4 hours
   - ☐ about every 3–4 hours
   - ☐ about every 2–3 hours
   - ☐ about every 1–2 hours
   - ☐ at least once an hour

2. How many times do you usually urinate at night (from the time you go to bed until the time you wake up for the day)?
   - ☐ 0–1 times
   - ☐ 2 times
   - ☐ 3 times
   - ☐ 4 times
   - ☐ 5 or more times

3. What is the reason that you usually urinate?
   - ☐ out of convenience (no urge or desire)
   - ☐ because I have a mild urge or desire (but can delay urination for over an hour if I have to)
   - ☐ because I have a moderate urge or desire (but can delay urination for more than 10 but less than 60 minutes if I have to)
   - ☐ because I have a severe urge or desire (but can delay urination for less than 10 minutes if I have to)
   - ☐ because I have desperate urge or desire (must stop what I am doing and go immediately)

4. Once you get the urge or desire to urinate, how long can you usually postpone it comfortably?
   - ☐ more than 60 minutes
   - ☐ about 30–60 minutes
   - ☐ about 10–30 minutes
   - ☐ a few minutes (less than 10 minutes)
   - ☐ must go immediately

5. How often do you get a sudden urge or desire to urinate that makes you want to stop what you are doing and rush to the bathroom?
   - ☐ never
   - ☐ rarely
   - ☐ a few times a month
   - ☐ a few times a week
   - ☐ at least once a day

6. How often do you get a sudden urge or desire to urinate that makes you want to stop what you are doing and rush to the bathroom but you do not get there in time (ie you leak urine or wet pads)?
   - ☐ never
   - ☐ rarely
   - ☐ a few times a month
   - ☐ a few times a week
   - ☐ at least once a day

7. In your opinion how good is your bladder control?
   - ☐ perfect control
   - ☐ very good
   - ☐ good
   - ☐ poor
   - ☐ no control at all

From Blaivas JG, Panagopoulos G, Weiss JP, et al. Validation of the Overactive Bladder Symptom Score. J Urol 2007;178:543; with permission.

Display box

Urgency Perception Score (same as question #3 of OAB Symptom Score Questionnaire above)[3]

"What is the reason you usually urinate?"

0   Convenience (no urge)

1   Mild urge (can hold greater than 1 hr)

2   Moderate urge (can hold greater than 10–60 mins)

3   Severe urge (can hold less than 10 mins)

4   Desperate urge (must go immediately)

From Blaivas JG, Panagopoulos G, Weiss JP, et al. The urgency perception score: validation and test-retest. J Urol 2007;177:199; with permission.

Display box

Patient Global Impression of Improvement[5]

Check the one number that best describes how your urinary tract condition is now, compared with how it was before you began taking medication in this study.

1.   Very much better

2.   Much better

3.   A little better

4.   No change

5.   A little worse

6.   Much worse

7.   Very much worse

From Yalcin I, Bump R. Validation of two global impression questionnaires for incontinence. Am J Obstet Gynecol 2003;189:98–101; with permission.

The King's Health Questionnaire Assessment (KHQ)[6,7]

1. How would you describe your health at the present?

Very good, Good, Fair, Poor, Very poor

2. How much do you think your bladder problem affects your life?

Not at all, A little, Moderately, A lot

Below are some daily activities that can be affected by bladder problems.

How much does your bladder problem affect you?

	1	2	3	4
3. ROLE LIMITATIONS	Not at all	Slightly	Moderately	A lot

A. Does your bladder problem affect your

   household tasks?

   (cleaning, shopping etc)

B. Does your bladder problem affect your

   job, or your normal daily activities

   outside the home?

	1	2	3	4
4. PHYSICAL/SOCIAL LIMITATION	Not at all	Slightly	Moderately	A lot

A Does your bladder problem affect

   your physical activities (e.g. going

   for a walk, running, sport, gym etc)?

B. Does your bladder problem affect

   your ability to travel?

C. Does your bladder problem limit

   your social life?

D. Does your bladder problem limit

   your ability to see and visit friends?

	0	1	2	3	4
5. PERSONAL RELATIONSHIPS	Not Applicable	Not at all	Slightly	Moderately	A lot

A. Does your bladder problem

   affect your relationship with

   your partner?

B. Does your bladder problem

   affect your sex life?

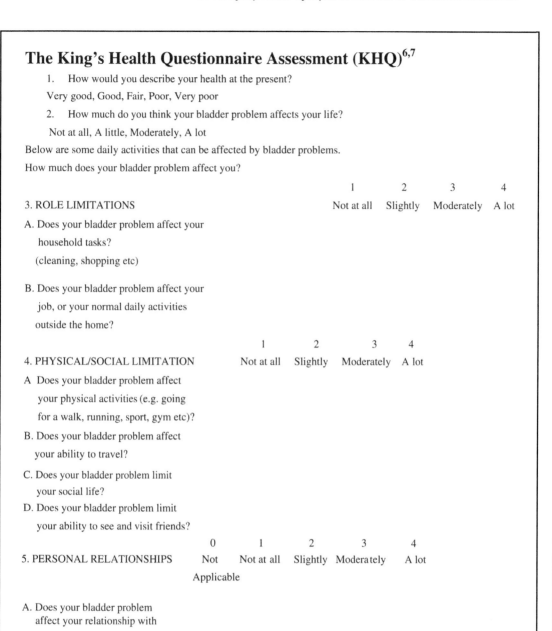

C. Does your bladder problem
affect your family life?

	1	2	3	4
6. EMOTIONS	Not at all	Slightly	Moderately	Very much

A. Does your bladder problem make
you feel depressed?

B. Does your bladder problem make
you feel anxious or nervous?

C. Does your bladder problem make
you feel bad about yourself?

	1	2	3	4
7.SLEEP/ENERGY	Never	Sometimes	Often	All the time

A. Does your bladder problem
affect your sleep?

B. Does your bladder problem make
you feel worn out and tired ?

8.Do you do any of the following?   If so how much?

	1	2	3	4
	Never	Sometimes	Often	All the time

A. Wear pads to keep dry?

B. Be careful how much
fluid you drink ?

C. Change your underclothes
because they get wet?

D. Worry in case you smell?

We would like to know what your bladder problems are and how much
they affect you ? From the list below choose only those problems that
you have at present. Leave out those that don't apply to you.

How much do they affect you?

FREQUENCY: going to the toilet very often
1. A little   2.Moderately   3. A lot
NOCTURIA: getting up at night to pass urine
1. A little   2.Moderately   3. A lot
URGENCY: a strong and difficult to control desire to pass urine
1. A little   2.Moderately   3. A lot
URGE INCONTINENCE: urinary leakage associated with a strong desire to pass urine
1. A little   2.Moderately   3. A lot
STRESS INCONTINENCE: urinary leakage with physical activity eg. coughing, running
1. A little   2.Moderately   3. A lot
NOCTURNAL ENURESIS: wetting the bed at night
1. A little   2.Moderately   3. A lot
INTERCOURSE INCONTINENCE: urinary leakage with sexual intercourse
1. A little   2.Moderately   3. A lot
WATERWORKS INFECTIONS
1. A little   2.Moderately   3. A lot
BLADDER PAIN
1. A little   2.Moderately   3. A lot

From Kelleher CJ, Cardozo LD, Khullar V, Salvatore S. A new questionnaire to assess the quality of life of urinary incontinent women. Br J Obstet Gynaecol 1997;104:1374–9; with permission.

The Pittsburgh Sleep Quality Index (PSQI)[8]

Name_____ ID#_____ Date_____ Time____ $\begin{array}{l}\text{AM}\\ \text{PM}\end{array}$

PITTSBURGH SLEEP QUALITY INDEX

INSTRUCTIONS:

The following questions relate to your usual sleep habits during the past month only. Your answers should indicate the most accurate reply for the majority of days and nights in the past month. Please answer all questions.

1. During the past month, what time have you usually gone to bed at night?

> BED TIME _____

2. During the past month, how long (in minutes) has it usually taken you to fall asleep each night?

> NUMBER OF MINUTES _____

3. During the past month, what time have you usually gotten up in the morning?

> GETTING UP TIME _____

4. During the past month, how many hours of actual sleep did you get at night? (This may be different than the number of hours you spent in bed.)

> HOURS OF SLEEP PER NIGHT _____

For each of the remaining questions, check the one best response. Please answer all questions.

5. During the past month, how often have you had trouble sleeping because you . . .

a) Cannot get to sleep within 30 minutes

Not during the   Less than   Once or twice   Three or more
past month_____   once a week_____   a week_____   times a week_____

b) Wake up in the middle of the night or early morning

Not during the   Less than   Once or twice   Three or more
past month_____   once a week_____   a week_____   times a week_____

c) Have to get up to use the bathroom

Not during the   Less than   Once or twice   Three or more
past month_____   once a week_____   a week_____   times a week_____

d) Cannot breathe comfortably

Not during the   Less than   Once or twice   Three or more
past month_____   once a week_____   a week_____   times a week_____

e) Cough or snore loudly

Not during the   Less than   Once or twice   Three or more
past month_____   once a week_____   a week_____   times a week_____

f) Feel too cold

Not during the   Less than   Once or twice   Three or more
past month_____   once a week_____   a week_____   times a week_____

g) Feel too hot

Not during the   Less than   Once or twice   Three or more
past month_____   once a week_____   a week_____   times a week_____

h) Had bad dreams

Not during the   Less than   Once or twice   Three or more
past month_____   once a week_____   a week_____   times a week_____

i) Have pain

Not during the   Less than   Once or twice   Three or more
past month_____   once a week_____   a week_____   times a week_____

j) Other reason(s), please describe_____

How often during the past month have you had trouble sleeping because of this?

Not during the   Less than   Once or twice   Three or more
past month____   once a week____   a week____   times a week____

6. During the past month, how would you rate your sleep quality overall?

Very good _____
Fairly good _____
Fairly bad _____
Very bad _____

7. During the past month, how often have you taken medicine to help you sleep (prescribed or "over the counter")?

Not during the   Less than   Once or twice   Three or more
past month____   once a week____   a week____   times a week____

8. During the past month, how often have you had trouble staying awake while driving, eating meals, or engaging in social activity?

Not during the   Less than   Once or twice   Three or more
past month____   once a week____   a week____   times a week____

9. During the past month, how much of a problem has it been for you to keep up enough enthusiasm to get things done?

No problem at all _____
Only a very slight problem _____
Somewhat of a problem _____
A very big problem _____

10. Do you have a bed partner or room mate?

No bed partner or room mate _____
Partner/room mate in other room _____
Partner in same room, but not same bed _____
Partner in same bed _____

If you have a room mate or bed partner, ask him/her how often in the past month you have had . . .

a) Loud snoring

Not during the   Less than   Once or twice   Three or more
past month____   once a week____   a week____   times a week____

b) Long pauses between breaths while asleep

Not during the   Less than   Once or twice   Three or more
past month____   once a week____   a week____   times a week____

c) Legs twitching or jerking while you sleep

Not during the   Less than   Once or twice   Three or more
past month____   once a week____   a week____   times a week____

d) Episodes of disorientation or confusion during sleep

Not during the   Less than   Once or twice   Three or more
past month____   once a week____   a week____   times a week____

e) Other restlessness while you sleep; please describe_____

Not during the   Less than   Once or twice   Three or more
past month____   once a week____   a week____   times a week____

From Buysse DJ, Reynolds CF 3rd, Monk TH, et al. The Pittsburgh Sleep Quality Index: a new instrument for psychiatric practice and research. Psychiatry Res 1989;2:193; with permission.

The LUTS Outcome Score (LOS)[9]

1) Subjective Response:

	Cured	Improved	Same/Worse
Score:	*0*	*1*	*2*

2) Number of voids per day:

	<8	8-11	>11
Score:	*0*	*1*	*2*

3) Maximum voided volume (MVV) (cc):

	>250	150-250	<150
Score:	*0*	*1*	*2*

4) Measured Peak Flow Rate (cc/sec):

	>15	10-15	<10
Score:	*0*	*1*	*2*

5) Post-Void Residual (cc):

	<50	50-200	>200
Score:	*0*	*1*	*2*

6) Urgency (#4 on AUA-SS):

	0-1	2-3	4-5
Score:	*0*	*1*	*2*

7) Nocturia (#7 on AUA-SS):

	0-1	2-3	4-5
Score:	*0*	*1*	*2*

8) Voiding Difficulty (#1,3,5,6 on AUA-SS)

	0-1	2-3	4-5
Score #1:	*0*	*1*	*2*
Score #3:	*0*	*1*	*2*
Score #5:	*0*	*1*	*2*
Score #6:	*0*	*1*	*2*

Sum of above four scores is divided by 4.

*If patient is currently requiring catheterization, then a LOS of 16 is given automatically.

Total Possible Score: 16

From Weiss JP, Blaivas JG, Tash Anger JA, et al. Development and validation of a new treatment outcome score for men with LUTS. Neurourol Urodyn 2004;23(2):88; with permission.

Urgency Perception Scale [4]

Describe your typical experience when you feel the desire to urinate.

1- **I am usually not able to hold urine.**

2- **I am usually able to hold urine until I reach the toilet if I go immediately.**

3- **I am usually able to finish what I am doing before going to the toilet.**

From Cardozo L, Coyne KS, Versi E. Validation of the urgency perception scale. BJU Int 2005;95(4):591; with permission.

BLADDER DIARY

Name: _____ Date: _____

Time of Day Diary Started: _____ AM   PM

Time you went to bed _____ Time you got up for the day _____

Time of Urination and /or Incontinence episode	Why did you urinate at this time ? (see question # (a) for responses)	Amount of Urination (measure with a cup in cc's, ml's or ounces)	Incontinence grad e (see question # (b) below for responses)
1			
2			
3			
4			
5			
6			
7			
8			
9			
10			
11			
12			
13			
14			
15			

Please select the number next to your answer and use it for your response to the above questions.

(a) **Why did you urinate?**   (b) **Incontinence grade.**

(0)   out of convenience(no urge or desire)   **(0)** Grade 1 - some drops

(1)   because I have a mild urge   **(1)** Grade 2 - moderate loss(wet underpants)

          (but can delay urination for over   **(2)** Grade 3 - extensive loss (wet outer clothes)

          an hour if I have to)

(2)   because I have a moderate urge

          (b ut can delay urination for more than

          10 but less than 60 minutes if I have to)

(3)   because I have a severe urge

          (but can delay urination for less than 10 minutes)

(4)   because I have desperate urge
          (must stop what I am doing and go immediately)

OFFICE USE

Total 24 hrs output _____   **# of voids** _____ **MVV =** _____

Day volume _____ **# voids**   **Night volume** _____ **# voids** _____ **NPI** _____

Role of Invasive Urodynamic Testing in Benign Prostatic Hyperplasia and Male Lower Urinary Tract Symptoms

Jennifer L. Mehdizadeh, MD[a], Gary E. Leach, MD[b],*

KEYWORDS

• Urodynamics • Prostatic hyperplasia • Evaluation studies

The goals of treatment of lower urinary tract symptoms (LUTS) and benign prostatic hyperplasia (BPH) are improvement of patient quality of life through relief of symptom-related bother and prevention of morbidities, including retention, urinary tract infections (UTIs), obstructive uropathy, and stones. When evaluating LUTS, it is helpful to divide them into storage-related issues (urinary frequency, urgency, incontinence, or nocturia) and emptying-related issues (slow stream, intermittency, hesitancy, straining, feeling of incomplete emptying, or retention). The bladder outlet obstruction caused by BPH is responsible for only a portion of the symptoms related to BPH, however. Other possible causes of LUTS in the setting of BPH include detrusor overactivity (DO), increased bladder sensation, poor compliance, and impaired detrusor contractility. The majority of the treatments for BPH, however, focus on the relief of the possible outlet obstruction. There is also general consensus that patients with proved bladder outlet obstruction have a higher success rate after treatment of BPH than those that do not. The questions raised are (1) How is the degree of outlet obstruction assessed? and (2) How are patients counseled in regards to expectations for treatment outcomes with or without the diagnosis of bladder outlet obstruction?

The American Urological Association (AUA) guidelines for treatment of BPH recommend that initial evaluation of patients includes a history and focused physical, including digital rectal examination, urinalysis, prostate-specific antigen in selected patients, and an AUA/international prostate symptom score (IPSS). Optional diagnostic testing includes uroflow and postvoid residual (PVR).[1] These investigative tools may suggest bladder outlet obstruction, but the gold standard for diagnosis of obstruction is a pressure-flow study. Several studies have shown that only 40% to 60% of patients with suspected outlet obstruction, based on history or symptom index score, actually demonstrate true obstruction on pressure-flow studies.[2–4] Also, filling cystometry during urodynamics can reveal other bladder storage dysfunction that can explain the patient symptoms that may or may not be related to obstruction. The follow-up question is, Can patients be treated empirically for BPH with medical therapy or surgical intervention without an accurate diagnosis of bladder outlet

Dr. Leach is a paid consultant for Coloplast.
[a] Tower Urology, CA, USA
[b] Institute for Continence, Tower Urology, Cedars-Sinai Medical Office Towers, 8635 West Third Street, Suite 1 West, Los Angeles, CA 90048, USA
* Corresponding author.
E-mail address: drdorado@aol.com (G.E. Leach).

Urol Clin N Am 36 (2009) 431–441
doi:10.1016/j.ucl.2009.07.002

obstruction, or does the improvement in treatment outcome sufficiently justify the cost and invasiveness of a urodynamic evaluation?

The aim of this article is to describe the role of urodynamics in the evaluation of BPH, including illustration of existing urodynamic techniques, reviewing best practice guidelines and current literature, and providing recommendations for use of urodynamics in clinical practice.

PRINCIPLES OF URODYNAMICS

Multichannel urodynamic studies (UDS), including filling cystometry and detrusor pressure–uroflow study, can provide important pathophysiologic information about bladder function and outlet obstruction, particularly in the setting of BPH. Bates and colleagues stated, "the bladder is an unreliable witness,"[5] and many urologists acknowledge the difficulty in assessing men with lower urinary tract dysfunction by history and physical examination alone. Therefore, urodynamics can provide invaluable information regarding the origin and, sometimes, a better definition of a patient's true symptoms. These studies, however, are invasive, expensive, time consuming, and bothersome for patients and, therefore, should be undertaken in a thoughtful manner with excellent quality control. The International Continence Society (ICS) outlined good urodynamic practice consisting of

- Appropriate patient selection with a clear question to be answered and clear indication for obtaining certain measurements
- Precise measurements with complete documentation and data quality control
- Accurate analysis with correlation of findings with patient symptoms[6]

The first step in deciding to perform urodynamics is to formulate the urodynamic questions from the standard noninvasive urologic investigations, including history and physical, symptom scores, uroflowmetry, urinalysis, diary, and PVR volume. The patients' recorded bladder diary and serial flow rates with volumes greater than 150 mL can also aid in identification of abnormal voiding patterns. These tools alone may strongly suggest the probability of bladder outlet obstruction. There may be other contributing factors, however, such as patient-reported sensation during filling, contractility, compliance, or urethral stricture disease, that are not obvious on noninvasive testing but may be suspected and, therefore, warrant further investigation. Once there exists a clear indication for UDS, the procedure is focused to allow for the collection of objective data to explain the clinical presentation.

Because the purpose of urodynamics is to identify the pathophysiology of LUTS, it is important that the study be performed interactively with patients, who are encouraged to communicate when their symptoms are reproduced. The study is also dynamic, with continuous observation of bladder pressures as they are collected and correlation of these pressures with subjective symptoms. With this in mind, the person performing UDS must have an understanding of the physics of the measurements; practical experience with the equipment, including the ability to troubleshoot problems; an understanding of quality control of signals; and the ability to analyze resulting data.[6]

Once the indications and directed urodynamic questions are established, patients should be counseled regarding the procedure itself, including catheter placement and morbidity related to the procedure. The primary morbidity of UDS is physical discomfort. Previous studies report a risk of UTI after urodynamics with the use of prophylactic antibiotics ranging from 4% to 16%.[7–10] Latthe and colleagues[11] performed a systematic review of randomized controlled trials performed through March 2007 comparing effectiveness of prophylactic antibiotics with placebo or nothing for reducing bacteriologically proved UDS-related UTI. Eight trials with 995 patients, primarily women, were included and the investigators found a 40% reduction in risk of significant bacteriuria (colony count $>10^5$/mL). The antibiotics used included nitrofurantoin, floroquinolones, augmentin, trimethoprim, and cotrimazole and most were given before the study. Patients have also reported low rates of transient micturition pain and difficulty voiding, which is usually more pronounced in men than women; hematuria; cloudy urine; and fever.[9,12] Despite these morbidities, when patient-reported discomfort, embarrassment, and apprehension were investigated, 33% to 70% of men reported only mild pain and 74% to 95% of men reported they would undergo urodynamics again if medically indicated.[12,13] Important factors that have been identified to reduce patient discomfort and anxiety include the ability of a physician to communicate and explain during the procedure and the level of expertise in technique when performing UDS.

In preparation for urodynamic evaluation, a 7 to 10F transurethral dual lumen catheter is placed into the bladder and connected to an external pressure transducer to measure bladder pressure (Pves). A separate rectal balloon catheter is placed for the measurement of abdominal pressure (Pabd). True detrusor pressure (Pdet) is a calculation subtracting Pabd from Pves and represents a true rise in detrusor pressure independent of the effect of increased abdominal pressure (ie, during Valsalva's maneuver). "Zero pressure" should be the value recorded when the open end of the fluid-filled bladder catheter, connected to the transducer, is at the same vertical level as the transducer. The transducer should be set at the reference height, which is at the level of the upper edge of the symphysis pubis. Patients can be catheterized in the supine position, but the test should be performed in the upright position if patients are able to stand, to mimic the stresses on the bladder when patients are vertical. Also, whatever activity precipitates a patient's symptoms, including change of position, hearing water run, and so forth, should be replicated during the study.

INDICATIONS FOR URODYNAMICS

The role of urodynamics in the evaluation of LUTS in men with BPH remains controversial despite its provision of potentially useful information regarding bladder function and outlet obstruction. This controversy is primarily based on outcome studies that have confirmed men without proved bladder outlet obstruction may still benefit from relaxation of the bladder outlet with medication or surgical resection. There is evidence that men with obstruction fare better in symptom reduction, including decreased bother impact and improvement in quality of life after ablative prostate surgery than those without obstruction.[14–18] The difference in surgical success rates for men with demonstrable outlet obstruction is 15% to 29% higher than in those patients without obstruction.[14,17] Despite this, unobstructed men do not always fail, with moderate success rates of 55% to 78%. Tanaka and colleagues[19] studied the predictive value of UDS regarding efficacy of transurethral resection of prostate (TURP) at 3 months based on IPSS, quality-of-life questionnaires, and improvement of maximum flow rate (Qmax). Their finding was that as the degree of outlet obstruction worsened, TURP efficacy improved. Unobstructed patients with DO improved only minimally after TURP. Jensen and colleagues[15] also studied the predictive value of UDS for the outcome of prostatic surgery in 130 men, finding that at 6 months the success rate was 93% as opposed to 78% in unobstructed patients ($P<.02$). These investigators followed up on the same patients 8 years later and reviewed their symptom score analysis, uroflowmetry, and subjective evaluation of outcome. The difference in success rates was less impressive but persisted in long-term outcomes at 8 years: 83% in obstructed men versus 72% in men with no obstruction.[16]

Urodynamic evaluation, therefore, can be a valuable tool in the evaluation of BPH in providing a pathophyisiologic explanation of symptoms and guidance for therapeutic management. When counseling patients for treatment outcome expectations, urodynamics can also help predict response to various treatments. When symptoms and initial evaluation strongly suggest that obstruction is present (ie, low flow rate, large prostate on digital rectal examination, primarily obstructive complaints on the AUA/IPSS scoring, and elevated PVRs), then patients may be treated for obstruction on an empiric basis (ie, omitting UDS from the evaluation). If patients have other health-related issues affecting voiding function, however (eg, diabetes; cerebrovascular disease; other neurologic disorders, such as multiple sclerosis or Parkinson's disease; or history of pelvic radiation), urodynamic evaluation seems prudent. The authors agree with European Association of Urology (EAU) guidelines recommending pressure-flow studies before prostatectomy under the following circumstances:

- Voided volume <150 mL or Qmax >15 mL, particularly if patients are elderly
- Younger men (ie, <50 years old)
- Elderly men (ie, >80 years old)
- PVR >300 mL
- Suspicion of neurogenic bladder (ie, Parkinson's disease)
- After radical pelvic surgery
- Previous unsuccessful invasive treatment[20]

The urodynamic evaluation is a tool in a urologist's armamentarium that must be used in perspective of the complete picture. Urologists should be wary of making decisions based on a single office visit and urodynamic findings (essentially a snapshot of a particular patient) because BPH is a dynamic process that may change with time.

One situation in which urodynamic evaluation is imperative is in men with significant LUTS persisting after TURP. The majority of these symptoms are related to detrusor dysfunction and not obstruction and, therefore, may require strategies other than those treating the bladder outlet. Nitti and colleagues[21] and Thomas and colleagues[22] found only a small percentage of men (12%–16%) who returned after TURP had persistent obstruction. Detrusor dysfunction may be in the form of involuntary detrusor activity during filling or detrusor underactivity that only is elucidated during a urodynamic study. LUTS persisting or recurring after TURP are explained by DO in the absence of obstruction 50% of the time in patients with concomitant neurologic disorders. Detrusor underactivity, alternatively, may be related to long-term obstruction or age-related changes, which may have been present before intervention and continue to progress despite relief of obstruction. In studying factors predictive of detrusor underactivity after TURP, Thomas and colleagues[22] only identified lower preoperative voiding pressures, similar to the findings of Neal and colleagues.[23] When this information is obtained before initial resection or after a patient returns with persistent symptoms, a urologist can better direct therapy and expectations.

FILLING CYSTOMETRY

This portion of the urodynamic evaluation is integral for the detection of abnormal bladder compliance, increased bladder sensation, and DO. Approximately 20% to 40% of men with BPH have demonstrable DO,[24–26] possibly related to long-term obstruction or age-associated detrusor changes.

Cystometry should be performed only as a part of a pressure-flow study when evaluating men with LUTS/BPH and not as a stand-alone test. The procedure involves filling the bladder with room temperature (22 °C) or body temperature (37 °C) sterile water or saline at a rate of 10 to 50 mL/min (depending on voided volumes as gleaned by voiding diary analysis) while bladder and abdominal pressures are simultaneously recorded. The first sensation of filling, first desire to void, and

strong desire to void should be recorded to reflect presence or absence of sensation reduction or amplification (first sensation of filling <100 mL). Changes in bladder pressure during filling should be noted as to correspondence with urgency or other symptoms.

Normally, the bladder should store urine at low pressure without involuntary detrusor contractions and normal compliance (>40 mL/cm H_2O). **Fig. 1**[27] demonstrates involuntary detrusor contraction during filling (DO). DO in men with BPH has been shown to be independently associated with aging and degree of obstruction. Oelke and colleagues[28] studied 1481 men with BPH and LUTS; after age adjustment, the odds ratios of DO compared with Schäfer's obstruction grade (0–VI) were: 1.2 for grade I, 1.4 for grade II, 1.9 for grade III, 2.5 for grade IV, 3.4 for grade V, and 4.7 for grade VI. Furthermore, men with BPH and DO tend to have decreased compliance and capacity. Gomes and colleagues[29] measured a difference of 31 mL/cm H_2O in bladder compliance and 120 mL in mean capacity between men with and without DO having undergone UDS for evaluation of BPH, both statistically significant differences. Men with DO have a higher risk of failure to improve symptom-related bother after prostatectomy than those that do not, particularly if no bladder outlet obstruction is identified.[18,19] When a patient reports significant storage-related symptoms and when DO and bladder outlet obstruction are present on UDS, a urologist may counsel the patient that these symptoms resolve

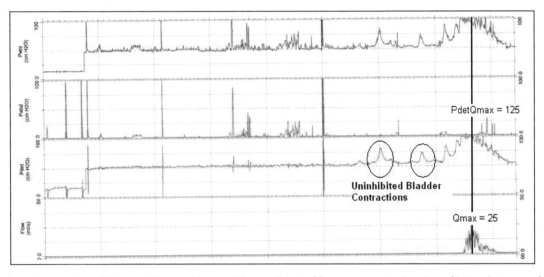

Fig. 1. Detrusor instability in a 68-year-old man with complaints of frequency, nocturia × 3, and intermittency and occasional urge incontinence. Initial filling cystometrogram demonstrates two uninhibited bladder contractions without incontinence. During micturition, the tracings suggest obstruction, given Pdet reaches 125 cm H_2O with Qmax = 25, giving a BOOI of 51. BOOI = PdetQmax − (2 × Qmax).

approximately two thirds of the time after outlet-reducing surgery. If DO persists, the patient may require further treatment with anticholinergic medication or other lower urinary tract rehabilitation to reduce bladder overactivity.

PRESSURE-FLOW STUDIES

A detrusor pressure–uroflow study is the most definitive study for illustrating the true degree of bladder outlet obstruction. A pressure-flow study can also identify patients in whom a low flow rate is due to poor detrusor contractility. When a patient expresses a strong desire to void during filling cystometry, the inflow is stopped and the patient asked to empty. On multichannel urodynamics, the rhabdosphincter and pelvic floor should relax on the electromyography and the pressure tracings should demonstrate an adequate detrusor contraction to produce a strong urinary stream. The ICS definition of detrusor underactivity is a contraction of inadequate magnitude or duration, or both, to empty the bladder within a normal time span.[30] Impaired detrusor contractility is present in 25% to 35% of men with LUTS but does not contraindicate outlet reduction therapy.[31,32] Han and colleagues[31] compared IPSS, quality of life, Qmax, and PVRs in men with obstruction versus men with weak bladder contractility with a mean follow-up of 19 months after TURP and found significant improvement in both groups. The men with obstruction exhibited greater improvement than did those without, but those with detrusor underactivity still improved their IPSS from 27.2 to 18.5 and IPSS quality of life from 5.4 to 3.2 on a scale from 0 to 6 (0 = delighted and 6 = terrible) and decreased their PVR from 167 mL to 74 mL.[31] Likewise, a normal or high flow rate does not exclude bladder outlet obstruction, because approximately 13% to 53% of men with a maximum urinary flow rate greater than 10 mL/s have obstruction on pressure-flow studies. **Fig. 2**[33,34] illustrates the difference between a patient with severe obstruction and a patient with a weak and poorly sustained detrusor contraction. Note that the Qmaxs are approximately the same despite the difference in pathophysiology.

There are several nomograms that have been developed (Abrams-Griffiths, ICS, Schäfer's, and so forth) to classify obstruction, based on Pdet and Qmax. The models generally agree in their definition of obstruction (ie, the line separating class II and class III on the Schäfer's nomogram is essentially the same as the line separating obstruction and equivocal in the Abrams-Griffiths nomogram). The ICS nomogram incorporates the similarities of the two other models and makes the equivocal zone smaller.[35] The obstruction category of a patient is determined by choosing the point of Qmax on an X-Y plot of detrusor pressure versus uroflow on the nomogram (**Fig. 3**).

Additionally, a continuous grading of outlet obstruction can be calculated by the bladder outlet obstruction index (BOOI), formerly known as the Abrams-Griffiths number. BOOI is calculated from the pressure in the bladder at the maximum flow (PdetQmax) minus twice the Qmax ($2 \times$ Qmax). Men with a BOOI greater than 40 are considered obstructed, between 20 and 40 equivocally obstructed, and less than 20 unobstructed. Many patients also increase their intra-abdominal pressures with straining and Valsalva's maneuvers in attempt to empty their bladder; this can be seen on a pressure-flow tracing as a series of hills and valleys on the Pabd tracing. **Fig. 4** illustrates a patient with poor detrusor contraction but who retains the ability to completely empty through abdominal straining.

ROLE OF VIDEOURODYNAMICS

Videourodynamics is the term used when fluid infused into the bladder is radiocontrast material and simultaneous fluoroscopic visualization of the lower urinary tract is obtained during a pressure-flow study. The illustration of bladder, prostate, and urethral anatomy during the filling and emptying stages of urodynamics can enhance understanding of patients' pathophysiologic explanations of their symptoms. The images provided by videourodynamics are not necessary for the diagnosis of bladder outlet obstruction but may provide information as to the cause or location of the obstruction, such as prostatic projection into the outflow tract, urethral stricture disease, or failure of relaxation of the bladder neck/internal sphincter. The narrowest point of the urethra or bladder neck during the point of maximum flow is assumed to be the locus of obstruction during video-UDS. Videourodynamics can also demonstrate complicating features, such as bladder diverticula and vesicoureteral reflux. The authors do not recommend videourodynamics in the initial evaluation of men with BPH, unless there is a strong suspicion of anatomic variations of the lower urinary tract or in men with neurologic disease.

CYSTOSCOPY

For the sake of completion, the use of urethrocystoscopy for the evaluation of BPH is discussed briefly. The AUA BPH treatment guidelines place

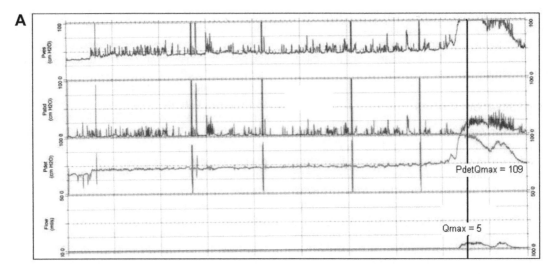

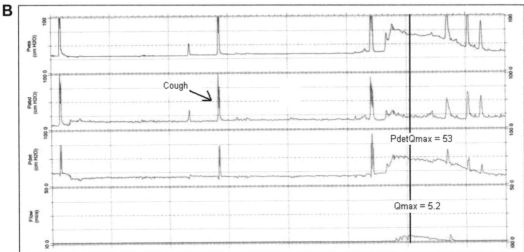

Fig. 2. (A) Obstructed voiding pattern of a 54-year-old man with frequency, urgency, and weak stream. Filling cystometrogram stable, but the pressure-flow study is suggestive of obstruction because Pdet is 109 cm H_2O at Qmax of 5 mL/s. PVR = 95 mL. BOOI = 91. (B) Poor detrusor contraction of a 62-year-old man complaining of weak streak, hesitancy, and nocturia. Bladder is stable during filling and during micturition there is a nominal contraction of the detrusor, illustrated by PdetQmax = 53 cm H_2O and Qmax = 5.2 mL/s. PVR = 56 mL. BOOI = 33.

this evaluation tool in the same category as pressure-flow studies and prostate ultrasound—to be used at the discretion of a urologist before performance of any type of surgical procedure on the lower urinary tract.[1] EAU guidelines further direct the use of cystoscopy particularly if the treatment depends on prostate shape (ie, presence of a middle lobe) or if a patient has a history of hematuria, urethral stricture, bladder cancer, or prior lower urinary tract surgery.[20] Urethrocystoscopy can give additional information regarding prostatic obstruction, prostate length, intravesical protrusion of prostate, visualization of urethra and bladder neck, and presence of bladder stones,

trabeculations, diverticula, or mucosal lesions. When a patient has a significant history of urethral instrumentation and the pressure-flow study demonstrates obstruction, it is prudent to visualize the urethra and rule out stricture disease before initiation of BPH therapy. Urethral strictures can also be diagnosed with retrograde urethrograms or sonourethrography.[36]

OTHER NONINVASIVE METHODS FOR THE DIAGNOSIS OF BLADDER OUTLET OBSTRUCTION

The AUA and EAU BPH treatment guidelines recommend that a PVR measurement and

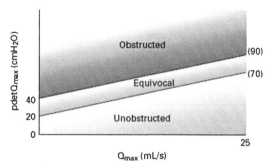

Fig. 3. The provisional ICS nomogram for the analysis of voiding with each category defined by the BOOI. *From* Abrams P. Bladder outlet obstruction index, bladder contractility index and bladder voiding efficiency: three simple indices to define bladder voiding function. BJU Int 1999;84:14; with permission.)

uroflowmetry be obtained as part of the initial evaluation of men with LUTS.[1,20] The uroflowmeter measures volumetric flow rate during micturition and the accumulated volume. Because normal uroflow is a bell-shaped curve, when the flow rate is reduced or the pattern is altered, there is a suggestion of outflow obstruction or decreased bladder contractility. Most uroflowmeters are calibrated for water, and variations in the specific gravity of the fluid (ie, urine or contrast) may result in the overestimation of the flow rate.[37] PVR volume is the volume remaining in the bladder after normal micturition as calculated by transabdominal ultrasound measurement. Elevation of PVR

indicates a problem with emptying, but a third of patients with bladder outlet obstruction do not have significant PVR.[38,39] Given the circadian variability of these measurements,[40] up to two SDs in men with BPH,[41] it is important to confirm suspicion of bladder dysfunction with urodynamic evaluation or serial measurements.

Several studies have looked at single ultrasound measurements, such as prostate size, prostate shape (ie, presumed circle area ratio [PCAR] = measures the degree to which the transverse image of the prostate approaches a circular shape), intravesical prostatic protrusion (IPP), bladder wall thickness, bladder weight, and the prostatic or detrusor resistant index to aid in the diagnosis of bladder outlet obstruction. All of these measurements correlate somewhat to degree of obstruction (strengthened when used in conjunction with one another) but their reproducibility and ability to predict treatment outcomes has not been proved. **Table 1** summarizes recent studies looking at noninvasive methods of diagnosing bladder outlet obstruction.[34,42–48]

Tests with high sensitivity but low specificity (ie, PVR and detrusor resistive index) detect obstruction, but have a high false-positive rate. Tests with high specificity/low sensitivity (ie, PCAR and IPP) efficiently exclude nonobstructed patients, but have a high false-negative rate. Given the shortcomings of individual measurements, several investigators have studied various combinations of these parameters in a logistic regression model

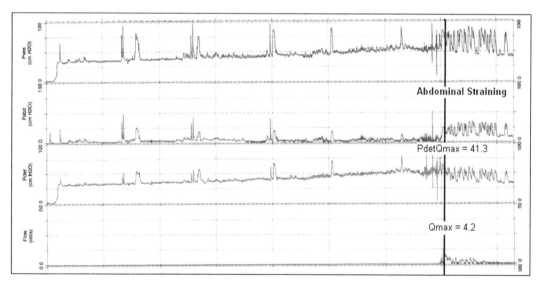

Fig. 4. Impaired detrusor contractility in 78-year-old-man with hesitancy, intermittency, and weak stream. The cystometrogram is normal during filling to a capacity of 450 mL. Qmax = 4.2 mL/s is achieved with a negligible detrusor contraction and multiple Valsalva's maneuver efforts as depicted by hills and valleys pattern of Pabd and Pves with PdetQmax = 41.3 cm H_2O and PVR of 55 mL.

Table 1
Accuracy of noninvasive techniques for diagnosing bladder outlet obstruction index

Study	Year	Measurement	Obstructed	No. Patients	Sensitivity	Specificity
28	1979	PVR	≥ 50 mL	117	87.5	35
29	1995	Prostate volume	≥ 40 g	571	49	32
30	1997	Bladder weight	>35 g	65	85	87
31	1997	Prostate roundness (PCAR)	≥ 0.8	174	54	92
32	2003	IPP	Grade 1	200	7	56
			Grade 2		17	53
			Grade 3		76	92
33	2000	Detrusor resistive index[a]	>0.7	57	85	46
34	1998	Uroflowmetry	>10 mL/sec	1271	47	70
			>15 mL/sec		82	38
35	2007	Detrusor wall thickness	≥ 2 mm	160	83	95

[a] Index of change in blood flow calculated by maximum velocity (Vmax) – [minimum velocity (Vmin)/Vmax].

to develop an algorithm diagnosis of bladder outlet obstruction. Unfortunately, these equations become more complex and difficult to use as more measurements are included. When using these equations, urologists should keep in mind the population group used to create the algorithm and their general limitations. The combination with the highest specificity published to date uses Qmax and total prostate volume to calculate a predicted BOOI (predicted BOOI = [2.21 − 0.5 log Qmax + 0.18 log total prostate volume] − 50) yielding a 92% positive predictive value of equivocal or worse obstruction in men whose predicted BOOI greater than 40.[49]

Another method of estimating outlet obstruction without an intubated pressure-flow study uses an external penile cuff measuring isovolumetric bladder pressure. The cuff obstructs flow during micturation; the pressure required to interrupt flow is used to estimate detrusor pressure. Griffiths and colleagues[50] created a modified nomogram using the cuff interruption pressure measurement from a noninvasive cuff test and the highest value of steady state flow recorded during the cuff deflation/inflation cycle. The sensitivity for predicting obstruction using this method and nomogram was 73% with a specificity of 75%.

RELIABILITY OF URODYNAMICS

When urodynamics are used in the evaluation of BPH, therapeutic decisions are usually made based on a single urodynamic study because the tests are invasive, expensive, and time consuming. It is, therefore, important to be aware of the physiologic variability of these measurements. When sequential pressure-flow studies are performed on individual patients during the same office visit, pdetQmax tend to decrease with subsequent voids. The intraindividual variability can be significant enough to change obstruction classification in up to 7% of patients.[51,52] A possible hypothesis for this difference is a reduction of the outlet resistance secondary to an increase in the stretch in urethra after repeat voids without the opportunity to return to baseline. When test-retest reliability was investigated in 121 men with BPH after 6 months of watchful waiting, Witjes and colleagues[53] found similar decreases in pdetQmax but an insignificant difference in the theoretical cross-sectional urethral lumen, arguing against the latter hypothesis.

There is a general consensus that transurethral catheters used during pressure-flow studies tend to increase perceived obstruction by creating some degree of urethral obstruction on their own. This is believed especially true in men with so-called constrictive BPH as opposed to compressive BPH. Klingler and colleagues[54] demonstrated a significant difference in Qmax, pdetQmax, and the degree of obstruction when various catheter sizes (5F–15F) were used. Walker and colleagues[55] performed pressure-flow studies with a suprapubic catheter and 10F transurethral catheter in 35 men with BPH and suspected bladder outlet obstruction. They found statistically significant decreases in Qmax, and increases in pdetQmax and obstruction classification. UDS, therefore, should be performed with the smallest transurethral catheter available that provides accurate measurements. There is also the question of other urethral instrumentation (ie, catheterization or urethrocystoscopy) during an office evaluation for BPH causing alteration in the urodynamic parameters. Walker and colleagues[56] studied the changes in pressure-flow variables in 72 men who underwent suprapubic pressure monitoring, then sequential pressure-flow studies after urethral instrumentation with a 12F catheter, and then after a 17F cystoscope and found no clinically significant change in pressure/flow variables after instrumentation.

SUMMARY

Urodynamics is a valuable tool in the evaluation of LUTS in men with BPH. It is an invasive procedure that can cause transient discomfort and anxiety and carries a small risk of minimal morbidity, such as UTI and hematuria; but, as discussed previously, many patients are willing to accept these risks, particularly if they can benefit their care. Straightforward patients may not require the information provided by pressure-flow studies to be successfully treated, particularly in selection of watchful-waiting or medical therapy. In more complex patients or those patients for whom surgical intervention is considered, however, the authors recommend UDS be performed before treatment. Diagnoses of increased bladder sensation, DO, decreased compliance, urethral disease, and detrusor underactivity all have important implications on efficiency of prostate resection in relieving symptoms. Videourodynamics may be required when there is a strong suspicion of anatomic variation of the lower urinary tract or in a patient whose neurologic disease may affect bladder neck function. Other noninvasive modalities have been studied to replace the pressure-flow study in the diagnosis of outlet obstruction, and it seems that the combination of some of these parameters, in particular Qmax and prostate volume, can approximate obstruction categorization by urodynamics. Information regarding detrusor stability during filling and contractility during emptying, however, is not obtained with these modalities. It is the authors' opinion that if information is needed regarding bladder function and voiding efficiency, a urodynamic study is recommended as the most comprehensive test available with minimal risk of morbidity.

REFERENCES

1. Kaplan SA. Update on the American Urological Association guidelines for the treatment of benign prostatic hyperplasia. Rev Urol 2006;8(Suppl 4):S10.

2. Ezz el Din K, Kiemeney LA, de Wildt MJ, et al. Correlation between uroflowmetry, prostate volume, post-void residue, and lower urinary tract symptoms as measured by the International Prostate Symptom Score. Urology 1996;48:393.

3. Knutson T, Schafer W, Fall M, et al. Can urodynamic assessment of outflow obstruction predict outcome from watchful waiting? A four-year follow-up study. Scand J Urol Nephrol 2001;35:463.

4. Schafer W. Principles and clinical application of advanced urodynamic analysis of voiding function. Urol Clin North Am 1990;17:553.

5. Bates CP, Whiteside CG, Turner-Warwick R. Synchronous cine-pressure-flow-cysto-urethrography with special reference to stress and urge incontinence. Br J Urol 1970;42:714.

6. Schafer W, Abrams P, Liao L, et al. Good urodynamic practices: uroflowmetry, filling cystometry, and pressure-flow studies. Neurourol Urodyn 2002;21:261.

7. Carter PG, Lewis P, Abrams P. Urodynamic morbidity and dysuria prophylaxis. Br J Urol 1991; 67:40.

8. Harari D, Malone-Lee J, Ridgway GL. An age-related investigation of urinary tract symptoms and infection following urodynamic studies. Age Ageing 1994;23:62.

9. Klingler HC, Madersbacher S, Djavan B, et al. Morbidity of the evaluation of the lower urinary tract with transurethral multichannel pressure-flow studies. J Urol 1998;159:191.

10. Porru D, Madeddu G, Campus G, et al. Evaluation of morbidity of multi-channel pressure-flow studies. Neurourol Urodyn 1999;18:647.

11. Latthe PM, Foon R, Toozs-Hobson P. Prophylactic antibiotics in urodynamics: a systematic review of effectiveness and safety. Neurourol Urodyn 2008;27:167.

12. Yokoyama T, Nozaki K, Nose H, et al. Tolerability and morbidity of urodynamic testing: a questionnaire-based study. Urology 2005;66:74.

13. Scarpero HM, Padmanabhan P, Xue X, et al. Patient perception of videourodynamic testing: a questionnaire based study. J Urol 2005;173:555.

14. Jensen KM, Jorgensen JB, Mogensen P. Urodynamics in prostatism. I. Prognostic value of uroflowmetry. Scand J Urol Nephrol 1988;22:109.

15. Jensen KM, Jorgensen JB, Mogensen P. Urodynamics in prostatism. II. Prognostic value of pressure-flow study combined with stop-flow test. Scand J Urol Nephrol Suppl 1988;114:72.

16. Jensen KM, Jorgensen TB, Mogensen P. Long-term predictive role of urodynamics: an 8-year follow-up of prostatic surgery for lower urinary tract symptoms. Br J Urol 1996;78:213.

17. Robertson AS, Griffiths C, Neal DE. Conventional urodynamics and ambulatory monitoring in the definition and management of bladder outflow obstruction. J Urol 1996;155:506.

18. Van Venrooij GE, Van Melick HH, Eckhardt MD, et al. Correlations of urodynamic changes with changes in symptoms and well-being after transurethral resection of the prostate. J Urol 2002;168:605.

19. Tanaka Y, Masumori N, Itoh N, et al. Is the short-term outcome of transurethral resection of the prostate affected by preoperative degree of bladder outlet obstruction, status of detrusor contractility or detrusor overactivity? Int J Urol 2006;13:1398.

20. Madersbacher S, Alivizatos G, Nordling J, et al. EAU 2004 guidelines on assessment, therapy and follow-up of men with lower urinary tract symptoms suggestive of benign prostatic obstruction (BPH guidelines). Eur Urol 2004;46:547.

21. Nitti VW, Kim Y, Combs AJ, et al. Voiding dysfunction following transurethral resection of the prostate: symptoms and urodynamic findings. J Urol 1997; 157:600.

22. Thomas AW, Cannon A, Bartlett E, et al. The natural history of lower urinary tract dysfunction in men: minimum 10-year urodynamic followup of transurethral resection of prostate for bladder outlet obstruction. J Urol 1887;174:2005.

23. Neal DE, Ramsden PD, Sharples L, et al. Outcome of elective prostatectomy. BMJ 1989;299:762.

24. Ameda K, Sullivan MP, Bae RJ, et al. Urodynamic characterization of nonobstructive voiding dysfunction in symptomatic elderly men. J Urol 1999;162: 142.

25. Fusco F, Groutz A, Blaivas JG, et al. Videourodynamic studies in men with lower urinary tract symptoms: a comparison of community based versus referral urological practices. J Urol 2001;166:910.

26. Madersbacher S, Pycha A, Klingler CH, et al. Interrelationships of bladder compliance with age, detrusor instability, and obstruction in elderly men with lower urinary tract symptoms. Neurourol Urodyn 1999;18:3.

27. Abrams P. Urodynamic techniques. In: Abrams P, editor. Urodynamics. 2nd edition. London: Springer-Verlag; 1997. p. 17.

28. Oelke M, Baard J, Wijkstra H, et al. Age and bladder outlet obstruction are independently associated with detrusor overactivity in patients with benign prostatic hyperplasia. Eur Urol 2008;54:419.

29. Gomes CM, Nunes RV, Araujo RM, et al. Urodynamic evaluation of patients with lower urinary tract symptoms and small prostate volume. Urol Int 2008;81:129.

30. Abrams P, Cardozo L, Fall M, et al. The standardisation of terminology of lower urinary tract function: report from the Standardisation Sub-committee of the International Continence Society. Neurourol Urodyn 2002;21:167.

31. Han DH, Jeong YS, Choo MS, et al. The efficacy of transurethral resection of the prostate in the patients with weak bladder contractility index. Urology 2008; 71:657.

32. Rollema HJ, Van Mastrigt R. Improved indication and followup in transurethral resection of the prostate using the computer program CLIM: a prospective study. J Urol 1992;148:111.

33. Porru D, Jallous H, Cavalli V, et al. Prognostic value of a combination of IPSS, flow rate and residual urine volume compared to pressure-flow studies in the preoperative evaluation of symptomatic BPH. Eur Urol 2002;41:246.

34. Reynard JM, Yang Q, Donovan JL, et al. The ICS-'BPH'Study: uroflowmetry, lower urinary tract symptoms and bladder outlet obstruction. Br J Urol 1998;82:619.

35. Griffiths D, Hofner K, van Mastrigt R, et al. Standardization of terminology of lower urinary tract function: pressure-flow studies of voiding, urethral resistance, and urethral obstruction. International Continence Society Subcommittee on Standardization of Terminology of Pressure-Flow Studies. Neurourol Urodyn 1997;16:1.

36. Morey AF, McAninch JW. Sonographic staging of anterior urethral strictures. J Urol 2000;163:1070.

37. Peterson AC, Webster GD. Urodynamic and videourodynamic evaluation of voiding dysfunction. In: Wein AJ, editor, Campbell-Walsh Urology. 9th edition. Philadelphia: Saunders Elsevier; 2007, vol. 3, p. 1986.

38. Kranse R, van Mastrigt R. Weak correlation between bladder outlet obstruction and probability to void to completion. Urology 2003;62:667.

39. Turner-Warwick R, Whiteside CG, Worth PH, et al. A urodynamic view of the clinical problems associated with bladder neck dysfunction and its treatment by endoscopic incision and trans-trigonal posterior prostatectomy. Br J Urol 1973;45:44.

40. Rule AD, Jacobson DJ, McGree ME, et al. Longitudinal changes in post-void residual and voided volume among community dwelling men. J Urol 2005;174:1317.

41. Golomb J, Lindner A, Siegel Y, et al. Variability and circadian changes in home uroflowmetry in patients with benign prostatic hyperplasia compared to normal controls. J Urol 1992;147:1044.

42. Abrams PH, Griffiths DJ. The assessment of prostatic obstruction from urodynamic measurements and from residual urine. Br J Urol 1979;51:129.

43. Chia SJ, Heng CT, Chan SP, et al. Correlation of intravesical prostatic protrusion with bladder outlet obstruction. BJU Int 2003;91:371.

44. Kojima M, Inui E, Ochiai A, et al. Noninvasive quantitative estimation of infravesical obstruction using ultrasonic measurement of bladder weight. J Urol 1997;157:476.

45. Kojima M, Ochiai A, Naya Y, et al. Doppler resistive index in benign prostatic hyperplasia: correlation with ultrasonic appearance of the prostate and infravesical obstruction. Eur Urol 2000;37:436.

46. Kojima M, Ochiai A, Naya Y, et al. Correlation of presumed circle area ratio with infravesical obstruction in men with lower urinary tract symptoms. Urology 1997;50:548.

47. Oelke M, Hofner K, Jonas U, et al. Diagnostic accuracy of noninvasive tests to evaluate bladder outlet obstruction in men: detrusor wall thickness, uroflowmetry, postvoid residual urine, and prostate volume. Eur Urol 2007;52:827.

48. Rosier PF, de la Rosette JJ. Is there a correlation between prostate size and bladder-outlet obstruction? World J Urol 1995;13:9.

49. Ockrim JL, Laniado ME, Patel A, et al. A probability based system for combining simple office parameters as a predictor of bladder outflow obstruction. J Urol 2001;166:2221.

50. Griffiths CJ, Harding C, Blake C, et al. A nomogram to classify men with lower urinary tract symptoms using urine flow and noninvasive measurement of bladder pressure. J Urol 2005;174:1323.

51. Rosier PF, de la Rosette JJ, Koldewijn EL, et al. Variability of pressure-flow analysis parameters in repeated cystometry in patients with benign prostatic hyperplasia. J Urol 1995;153:1520.

52. Tammela TL, Schafer W, Barrett DM, et al. Repeated pressure-flow studies in the evaluation of bladder outlet obstruction due to benign prostatic enlargement. Finasteride Urodynamics Study Group. Neurourol Urodyn 1999;18:17.

53. Witjes WP, de Wildt MJ, Rosier PF, et al. Variability of clinical and pressure-flow study variables after 6 months of watchful waiting in patients with lower urinary tract symptoms and benign prostatic enlargement. J Urol 1996;156:1026.

54. Klingler HC, Madersbacher S, Schmidbauer CP. Impact of different sized catheters on pressure-flow studies in patients with benign prostatic hyperplasia. Neurourol Urodyn 1996;15:473.

55. Walker RM, Di Pasquale B, Hubregtse M, et al. Pressure-flow studies in the diagnosis of bladder outlet obstruction: a study comparing suprapubic and transurethral techniques. Br J Urol 1997;79:693.

56. Walker RM, Patel A, St Clair Carter S. Is there a clinically significant change in pressure-flow study values after urethral instrumentation in patients with lower urinary tract symptoms? Br J Urol 1998;81:206.

Established Medical Therapy for Benign Prostatic Hyperplasia

Gregory B. Auffenberg, MD, Brian T. Helfand, MD, PhD,
Kevin T. McVary, MD, FACS*

KEYWORDS

- Benign prostatic hyperplasia
- 5-alpha reductase inhibitor • Alpha-blocker
- Anti-cholinergic • Phytotherapeutics

As noted in other articles in this issue, benign prostatic hyperplasia (BPH) is a histologic diagnosis that refers to the proliferation of smooth muscle and epithelial cells within the prostatic transition zone.[1,2] The enlarged gland is thought to lead to disease manifestations via two routes: (1) static component: direct bladder outlet obstruction (BOO) from enlarged tissue, and (2) dynamic component: from increased smooth muscle tone and resistance within the enlarged gland. This most common manifestation of BPH is the collection of symptoms described as lower urinary tract symptoms (LUTS). LUTS are any combination of urinary symptoms, including voiding symptoms (hesitancy, weak stream, intermittency, terminal dribbling, and feeling of incomplete emptying) and storage symptoms (frequency, urgency, and nocturia). Voiding symptoms are often attributed to, but not pathognomonic for, the physical presence of BOO. Longstanding BOO and bladder overdistension may cause fibrotic changes of the bladder wall leading to changes in detrusor function (ie, detrusor instability). Detrusor instability is thought to be a contributor to the storage symptoms seen in LUTS.[3] Less frequently, BPH has been associated with other comorbidities including acute urinary retention (AUR), renal insufficiency, development of bladder calculi, urinary incontinence, and recurrent urinary tract infection.[4,5] Therapy for BPH typically targets one or both of the disease components (static or dynamic) to provide relief.

For years, the primary treatment options for BPH were surgical; however the number of prostatectomies performed for BPH-related disease has decreased from 250,000 in the mid 1980s to 88,000 in 1997.[6,7] This decrease in rate of prostatectomy in the face of increasing BPH diagnoses is likely attributable to a variety of factors. One major factor is a paradigm shift to a treatment strategy focused on medical treatment of BPH in favor of surgery.[8] The development of safe, effective medical therapies for BPH is largely responsible for this change in treatment approach.

Traditionally, the primary goal of treatment has been to alleviate bothersome LUTS that result from prostatic enlargement. More recently, treatment has additionally been directed toward alteration of disease progression and prevention of the comorbidities that can be associated with BPH. A variety of medication classes are used in BPH therapy including alpha-adrenergic antagonists, 5-alpha reductase inhibitors (5-ARI), antimuscarinics, phytotherapeutics, and the more recently explored phosphodiesterase inhibitors, intraprostatic neurotoxins, and luteinizing hormone releasing hormone (LHRH) analogs. Choosing the correct medical treatment for BPH is complex and ever changing. This article focuses on the most established medical therapies for the

Department of Urology, Feinberg School of Medicine, Northwestern University, 303 East Chicago Avenue, Tarry 16-703, Chicago, IL 60611-3008, USA
* Corresponding author.
E-mail address: k-mcvary@northwestern.edu (K. McVary).

Urol Clin N Am 36 (2009) 443–459
doi:10.1016/j.ucl.2009.07.004
0094-0143/09/$ – see front matter © 2009 Elsevier Inc. All rights reserved.

treatment of symptomatic BPH, and the article that follows discusses newer medical interventions.

ALPHA-ADRENERGIC ANTAGONISTS

As mentioned previously, symptomatic BPH has been attributed, with various levels of evidence, to arise from two major components: static and dynamic, with an increase in prostatic smooth muscle tone believed to be largely responsible for the latter. Noradrenergic sympathetic nerves have been demonstrated to effect the contraction of prostatic smooth muscle.[9] The prostate gland contains high levels of both α_1- and α_2-adrenergic receptors (ARs).[10–13] Ninety-eight percent of α_1-adrenoreceptors are associated with the stromal elements of the prostate and are thus thought to have the greatest influence on prostatic smooth muscle tone.[11] Activation of these receptors and the subsequent increase in prostatic smooth muscle tone with urethral constriction and impaired flow of urine is thought to be a major contributor to the pathophysiology of symptomatic BPH. In addition, there is evidence that ARs further mediate the symptoms of BPH via their activation within the central nervous system (CNS) and bladder.[14,15]

Alpha-ARs are not unique to the prostate. The two basic subtypes of α-receptors (α_1 and α_2) are distributed ubiquitously throughout the human body. In general, α_2-receptors are typically located presynaptically and down-regulate norepinephrine release via a negative feedback mechanism. If stimulated, one expects resultant smooth muscle relaxation. α_1-Receptors are the postsynaptic receptors that affect a response to neurotransmitter release. Several subtypes of the α_1-adrenoreceptors have been identified and classified into three groups: α_{1A}, α_{1B}, and α_{1D}.[16–18]

Both α_{1A} and α_{1B}-adrenoreceptors have been identified within the prostate. The α_{1A} receptors are the predominant adrenoreceptors expressed by stromal smooth muscle cells.[11] In contrast, the α_{1B} receptors are predominantly located in the smooth muscle of arteries and veins, including the microvasculature contained within the prostate gland.[18] Within the genitourinary system, α_{1D}-adrenoreceptors are mainly located in the bladder body and dome.[19] α_{1D}-receptors are also located in the spinal cord where they are presumed to play a role in the sympathetic modulation of parasympathetic activity.[20] The α_{1D}-receptor has been proposed to mediate the irritative components of LUTS.

The importance of the α_1-ARs in the normal and functionally disturbed detrusor has been discussed for decades. There seems to be a general agreement that in the normal human detrusor the number of α_1-ARs is low, and that the contractile function is almost negligible.[21] However, the questions raised have been: do the numbers or types of α_1-ARs and/or their function change in outflow obstruction? In the human detrusor, Malloy and colleagues[19] found mRNA expression of both α_{1D}- and α_{1A}-receptor subtypes but no expression of α_{1B}. The relation between the former subtypes was α_{1D}: 66% and α_{1A}: 34%. In rats, Hampel and colleagues[22] found that 70% of α_1-AR mRNA was the α_{1A} subtype, 5% were α_{1B} and 25% were α_{1D}. Although bladder α_1-AR density did not increase overall with obstruction, striking changes in α_1-AR subtype expression occurred: α_1-AR expression changed to 23% α_{1A}, 2% α_{1B}, and 75% α_{1D}. No functional correlates were reported. In another study from the same group, however, Gu and colleagues[23] found evidence supporting the hypothesis that the α_{1D}-ARs are mechanistically involved in the development of irritative symptoms in rats and that they may be plausible targets for therapeutic intervention. In the human detrusor, Nomiya and Yamaguchi[24] demonstrated that there was no up-regulation of any of the ARs (α- or β-AR mRNA) with obstruction. In addition, in functional experiments they confirmed previous functional results, showing that the human detrusor has a low sensitivity to α-AR stimulation—phenylephrine at high drug concentrations produced a weak contraction with no difference between normal and obstructed bladders. Thus, in the obstructed human bladder, there seems to be no evidence for α-AR up-regulation or change in subtype. This would mean that it is unlikely that the α_{1D}-ARs in the detrusor muscle are responsible for detrusor overactivity or the overactive bladder syndrome. This does not exclude that the α-ARs on eg, bladder vascular smooth muscle may have important roles in the changes in bladder function found after outflow obstruction.[25,26]

Knowledge of α_1-receptor subtype location and action has been instrumental in targeting BPH therapy to the correct location. Given their location, α_{1A}-adrenoreceptors are ideal targets for therapy. Blockade of the α_{1A}-adrenoreceptors has been shown to reduce prostatic tone and improve the dynamic aspects of voiding.[27] Blockade of α_{1B}-receptors leads to venous and arterial dilation as smooth muscle cells in the vessel walls relax. In some patients this can cause dizziness and hypotension because of decreased total peripheral resistance, potentially serious side effects. Stimulation of α_{1D}-receptors can lead to detrusor overactivity, and blockade of these receptors has been shown in animal models to reduce irritative voiding symptoms.[19] Taken together, it appears that combined antagonism of α_{1A}- and α_{1D}-receptors is, in theory, a great option for the management of BPH as it combines a reduction of prostatic smooth muscle tone with decreased detrusor instability and avoids the possible cardiovascular side effects of α_{1B}-receptor blockade.

As the knowledge of receptor subtypes has advanced, medications have been engineered to attempt to provide the optimal benefit of specific alpha-blockade while reducing side effects. This has led to the development of three generations of alpha-blocking medications with increasing specificity for the most desirable receptors. Following is a listing of many of the most common alpha-blocking medications with their receptor specificity profiles (**Table 1**).

The first generation of specific alpha-blocking agents explored and found to be useful for relief of BPH symptoms was phenoxybenzamine. Phenoxybenzamine is a nonselective α_1/α_2-receptor blocker that was one of the earliest alpha-blocking medications found to be effective in the therapy of BPH.[28–31] The utility of this medication was limited by the frequently encountered side effects of syncope, orthostatic hypotension, reflex tachycardia, cardiac arrhythmias, and retrograde ejaculation.[28,31] Most of these side effects were attributed to α_2-receptor blockade.

In an effort to minimize side effects, second-generation alpha-blocking agents (eg, prazosin, terazosin, doxazosin, alfuzosin) were developed that were specific to α_1-receptors and had reduced activity at α_2-receptors. Therefore, they improve LUTS with fewer vasodilatory-related effects.

Third-generation α_1-adrenergic antagonists (eg, tamsulosin, silodosin) are thought to be more selective antagonists for prostatic α_{1A}-receptors.[32–34] These drugs selectively target the smooth muscle cells contained within the prostate gland and exert lesser effects on the other α-adrenergic receptor subtypes that regulate blood pressure. Therefore, these agents theoretically act in the location that will have the greatest benefit for symptoms with the fewest side effects.[35] Second- and third-generation alpha-blocking agents remain a mainstay of BPH therapy and several will be discussed individually in the following sections.

Second Generation: Terazosin, Doxazosin, and Alfuzosin

Terazosin is an α_1-selective antagonist with a relatively long half-life that allows for once-daily dosing. The Hytrin Community Assessment Trial demonstrates the effectiveness of this medication.[36] In this study, 2084 men 55 years of age or older with moderate to severe urinary symptoms were randomized to receive treatment with terazosin or placebo. Terazosin was significantly superior to placebo in all measurements of efficacy; in the terazosin group, the American Urological Association International Prostate Symptom Score (AUA-IPSS) improved by 37.8%, compared with 18.4% in the placebo. The mean change from baseline in peak urinary flow rate (Qmax) was 2.2 mL/s for terazosin compared with 0.8 mL/s for placebo. Treatment failure occurred in approximately 11% of the terazosin study group, compared with approximately 25% in the placebo group. Withdrawal from the study owing to adverse effects of treatment occurred in 20% of the terazosin group and 15% of placebo patients. Terazosin is thus an effective medical treatment for reducing LUTS and the impairment of quality of life because of urinary symptoms created by BPH.

Doxazosin, a long-acting, α_1-selective antagonist also allows for once-daily dosing. Clinical trials have demonstrated that doxazosin increases Qmax by 23% to 28% and decreases symptom scores by 16.4% versus 9.8% in placebo groups in men with symptomatic BPH.[37,38] It has been shown that the response to doxazosin is dose dependent. The side-effect profile has also been shown to be dose dependent. To minimize the frequency of side effects (ie, postural hypotension and syncope), doxazosin is typically initiated at

Table 1
Variable receptor affinities for α-adrenergic antagonists

	Rank Order of Receptor Selectivity
Prazosin	$\alpha_{1A} = \alpha_{1B} = \alpha_{1D}$
Doxazosin	$\alpha_{1A} = \alpha_{1B} = \alpha_{1D}$
Terazosin	$\alpha_{1B} = \alpha_{1D} > \alpha_{1A}$
Alfuzosin	$\alpha_{1A} = \alpha_{1B} = \alpha_{1D}$
Tamsulosin	$\alpha_{1A} = \alpha_{1D} > \alpha_{1B}$
Silodosin	$\alpha_{1A} > \alpha_{1D} \gg \alpha_{1B}$

Data from Shibata K, Foglar R, Horie K, et al. KMD-3213, a novel, potent, alpha 1a-adrenoceptor-selective antagonist: characterization using recombinant human alpha 1-adrenoceptors and native tissues. Mol Pharmacol 1995;48(2):250–8; Lyseng-Williamson KA, Jarvis B, Wagstaff AJ. Tamsulosin: an update of its role in the management of lower urinary tract symptoms. Drugs 2002;62(1):135–67.

a dose of 1 mg administered once daily. Depending on response to therapy and tolerability, the dosage may be increased to 8 mg/d. Doxazosin is an effective therapy for symptomatic BPH, which like terazosin, has been shown to relieve symptoms and improve urinary flow rates.[37–39]

Alfuzosin, another second-generation α_1-adrenoreceptor antagonist, is indicated for the management of moderate to severe BPH symptoms. Alfuzosin has been shown to improve bothersome urinary symptoms and increase urine flow rates with efficacy similar to other second-generation α_1-adrenoreceptor antagonists.[33,35,40,41] Additionally, in alfuzosin trials the incidence of cardiovascular side effects are lower when compared with separate trials conducted with terazosin and doxazosin (**Table 2**).[36–41] Although a comparison across different trials does not provide the most solid evidence, this speaks to a safety profile for alfuzosin with lesser cardiovascular effects than its other second-generation counterparts. The mechanistic origin of the lesser cardiovascular effects is not entirely known, but decreased blood brain barrier penetration, preferential distribution to the prostate, and pharmacokinetic differences have been theorized to contribute. This medication comes in three formulations: immediate release (requires 2–3 daily doses), extended release (XL), and sustained-release with the latter two only requiring 1 daily dose.

Third Generation: Tamsulosin, Silodosin

Tamsulosin is a third-generation alpha-blocker with greater specificity for the α_{1A}-adrenoreceptor in relation to the α_{1B}-adrenoreceptor. Clinical trials suggest that tamsulosin provides relatively rapid symptom improvement and improvement in peak urinary flow rate.[42] Early clinical trials suggested that tamsulosin increased Qmax by approximately 1.5 mL/s and decreased AUA-IPSS scores by more than 35%. Long-term studies (up to 60 weeks) examining the effects of tamsulosin demonstrate its beneficial effects are sustained over time, as measured by maximal urinary flow rates and symptoms score.[43] The most common side effects reported with tamsulosin use are dizziness (~5%) and retrograde ejaculation (~8%). Clinical studies have also demonstrated that tamsulosin can be coadministered with antihypertensive medications such as nifedipine, enalapril, and atenolol without any increased risk of hypotensive or syncopal episodes.[44,45] Tamsulosin is thus, a safe and efficacious drug for the treatment of BPH with fewer documented cardiovascular side effects than the other available alpha-blocking medications.[41,46]

Silodosin, one of the most recently approved alpha-blocking medications for BPH, is a third-generation medication with reported α_{1A} versus α_{1B} affinity 38 times greater than tamsulosin.[34] There is limited published evidence to date as to the effectiveness of silodosin. This information hails from the phase 3 clinical trial performed in Japan using a lower dose of tamsulosin (0.2 mg) than available elsewhere.[47] This 12-week trial enrolled 457 men who met inclusion criteria and enrolled them in three groups: silodosin 4 mg twice daily, tamsulosin 0.2 mg once daily (standard Japanese dose), and placebo. Mean AUA-IPSS improvement was significantly better when compared with placebo (−8.3 vs −5.3) but there was not a significant improvement in AUA-IPSS when compared with tamsulosin. Across the three groups, there were 1.70 mL/s, 2.60 mL/s, and 0.26 mL/s improvements in Qmax in the silodosin, tamsulosin, and placebo groups, respectively ($P = .063$ vs tamsulosin; $P = .005$ vs placebo). There were −1.7, −1.4, and −1.1 improvements in quality of life (QOL) questions in the silodosin, tamsulosin, and placebo groups, respectively ($P = .052$ vs tamsulosin; $P = .002$ vs placebo). Adverse event rates were relatively similar with the exception that the rate of ejaculatory dysfunction in the silodosin group was 22.3% versus 1.6% in the tamsulosin group and 0% in the placebo group (no significance data provided). There were no clinically significant differences of blood pressure or heart rate and dizziness rates were 5.1% versus 7.3% (no significance data provided) between the silodosin and tamsulosin groups, respectively. Thus, this study provides evidence that silodosin is more effective than placebo but provides no evidence that silodosin is more effective than other alpha blockers. Given the lack of evidence for lesser side effects than tamsulosin, it cannot be currently concluded that the silodosin's increased α_{1A} versus α_{1B} affinity offers any additional significant clinical benefit. More data from longer-term studies would be useful in solidly establishing the true effectiveness of this medication as well as it side-effect profile.

Adverse Effects of α-Adrenergic Antagonists

Depending on dosage and selectivity, all α-adrenergic antagonists can be associated with adverse reactions (see **Table 2**). Dizziness is the most common side effect of α-adrenergic antagonists. Dizziness is thought to be caused by effects on the central nervous system or other unconventional drug mechanisms that may be unrelated to effects on the blood vessels themselves. This is supported by the finding that some dizziness can

Table 2
Adverse effects of α-adrenergic antagonists[4,36-41,46]

Effect	Phenoxybenzamine (%)	Prazosin (%)	Terazosin (%)	Doxazosin (%)	Tamsulosin (%)	Alfuzosin (%)	Silodosin (%)
Hypotension	15–20	10–15	2–8	1–2	<1	<1	<1
Dizziness	10–14	15–17	7–14	10–15	15	6–9	5
Headache	4–15	13–15	4–10	9–10	19	8–14	NR
Sexual dysfunction	5–8	NR	2–7	NR	8	1–2	22
Fatigue	10–15	10	4–8	1–2	8	1–7	NR
Syncope	NR	NR	<1	<1	<1	<1	NR
Nasal congestion	8	NR	2	NR	13	5–6	NR

Data in this table compiled from multiple trials with different patient cohorts. Data represent accurate complication rates for each individual agent as documented in those trials for the cohort studied in that trial. However, given data are from differently designed trials, they cannot be used to accurately compare the side effect rates between medications.
Abbreviation: NR, not reported.

be seen with tamsulosin (a selective α_{1A}-adrenergic antagonist), a medication thought to have a lesser effect on blood vessels than the other medications of this class. Hypotension decreases with longer-acting drugs, and occurs least with α_{1A}-adrenergic selective agents. Dizziness and hypotension are more common in those older than 65 years. Ejaculatory dysfunction may occur, and although not entirely understood, is thought to possibly result from medication interactions with the vas deferens.[38,41,43,48]

HORMONAL THERAPY

The exact mechanisms and molecular pathways that lead to the histologic development of BPH are yet to be fully explained. However, current theories assert BPH is a multifactorial process involving interactions between prostatic cells, the endocrine system, neural input, heredity, and environmental influences.[49] Although the full mechanistic pathways are not entirely known, a major contributor to the development of BPH has been shown to be the male androgen hormones testosterone and dihydrotestosterone (DHT).

Testosterone is the primary circulating androgen. Before testosterone can exert its effects on the prostatic cells, it undergoes local modification within the prostate to become DHT; 5α-reductase is responsible for this conversion. DHT then forms a complex with androgen receptors, and is transported to the nucleus. Within the nucleus, this complex acts to modify gene expression. The influence of androgens is vital to normal development and growth of the prostate gland. However, the effects of androgens have been shown to also play a role in the development of the prostatic overgrowth seen in BPH.[50] Androgens lead to overall enlargement of the gland contributing to the static component of BPH.

In an effort to curb the production of the active compound, DHT, medications have been developed that specifically target and inhibit the enzyme 5α-reductase. Finasteride and dutasteride are examples of available 5-ARIs. These compounds virtually eliminate the production of DHT, in turn inhibiting prostate growth. The blockade of DHT production has been associated with a reduction of prostatic volume with the maximal reduction coming within 6 months of therapy initiation.[51]

Finasteride

Finasteride is a competitive inhibitor of the type 2 isozyme of 5α-reductase. The North American

Finasteride trial was the first study to report the efficacy of finasteride.[51] This 1-year randomized, double-blind, placebo-controlled multicenter trial demonstrated that patients taking finasteride had a mean decrease in intraprostatic and circulating DHT levels of 80% that was sustained for the 12 months of treatment. There was no significant change in circulating serum testosterone levels in the treatment group, indicating there was not a positive feedback increase in testosterone levels as a result of lowered DHT. This study demonstrated Qmax increased by 1.6 mL/s, compared with 0.2 mL/s in the placebo group. The symptom score decreased an average of 2.7% in the finasteride group compared with 1.0% in the placebo group.

The Proscar Long-Term Efficacy and Safety Study (PLESS) trial is the largest clinical study to investigate finasteride therapy for BPH.[52] This double-blind, placebo-controlled, multicenter study conducted in the United States was composed of 3040 men with moderate to severe LUTS who were randomized to a finasteride group (5 mg/d) or a placebo group for the course of a 4-year trial. At the completion of the trial, the finasteride group showed a 2.0-point greater reduction from their pre-enrollment symptom scores than did the placebo group. The finasteride group also showed a 1.7 mL/s greater improvement in Qmax and displayed a 32% reduction in prostate volume. The greatest impact from this study came from the demonstration that over the course of 4 years, compared with placebo, the finasteride group had a 57% risk reduction for the development of acute urinary retention (AUR) and a 55% risk reduction in the need for BPH-related surgery. In men with a prostate larger than 55 cm^3 there was a 70% risk reduction for the development of AUR and/or need for surgery. These new findings suggested that long-term 5-ARI therapy could impact the progression of BPH by reducing the risk of AUR and the need for surgery. Given the findings of this trial, it is recommended that patients with a prostate larger than 30 g or with moderate to severe BPH symptoms consider a 5-ARI as it may alter the condition's natural history.

Dutasteride

Dutasteride is a dual inhibitor of both the type-1 and type-2 5α-reductase isozymes.[53] The major source of the DHT that plays a relevant role in the prostatic enlargement seen in BPH is thought to be the type-2 5α-reductase isozyme found mostly in the prostate; however, the type-1 5α-reductase in the liver, skin, and small amount in the prostate, may also play a role in prostatic enlargement.[54–56] Dutasteride was thus developed to block DHT production from both enzymatic sources.

Like finasteride, dutasteride has been shown to significantly suppress DHT levels (>90%) and has been associated with decreasing LUTS caused by BPH.[15,57] It has been associated with a significant decrease in prostate volume (~50%), increase in Qmax (~30%), decreased risk of AUR, and decreased risk of requiring BPH-related surgery compared with placebo. This provides evidence that like finasteride, dutasteride is useful in altering the disease course of BPH.[14,57]

Adverse Effects of 5-ARI Therapy

Side effects with finasteride and dutasteride are relatively infrequently encountered. The most common side effects are impotence, loss of libido, ejaculatory dysfunction, and gynecomastia (**Table 3**), but these occur with much less frequency than with other anti-androgenics that have larger effects on circulating androgens and will be discussed later (ie, LHRH antagonists).[58]

5-ARI Therapy and Prostate Cancer

Prostate-specific antigen (PSA) is an enzyme produced by the prostate gland detectable at low levels in the blood of all male patients. It has been shown that most men with prostate cancer have elevations of their PSA level.[59] The prostatic enlargement seen in BPH has also been associated with a rise in PSA, although it is thought that a slower rise with a milder total elevation is more typical of BPH than the elevations seen in cancer.[59,60] Because of its ability to enhance early detection of prostate cancer (albeit with some controversy over the specificity and thus utility of the test), PSA has become a commonly used screening technique for malignancy.[61]

Treatment with finasteride decreases serum PSA levels by approximately 50% over a 4- to 6-month time period.[62–64] This can lead to difficulty interpreting PSA values in a patient on a 5-ARI for BPH. Oesterling and colleagues[65] suggested a mathematical doubling of the serum PSA level approximates the true PSA to a level accurate enough for adequate use as a cancer screening tool in 5-ARI treated patients.

There are no official recommendations to screen 5-ARI–treated patients any differently from the general population. However, given the derangements of PSA seen on 5-ARI therapy, it is wise to obtain a baseline PSA before the start of therapy. On follow-up screening, any sustained increases in PSA levels during 5-ARI treatment should be

Table 3 Adverse effects of 5-ARI therapy[52]		
Effect	Finasteride (%)	Dutasteride (%)
Impotence	5.1	0.8–4.7
Loss of libido	2.6	0.3–3.0
Ejaculatory disorder	1.7	0.1–1.4
Gynecomastia	1.8	0.6–1.1

Data in this table compiled from multiple trials with different patient cohorts. Data represent accurate complication rates for each individual agent as documented in those trials for the cohort studied in that trial. However, given data are from differently designed trials, they cannot be used to accurately compare the side effect rates between medications.
Data from Physicians' Desk Reference 52, Montvale (NJ): Medical Economics Co; 1998.

carefully evaluated and consideration given for a prostate biopsy.

The role 5-ARI therapy plays on the natural course of prostate cancer has not been fully elucidated. The large multicenter Prostate Cancer Prevention Trial showed that daily finasteride therapy was accompanied by a statistically significant 24.8% reduction in prostate cancer prevalence over a 7-year period.[66] However, the same study also showed an increase (4.8% with high grade: placebo, 5.8% with high grade: finasteride) in the clinical grade of prostate cancer in patients who were taking finasteride.[66] This suggests that although finasteride therapy led to a lower prevalence of cancer, the cases that were discovered in patients on finasteride were of a higher clinical grade and thus potentially more aggressive. As a result, the authors of that study concluded it is important to weigh the benefit of lower cancer prevalence and improvement of urinary symptoms with the increased risk of high-grade prostate cancer. A follow-up report from several authors of this trial suggested finasteride may actually selectively inhibit low-grade cancer cells within a tumor, making the tumor appear to be of higher grade. They suggest this may account for the greater incidence of high-grade tumors with finasteride and not effects on tumor morphology leading to induction of high-grade tumors.[67]

A similar, yet to be published, study investigated the effect of Dutasteride on the incidence of prostate cancer in men with PSA between 2.5 and 10.0. The results of the REduction by DUtasteride of prostate Cancer Events trial were presented at the 2009 annual meeting of the American Urological Association (AUA) and are to be published later in 2009.[68] The preliminary summary released by the AUA reported a statistically significant 23% reduction in prostate cancer incidence over 4 years. Of important note there was no significant difference in tumor grade between the Dutasteride and placebo groups.

COMBINATION THERAPY

As explained previously, α-adrenergic blockade and 5-ARI therapy have become two key components of BPH therapy. Alpha-blockers and 5-ARIs are typically thought to separately address the dynamic and static components of the disease respectively. Multiple trials have been conducted to determine if there is any additional therapeutic benefit when medications from each class are combined.

The Veterans Administration (VA) Cooperative Trial was the first randomized, double-blind, placebo-controlled study investigating combination therapy using α-adrenergic antagonists and 5-ARIs.[69] The study was a 1-year randomized controlled trial (RCT) with 1229 patients randomized to one of four study arms: placebo, finasteride alone, terazosin alone, and combination therapy with finasteride and terazosin. End points were mean change from baseline in symptom score and mean change in Qmax. The terazosin alone and combination therapy arms both had significant improvements in the measured end points when compared with placebo. The combination therapy was no more effective than terazosin alone. Finasteride had no greater effect on either end point than did placebo. Finasteride did show the greatest change in prostate size, but that was not correlated with a measured change in symptoms. The authors of this study concluded terazosin therapy was effective while finasteride was not, and combination therapy, although effective, was no more effective than terazosin alone. The conclusion that finasteride was not an effective therapy for BPH differed from the conclusions of many of the major finasteride trials, and this is likely at least partially explained by a mean prostate size of 36.2 and 38.4 cm^3 in the VA study where many of the large finasteride trials had a greater portion of study patients with larger prostates.

The PREDICT trial examined the use of doxazosin, finasteride, and the combination of the two in comparison with placebo.[39] This study concluded that doxazosin was a superior treatment for symptomatic BPH compared with finasteride alone or placebo. The addition of finasteride to doxazosin did not provide any increased benefit compared with doxazosin alone.

Although the early studies for combination therapy appeared to suggest there was no benefit from the addition of a 5-ARI to alpha-blocker therapy, and that there may be little to no benefit to 5-ARI therapy alone, these results were explored further in subsequent trials. Significantly, these early trials only looked at improvement of symptoms. They did not monitor whether therapy had an effect on the progression of BPH symptoms. Additionally, issues were raised with the relatively short 1-year duration of the trials and enrollment of a disproportionate number of men with relatively small volume prostates.

The Medical Treatment of Prostatic Symptoms (MTOPS) trial was the first major trial to attempt to address some of the questions raised by the early combination therapy trials.[70,71] MTOPS was a multicenter, double-blind, randomized, placebo-controlled clinical trial. The study enrolled 3047 men across four arms (placebo, doxazosin, finasteride, and combination) and when published reported a mean of 4.5 years of follow-up. The primary measured outcome was overall clinical progression (defined as development of AUR, renal insufficiency, recurrent urinary tract infection, urinary incontinence, or an increase over baseline of at least 4 points in AUA-IPSS).[71] This was the first trial to investigate this outcome. Secondary outcomes were changes in AUA-IPSS and changes in Qmax. Other outcomes were incidence of invasive therapy for BPH, and change in PSA and prostate volume.

In regard to the primary outcome, all three treatment groups showed a significant risk reduction of clinical progression when compared with placebo (**Table 4**). The combination therapy group saw the largest risk reduction at 66%. The doxazosin group and finasteride group had risk reductions of 39% and 34%, respectively. The 4-year cumulative incidence of clinical progression was 17% in the placebo group, 10% in the doxazosin and finasteride groups, and 5% in the combination group. Each treatment group's decrease in incidence of progression achieved statistical significance. Pairwise comparison of the combination group with each of the three other groups showed it was significantly more effective in decreasing progression than either drug alone or placebo.

The results in regard to the secondary outcomes also favored all forms of therapy (see **Table 4**). Combination therapy was again the most favorable. All 3 active treatment groups showed significant 4-year mean reductions in AUA-IPSS when compared with placebo. When compared with one another in paired analysis, the symptom score improvement for the combination group was significantly greater than in the doxazosin group or the finasteride group (7.5 vs 6.6 vs 5.6, respectively). Qmax also was significantly improved compared with placebo with 4-year mean improvements of 5.1 mL/s, 4.0 mL/s, and 3.2 mL/s in combination, doxazosin, and finasteride groups, respectively.

The MTOPS trial showed a reduction in the need for invasive therapy for BPH in the combination therapy and finasteride monotherapy groups (see **Table 4**). In the placebo group, 40 men underwent invasive therapy. Risk reductions of 67% (*P*<.001) and 64% (*P*<.001) were seen in the combination group and finasteride group, respectively. Interestingly, the doxazosin monotherapy group had no significant reduction in the need for invasive surgery.

The incidence of adverse events in the MTOPS trial was similar to what had been seen in

Table 4
Results of the MTOPS trial

	4-y Cumulative Incidence of Clinical Progression	Clinical Progression (Risk Reduction)	Δ AUA-IPSS	Δ Qmax (mL/s)	Risk Reduction for Invasive Surgical Intervention
Placebo	17%	—	−4.9	NR	—
Finasteride	10%	34%	−5.6	3.2	64%
Doxazosin	10%	39%	−6.6	4	Non-significant
Combination	5%	66%	−7.4	5.1	67%

Abbreviations: NR, not reported; —, risk reductions calculated in comparison to placebo.
Data from McConnell JD, Roehrborn CG, Bautista OM, et al. The long-term effect of doxazosin, finasteride, and combination therapy on the clinical progression of benign prostatic hyperplasia. N Engl J Med 2003;349(25):2387–98.

preceding trials. In the doxazosin group, the most common adverse events were dizziness, postural hypotension, and asthenia. In the finasteride group the most common events were erectile dysfunction, decreased libido, and abnormal ejaculation. In the combination therapy group, the adverse event rate was similar to the rate in each monotherapy group combined. In the active therapy groups, the rates of discontinuation were 18% (discontinuation of both drugs) in the combination group, 27% in doxazosin group, and 24% in the finasteride group.

Given their findings, the authors of the MTOPS trial concluded that over a long-term treatment course, combination therapy is both safe and the most effective therapy for patients with LUTS secondary to BPH. Additionally, combination therapy is the best option in preventing disease progression.[71] The findings of this study made a strong case for the benefit of combination therapy and have led to this treatment option being a mainstay of BPH therapy.

The most recent major multicenter, long-term, placebo-controlled, randomized trial to investigate the utility of combination therapy is the on-going Combination of Avodart and Tamsulosin (CombAT) trial.[72] This study compares therapy with the 5-ARI dutasteride, the alpha-blocking medication Tamsulosin, and the two medications taken in combination. The CombAT trial was designed to address several outstanding issues that remain following the completion of the MTOPS trial, namely, (1) not all men in MTOPS were at a heightened risk for progression as determined by prostate volume and/or PSA thresholds, making analysis of the benefit of combination therapy in those at high risk for progression not possible; (2) owing to study design and patient monitoring there was little insight provided for the time of onset of benefit for combination therapy over monotherapies in MTOPS; and

(3) MTOPS used finasteride, a medication that suppresses DHT via the type 2–specific 5-AR enzyme only.

Men 50 years and older with BPH who met inclusion criteria were randomized to one of three groups: tamsulosin, dutasteride, and combination of tamsulosin and dutasteride. There was no placebo group. As mentioned, this study is currently ongoing; however, in 2008 a 2-year report of the results was published. The primary end point for the 2 year report was change in AUA-IPSS from baseline. Secondary end points reported were change in AUA-IPSS QOL response, Q-max, and prostate volume.

The CombAT trial reported significantly greater decrease in AUA-IPSS for the combination group than in either monotherapy group at 24 months (**Table 5**). The combination group displayed a significant decrease in AUA-IPSS (-6.2 vs -4.9 vs -4.3; combination vs dutasteride vs tamsulosin; $P<.001$). In the categories of improvement of QOL score by 25% or more, 2 or more points, and 3 or more points, a statistically significant higher percentage of patients from the combination therapy group met all three of the above benchmarks as compared with either monotherapy group. At 24 months, statistically significant Qmax improvements from baseline were reported in the combination group versus either monotherapy (improvement of 2.4 mL/s for combination therapy vs 1.9 and 0.9 mL/s for dutasteride and tamsulosin, respectively). Between the combination therapy and tamsulosin groups there was a significant difference in change in prostate size. However, there was no significant difference in change of prostate size between the combination group and the dutasteride group. Less than 5% of the men in each treatment group withdrew because of adverse events.

The 2-year report on the CombAT trial shows superiority of combination therapy over either

Table 5
Results of CombAT trial

	Δ AUA-IPSS	Quality of Life Survey Improvement			Δ Qmax (mL/s)	Δ Prostate VOLUME
		>25%	≥2 pts	≥3 pts		
Dutasteride	−4.9	59%	70%	65%	1.9	−28%[a]
Tamsulosin	−4.3	55%	68%	62%	0.9	0%
Combination	−6.2	67%	77%	75%	2.4	−27%

[a] No significant difference in paired comparison to combination.

Data from Roehrborn CG, Siami P, Barkin J, et al. The effects of dutasteride, tamsulosin and combination therapy on lower urinary tract symptoms in men with benign prostatic hyperplasia and prostatic enlargement: 2-year results from the CombAT study. J Urol 2008;179(2):616–21 [discussion 21].

5-ARI or alpha-blocker monotherapy in terms of improvement of urinary symptoms and urinary flow. Of note, this study is specific to men with moderate to severe LUTS *AND* prostatic enlargement (≥ 30 cm^2). It supports the findings of the MTOPS trial that there is indeed benefit from combination therapy for management of BPH.

ANTICHOLINERGICS

Anticholinergic medications act by blocking acetylcholine receptors within the body. These medications have been shown to be useful in providing relief from the symptoms of overactive bladder. This condition is characterized by frequency, nocturia, and urgency with or without urge incontinence that is not accounted for by other factors or disease entities.[73] These symptoms are often noted to be quite similar to the storage symptoms of LUTS attributed to BOO. Historically, regardless of the similarity between these two disorders, anticholinergics were considered contraindicated in the setting of LUTS attributable to BPH because of the perceived risk of AUR. Recently, several trials have been conducted to assess the utility of anticholinergics as therapy for BPH, either as an isolated agent or in combination with other medication classes.

In the largest RCT examining the safety of anticholinergics alone for the treatment of BPH with LUTS, 222 men older than 40 years with storage symptoms and BOO documented by urodynamics were randomized to receive tolterodine 2 mg twice a day or placebo.[74] Excluded from the study were men with postvoid residual volume (PVR) greater than 40% of maximum capacity as well as men with a history of urinary retention. After 12 weeks, repeat urodynamic evaluation revealed no significant difference in Qmax change from baseline between the treatment and placebo groups. Compared with the placebo group, within the tolterodine group PVR increased (+27 mL, $P = .004$), voiding efficiency decreased (-7, $P = .018$), and the Bladder Contractility Index decreased (-10, $P = .005$). There was only one event of AUR, occurring in the placebo group. The study authors concluded there was no signal that tolterodine aggravated preexisting voiding difficulties.

A 2007 meta-analysis evaluated 633 patients from four RCTs that studied the use of anticholinergics in men with LUTS.[75] This analysis found anticholinergics did not significantly alter Qmax (0.1 mL/s, 95% confidence interval (CI) 0.6–0.7). The PVR was increased by 11.6 mL (95% CI 4.5–18.6) with no significant difference between AUR rates. The AUA-IPSS scores were not significantly different, but there were improvements for AUA-IPSS storage subscores in one RCT. The AUR rate was 0.3% in 365 men at the 12-week follow-up point. Given these findings, the conclusions of the meta-analysis were that anticholinergic use in men with LUTS from BPH appears to be safe, and further studies are necessary to establish efficacy.

An additional RCT not included in the above meta-analysis evaluated 851 men 40 years or older who were randomized to four groups: placebo, tolterodine extended release (ER) 4 mg/d, tamsulosin 0.4 mg/d, or tolterodine plus tamsulosin at the previously mentioned doses.[76] Men with PVR greater than 200 mL or Qmax less than 5 mL/s were excluded from the trial. The study measured patient perception of treatment benefit, bladder diary variables, AUA-IPSS, and safety and tolerability (**Table 6**). Eighty percent receiving tolterodine ER plus tamsulosin reported treatment benefit by week 12 compared with 62% receiving placebo ($P<.001$). Patients receiving tolterodine ER plus tamsulosin compared with placebo experienced significant reductions in urgency urinary incontinence, urgency episodes without incontinence, micturitions per 24 hours, and micturitions per night. They also demonstrated significant improvements in AUA-IPSS and the quality of life item. In the tolterodine ER group, 65% reported benefit ($P = .48$ vs placebo). Patients in the latter group displayed a significant reduction in only the urgency urinary incontinence item in the bladder diary at 12 weeks. There were no significant differences between tolterodine ER and placebo on the total AUA-IPSS at any visit. In the tamsulosin alone group 71% reported benefit ($P = .06$ vs placebo). At 12 weeks there were no significant differences for any voiding diary variables versus placebo or the QOL score, but there was a significant improvement in total AUA-IPSS. All interventions were well tolerated. The incidence of AUR requiring catheterization was low (tolterodine ER plus tamsulosin, 0.4%; tolterodine ER, 0.5%; tamsulosin, 0%; and placebo, 0%). The conclusion of this study was that patients with LUTS including overactive bladder symptoms may not respond to monotherapy with either antimuscarinic agents or alpha-blocking agents, but combination therapy with tolterodine ER and tamsulosin shows a statistically and clinically significant benefit in such patients. Given the low complication rate they determined that all treatment options were safe.

Given the data available regarding the role of antimuscarinics in the management of BPH-related urinary storage symptoms, there is no true consensus or guideline. It appears that the

Table 6
Treatment benefit of tolterodine ER plus tamsulosin

	Patient-reported Treatment Benefit (%)	Significant Improvement Demonstrated with Therapy					
		Urgency Urinary Incontinence	Urgency	Micturitions/24 h	Micturitions/Night	AUA-IPSS	Quality-of-Life Item
Placebo	62	—	—	—	—	—	—
Tolterodine ER	65	Yes	No	No	No	No	No
Tamsulosin	71	No	No	No	No	Yes	No
Combination	80	Yes	Yes	Yes	Yes	Yes	Yes

Abbreviation: —, placebo is baseline for comparison.
Data from Kaplan SA, Roehrborn CG, Rovner ES, et al. Tolterodine and tamsulosin for treatment of men with lower urinary tract symptoms and overactive bladder: a randomized controlled trial. JAMA 2006;296(19):2319–28.

previously held perception that use of these agents in the setting of BOO should be contraindicated is unfounded, as multiple studies have shown safety in this circumstance. However, it is notable that nearly every study pertaining to antimuscarinics in this patient population excluded those with higher grade obstructions as evidenced by an elevated PVR or low Qmax. As a result, the risk of AUR in those with higher-grade BOO is unknown. No study has shown significant improvement in symptoms from the use of antimuscarinic agents alone. Recent evidence shows that when added to alpha-blocker therapy, this combination provides a statistically significant improvement in urinary symptoms.[76] This class of medication could be useful as an adjunct to alpha-blocker therapy in patients who continue to have storage urinary symptoms.

PHYTOTHERAPEUTICS

Phytotherapeutic products are food supplements derived from plants (typically extracts from roots, seeds, bark, or fruits), and patients with BPH and LUTS commonly use them as substitute for proven medications. A recent survey reported that 34% of patients with LUTS secondary to BPH were using a phytotherapeutic product either alone or along with more traditional medical therapy for management of their symptoms.[77] In a 2001 review, Lowe[78] attributes the widespread use of these products to (1) aggressive marketing to promote prostate health, (2) feelings that they are "natural" products (not medications), (3) the presumption they are safe (in many cases not proven), (4) ease of obtainability (no prescription needed), (5) thinking they may help avoid prostate surgery, and (6) hope that they prevent prostate cancer (assumed falsely). Although widely available and commonly used, in most cases these products have yet to be fully endorsed by traditional medicine. A major reason for this is the significant lack evidence for the mechanism of action of these compounds or of well-designed and executed clinical trials attesting to their safety and/or efficacy. Also, there is little regulation on the consistency of these compounds, meaning products from different manufacturers said to contain the same "active ingredient" are not subject to strict monitoring for strength, purity, or safety.

There are a vast number of phytotherapeutic agents marketed and sold to "promote prostate health." Commercially available formulations commonly contain two or more of these compounds, making comparison of products even more difficult. It is difficult to review all of these compounds due to their sheer number and little to no scientific evidence supporting their use. However, there are several compounds that have been studied in more formal investigations providing a small amount of evidence for their use. Three such compounds are reviewed here.

Saw Palmetto (Serenoa repens)

Saw palmetto is the most popular extract in terms of sales revenue and clinical trial involvement.[79] This agent is derived from the dried berry of the American dwarf palm. It is widely used in Europe and is an often reimbursed treatment in France and Germany.[80]

The action of saw palmetto is not known, but there are four proposed mechanisms that have been investigated including anti-inflammatory, anti-androgenic, pro-apoptotic, and alpha-blocking. In vitro studies have demonstrated saw palmetto inhibits the biosynthesis of cyclooxygenase and 5-lipoxygenase, leading to the anti-inflammatory theory.[81] Other studies have argued that saw palmetto may have action similar to 5-ARIs, blocking DHT production and thus acting as an anti-androgen. An in vitro study by Weisser and colleagues[82] argued that the IDS 89 extract from the saw palmetto plant inhibited 5α-reductase in a dose-dependant manner in the epithelium and stroma of human BPH. This result is challenged by several authors who state the 5-ARI effect of saw palmetto is either weak in comparison with finasteride or not present at a physiologic dose.[83,84] The pro-apoptotic theory arose from a group showing that S repens increased apoptotic activity by increasing the bax-to-bcl-2 expression ratio and increasing caspase-3 activity in patients with BPH.[85] However, a second study found no pro-apoptotic effect of S repens on in vitro prostate cell lines.[83] The fourth proposed mechanism originated from early in vitro experiments of Goepel and colleagues[86] that showed saw palmetto may possess α-adrenergic blocking capabilities. However, multiple subsequent in vivo studies have refuted this claim including a follow-up by Goepel and colleagues.[87,88]

A variety of trials have been conducted to attempt to prove the efficacy of saw palmetto in patients. Nearly every trial stating saw palmetto is an efficacious treatment option has been flawed in some way, lending difficulty in interpreting the results in a manner that would affect therapeutic recommendations. Common flaws include lack of randomization, lack of placebo control, nonstandard or difficult to determine concentration of study medication, short study duration, nonstandardized study end, and lack of blinded, placebo-controlled trials comparing saw palmetto to established medical therapies.

Much of the earliest data regarding the efficacy of saw palmetto has been summarized in two different meta-analyses.[89,90] These analyses both attempted to compile data from many studies with different designs and outcomes (ie, the duration of trials included in the two analyses ranged from 3 to 107 weeks). In spite of the difficulty analyzing the variety of trials, both meta-analyses concluded that saw palmetto showed evidence of statistically significant improvement of symptom scores, Qmax, and a reduction of nocturnal urinations versus placebo. A 2001 RCT not included in either meta-analysis randomized 85 patients to a placebo-controlled trial of 26 weeks' duration and reported significant improvement of AUA-IPSS in the saw palmetto group versus placebo.[91] However, two subsequent, well-designed, double-blind, placebo-controlled trials have reported no significant beneficial effects from the use of saw palmetto when compared with placebo.[92,93] The most recent and best designed RCTs have shown no significant effect from saw palmetto.[92,93] Although several trials and meta-analyses have reported significant positive effects from saw palmetto, inconsistencies in study design, type and duration of study, and outcomes reported cast a bit of question over their conclusions. In summary, given the available data, there are not sufficient and consistent enough data to recommend for or against the use of saw palmetto for the medical treatment of BPH.

Fortunately, under the guidance of the National Institute for Diabetes and Digestive and Kidney Diseases (NIDDK), a large multicenter trial is under way to evaluate the efficacy of saw palmetto. The Complimentary and Alternative Medicine for Urological Symptoms (CAMUS) trial is a randomized, long-term, double-blind, placebo-controlled study designed to evaluate the effects of saw palmetto in a manner similar to many of the trials used for evaluation of other pharmaceuticals used to treat BPH. The first results of this trial are expected in December 2010.[94]

African Prune Tree (Pygeum africanum)

P africanum is derived from an extract of the bark of the African prune tree. Similar to saw palmetto, the full mechanism of this phytotherapeutic is not known. Studies have argued this compound may play a role in BPH management via growth factor inhibition, anti-inflammation, anti-androgenic action, or via a protective effect on the obstructed bladder.[95–100]

P africanum has very little data from trials in regard to its efficacy. A 2000 meta-analysis evaluated 18 trials in which *P africanum* was investigated either as a single agent or given in combination with other phytotherapeutics.[101] Most of the studies included in this analysis suffered from many of the inconsistencies discussed with the saw palmetto trials, again making valuable conclusions difficult to reach. Nonetheless, this analysis reported a significant difference in physician-reported symptom improvement with 65% of patients taking *P africanum* improving in contrast to 30% on placebo (risk ratio 2.1, 95% CI 1.4–3.1).[101] Since the publication of this trial, there have been very few trials evaluating *P africanum*. A 2002 trial evaluated *P africanum* plus sting nettle extract versus placebo and concluded there was no significant change in end points versus placebo.[102] Given the absence of proper data, no recommendation or conclusion can be made concerning the efficacy of *P africanum*.

South African Star Grass (Hypoxis Rooperi)

South African star grass is an additional phytotherapeutic agent, whose active ingredient is a β-sitosterol extracted from the plant. Similar to the other agents, the mechanism of action is unknown with proposed actions including anti-inflammation, alteration of cholesterol metabolism, direct inhibition of prostate growth, antiandrogenic or antiestrogenic effects, and decreased sex-hormone–binding globulin availability.[103] The primary source of efficacy data is a 2000 Cochrane review meta-analysis evaluating four trials with 519 total patients.[104] The data from two of the studies evaluated reported an AUA-IPSS weighted mean difference of −4.9 when compared with placebo. If reproducible, this would represent quite a significant improvement in symptoms; however, there have been no trials to confirm these findings. The data available regarding South African star grass is encouraging, yet with such little data regarding its long-term efficacy, safety, and side effects, no recommendation can be made regarding its use.

Other Extracts

As mentioned previously, there are numerous phytotherapeutics on the market that list treatment of prostate disorders as one of their uses. The three reviewed previously are those with the most data concerning their effectiveness. Several other commonly available agents include stinging nettle (*Urtica dioica*), rye pollen (*Secale cereale*), pumpkin seed (*Cucurbita pepo*), cactus flower (*Opuntia*), pine flower (*Pinus*), and spruce (*Picea*).[59] Unfortunately, there are very little data to comment on the effectiveness of these agents.

SUMMARY

BPH is a common affliction in aging men with the most common symptom being LUTS. Treatment of this disorder has typically been aimed at relieving troubling LUTS, and more recently has had alteration of disease progression as a treatment goal in some cases. There are many treatment options available for this disorder (ie, medical, herbal, surgical); however, in recent years medical therapy has become the mainstay of first-line management. There are many options when choosing a medical regimen, most of which were outlined earlier in this article.

Watchful waiting is an appropriate option for patients with mild LUTS (AUA-IPSS ≤ 7). This strategy requires annual reassessment of a patient's symptoms with consideration of need for therapy. Behavioral modifications such as limiting nighttime fluid intake can be useful adjuncts in this method. In those patients whose symptoms progress to moderate or severe levels (AUA-IPSS >7), consideration of further therapy is warranted.

To summarize the data presented in this chapter: the use of alpha-blocking medications, 5-ARIs, and combination therapy (alpha-blocker plus 5-ARI) for BPH symptoms all have been supported by well-designed trials. The second- and third-generation alpha-blockers have been shown to provide relief of LUTS while limiting side effects and are especially useful in the patient experiencing symptoms without a markedly enlarged prostate. Therapy with 5-ARI alone is typically recommended for patients with an enlarged prostate (>50 g) and few urinary symptoms because of data that it is most effective in this patient subpopulation. Combination therapy is rapidly emerging as a mainstay of therapy, especially for patients with bothersome LUTS and an enlarged prostate. It has been shown that not only does combination therapy provide symptom relief, it is the only therapy shown to alter disease progression. Recent data have shown the previously held belief that anticholinergic therapy should be contraindicated in the setting of BOO is unfounded. Although more data are needed, anticholinergics can be useful when added to α-blocker therapy for the patient with mild to moderate BOO and storage urinary symptoms. Although many phytotherapeutic treatment options exist, there are not sufficient scientific data to recommend them as efficacious treatment options. With the results of the on-going CAMUS trial, the hope is a more definitive statement could be made about the use of saw palmetto for BPH therapy.

REFERENCES

1. Lee C, Kozlowski JM, Grayhack JT. Etiology of benign prostatic hyperplasia. Urol Clin North Am 1995;22(2):237–46.
2. Lee C, Kozlowski JM, Grayhack JT. Intrinsic and extrinsic factors controlling benign prostatic growth. Prostate 1997;31(2):131–8.
3. Reynard JM. Does anticholinergic medication have a role for men with lower urinary tract symptoms/benign prostatic hyperplasia either alone or in combination with other agents? Curr Opin Urol 2004;14(1):13–6.
4. Di Silverio F, Gentile V, Pastore AL, et al. Benign prostatic hyperplasia: what about a campaign for prevention? Urol Int 2004;72(3):179–88.
5. O'Leary MP. Lower urinary tract symptoms/benign prostatic hyperplasia: maintaining symptom control and reducing complications. Urology 2003;62(3 Suppl 1):15–23.
6. Gushchin GL, Jones CA, Nyberg LM. Decline in the surgical treatment of benign prostatic hyperplasia among black and white men in the United States: 1980 to 1994 [abstract]. J Urol 1997;157:311.
7. Wasson JH, Bubolz TA, Lu-Yao GL, et al. Transurethral resection of the prostate among Medicare beneficiaries: 1984 to 1997. For the Patient Outcomes Research Team for Prostatic Diseases. J Urol 2000;164(4):1212–5.
8. Baine WB, Yu W, Summe JP, et al. Epidemiologic trends in the evaluation and treatment of lower urinary tract symptoms in elderly male Medicare patients from 1991 to 1995. J Urol 1998;160(3 Pt 1):816–20.
9. Caine M, Raz S, Zeigler M. Adrenergic and cholinergic receptors in the human prostate, prostatic capsule and bladder neck. Br J Urol 1975;47(2):193–202.
10. Furuya S, Kumamoto Y, Yokoyama E, et al. Alpha-adrenergic activity and urethral pressure in prostatic zone in benign prostatic hypertrophy. J Urol 1982;128(4):836–9.
11. Kobayashi S, Tang R, Shapiro E, et al. Characterization and localization of prostatic alpha 1 adrenoceptors using radioligand receptor binding on slide-mounted tissue section. J Urol 1993;150(6):2002–6.
12. Lepor H, Laddu A. Terazosin in the treatment of benign prostatic hyperplasia: the United States experience. Br J Urol 1992;70(Suppl 1):2–9.
13. Yokoyama E, Furuya S, Kumamoto Y. [Quantitation of alpha-1 and beta adrenergic receptor densities in the human normal and hypertrophied prostate].

Nippon Hinyokika Gakkai Zasshi 1985;76(3):325–37 [in Japanese].
14. Roehrborn CG, Lukkarinen O, Mark S, et al. Long-term sustained improvement in symptoms of benign prostatic hyperplasia with the dual 5alpha-reductase inhibitor dutasteride: results of 4-year studies. BJU Int 2005;96(4):572–7.
15. Roehrborn CG, Marks LS, Fenter T, et al. Efficacy and safety of dutasteride in the four-year treatment of men with benign prostatic hyperplasia. Urology 2004;63(4):709–15.
16. Lepor H. Alpha blockade for the treatment of benign prostatic hyperplasia. Urol Clin North Am 1995;22(2):375–86.
17. Lepor H. Long-term efficacy and safety of terazosin in patients with benign prostatic hyperplasia. Terazosin Research Group. Urology 1995;45(3):406–13.
18. Price DT, Schwinn DA, Lomasney JW, et al. Identification, quantification, and localization of mRNA for three distinct alpha 1 adrenergic receptor subtypes in human prostate. J Urol 1993;150(2 Pt 1):546–51.
19. Malloy BJ, Price DT, Price RR, et al. Alpha1-adrenergic receptor subtypes in human detrusor. J Urol 1998;160(3 Pt 1):937–43.
20. Smith MS, Schambra UB, Wilson KH, et al. Alpha1-adrenergic receptors in human spinal cord: specific localized expression of mRNA encoding alpha1-adrenergic receptor subtypes at four distinct levels. Brain Res Mol Brain Res 1999;63(2):254–61.
21. Andersson K-E, Wein AJ. Pharmacology of the lower urinary tract—basis for current and future treatments of urinary incontinence. Pharmacol Rev 2004;56(4):581–631.
22. Hampel C, Dolber PC, Smith MP, et al. Modulation of bladder alpha1-adrenergic receptor subtype expression by bladder outlet obstruction. J Urol 2002;167(3):1513–21.
23. Gu B, Reiter JP, Schwinn DA, et al. Effects of alpha 1-adrenergic receptor subtype selective antagonists on lower urinary tract function in rats with bladder outlet obstruction. J Urol 2004;172(2):758–62.
24. Nomiya M, Yamaguchi O. A quantitative analysis of mRNA expression of alpha 1 and beta-adrenoceptor subtypes and their functional roles in human normal and obstructed bladders. J Urol 2003;170(2 Pt 1):649–53.
25. Das AK, Leggett RE, Whitbeck C, et al. Effect of doxazosin on rat urinary bladder function after partial outlet obstruction. Neurourol Urodyn 2002;21(2):160–6.
26. Pinggera G-M, Schuster A, Pallwein L, et al. Alpha-blockers increase vesical and prostatic blood flow and bladder capacity [abstract]. Eur Urol 2003;159(Suppl 2):628.

27. Beduschi MC, Beduschi R, Oesterling JE. Alpha-blockade therapy for benign prostatic hyperplasia: from a nonselective to a more selective alpha1A-adrenergic antagonist. Urology 1998; 51(6):861–72.

28. Abrams P, Hollister P, Lawrence J, et al. Bladder outflow obstruction treated with phenoxybenzamine. Preliminary note. Br J Urol 1982;54(5):530.

29. Caine M, Perlberg S, Meretyk S. A placebo-controlled double-blind study of the effect of phenoxybenzamine in benign prostatic obstruction. Br J Urol 1978;50(7):551–4.

30. Caine M, Perlberg S, Meretyk S. A placebo-controlled double-blind study of the effect of phenoxybenzamine in benign prostatic obstruction. 1978 [editorial]. J Urol 2002;167(2 Pt 2):1101.

31. Caine M, Perlberg S, Shapiro A. Phenoxybenzamine for benign prostatic obstruction. Review of 200 cases. Urology 1981;17(6):542–6.

32. Chapple CR, Wyndaele JJ, Nordling J, et al. Tamsulosin, the first prostate-selective alpha 1A-adrenoceptor antagonist. A meta-analysis of two randomized, placebo-controlled, multicentre studies in patients with benign prostatic obstruction (symptomatic BPH). European Tamsulosin Study Group. Eur Urol 1996;29(2):155–67.

33. Michel MC, Flannery MT, Narayan P. Worldwide experience with alfuzosin and tamsulosin. Urology 2001;58(4):508–16.

34. Shibata K, Foglar R, Horie K, et al. KMD-3213, a novel, potent, alpha 1a-adrenoceptor-selective antagonist: characterization using recombinant human alpha 1-adrenoceptors and native tissues. Mol Pharmacol 1995;48(2):250–8.

35. Lee M. Alfuzosin hydrochloride for the treatment of benign prostatic hyperplasia. Am J Health Syst Pharm 2003;60(14):1426–39.

36. Roehrborn CG, Oesterling JE, Auerbach S, et al. The Hytrin Community Assessment Trial study: a one-year study of terazosin versus placebo in the treatment of men with symptomatic benign prostatic hyperplasia. HYCAT Investigator Group. Urology 1996;47(2):159–68.

37. Kirby RS. Doxazosin in benign prostatic hyperplasia: effects on blood pressure and urinary flow in normotensive and hypertensive men. Urology 1995;46(2):182–6.

38. Roehrborn CG, Siegel RL. Safety and efficacy of doxazosin in benign prostatic hyperplasia: a pooled analysis of three double-blind, placebo-controlled studies. Urology 1996;48(3):406–15.

39. Kirby RS, Roehrborn C, Boyle P, et al. Efficacy and tolerability of doxazosin and finasteride, alone or in combination, in treatment of symptomatic benign prostatic hyperplasia: the Prospective European Doxazosin and Combination Therapy (PREDICT) trial. Urology 2003;61(1):119–26.

40. Roehrborn CG. Efficacy and safety of once-daily alfuzosin in the treatment of lower urinary tract symptoms and clinical benign prostatic hyperplasia: a randomized, placebo-controlled trial. Urology 2001;58(6):953–9.

41. Roehrborn CG, Van Kerrebroeck P, Nordling J. Safety and efficacy of alfuzosin 10 mg once-daily in the treatment of lower urinary tract symptoms and clinical benign prostatic hyperplasia: a pooled analysis of three double-blind, placebo-controlled studies. BJU Int 2003;92(3):257–61.

42. Abrams P, Schulman CC, Vaage S. Tamsulosin, a selective alpha 1c-adrenoceptor antagonist: a randomized, controlled trial in patients with benign prostatic 'obstruction' (symptomatic BPH). The European Tamsulosin Study Group. Br J Urol 1995;76(3):325–36.

43. Dunn CJ, Matheson A, Faulds DM. Tamsulosin: a review of its pharmacology and therapeutic efficacy in the management of lower urinary tract symptoms. Drugs Aging 2002;19(2):135–61.

44. Michel MC, Mehlburger L, Bressel HU, et al. Comparison of tamsulosin efficacy in subgroups of patients with lower urinary tract symptoms. Prostate Cancer Prostatic Dis 1998;1(6):332–5.

45. Michel MC, Mehlburger L, Bressel HU, et al. Tamsulosin treatment of 19,365 patients with lower urinary tract symptoms: does co-morbidity alter tolerability? J Urol 1998;160(3 Pt 1):784–91.

46. van Kerrebroeck P, Jardin A, Laval KU, et al. Efficacy and safety of a new prolonged release formulation of alfuzosin 10 mg once daily versus alfuzosin 2.5 mg thrice daily and placebo in patients with symptomatic benign prostatic hyperplasia. ALFORTI Study Group. Eur Urol 2000;37(3):306–13.

47. Kawabe K, Yoshida M, Homma Y. Silodosin, a new alpha1A-adrenoceptor-selective antagonist for treating benign prostatic hyperplasia: results of a phase III randomized, placebo-controlled, double-blind study in Japanese men. BJU Int 2006;98(5):1019–24.

48. Wilt TJ, Howe W, MacDonald R. Terazosin for treating symptomatic benign prostatic obstruction: a systematic review of efficacy and adverse effects. BJU Int 2002;89(3):214–25.

49. Partin AW. Etiology of benign prostatic hyperplasia. Philadelphia: WB Saunders Co; 2000. p. 95–100.

50. Coffey DS, Walsh PC. Clinical and experimental studies of benign prostatic hyperplasia. Urol Clin North Am 1990;17(3):461–75.

51. Gormley GJ, Stoner E, Bruskewitz RC, et al. The effect of finasteride in men with benign prostatic hyperplasia. The Finasteride Study Group. N Engl J Med 1992;327(17):1185–91.

52. McConnell JD, Bruskewitz R, Walsh P, et al. The effect of finasteride on the risk of acute urinary retention and the need for surgical treatment

among men with benign prostatic hyperplasia. Finasteride Long-Term Efficacy and Safety Study Group. N Engl J Med 1998;338(9):557–63.

53. Evans HC, Goa KL. Dutasteride. Drugs Aging 2003;12(20):905–16 [discussion: 17–18].

54. Gisleskog PO, Hermann D, Hammarlund-Udenaes M, et al. A model for the turnover of dihydrotestosterone in the presence of the irreversible 5 alpha-reductase inhibitors GI198745 and finasteride. Clin Pharmacol Ther 1998;64(6):636–47.

55. Shirakawa T, Okada H, Acharya B, et al. Messenger RNA levels and enzyme activities of 5 alpha-reductase types 1 and 2 in human benign prostatic hyperplasia (BPH) tissue. Prostate 2004; 58(1):33–40.

56. Thigpen AE, Davis DL, Milatovich A, et al. Molecular genetics of steroid 5 alpha-reductase 2 deficiency. J Clin Invest 1992;90(3):799–809.

57. Roehrborn CG, Boyle P, Nickel JC, et al. Efficacy and safety of a dual inhibitor of 5-alpha-reductase types 1 and 2 (dutasteride) in men with benign prostatic hyperplasia. Urology 2002;60(3):434–41.

58. Physician's Desk Reference. 62 nd edition. Montvale (NJ): Thompson Healthcare, Inc; 2008. p. 1375, 2083.

59. Lieber MM, Jacobsen SJ, Roberts RO, et al. Prostate volume and prostate-specific antigen in the absence of prostate cancer: a review of the relationship and prediction of long-term outcomes. Prostate 2001;49(3):208–12.

60. Oesterling JE, Jacobsen SJ, Chute CG, et al. Serum prostate-specific antigen in a community-based population of healthy men. Establishment of age-specific reference ranges. JAMA 1993; 270(7):860–4.

61. Boyle P, Gould AL, Roehrborn CG. Prostate volume predicts outcome of treatment of benign prostatic hyperplasia with finasteride: meta-analysis of randomized clinical trials. Urology 1996;48(3):398–405.

62. Guess HA, Heyse JF, Gormley GJ. The effect of finasteride on prostate-specific antigen in men with benign prostatic hyperplasia. Prostate 1993; 22(1):31–7.

63. Guess HA, Heyse JF, Gormley GJ, et al. Effect of finasteride on serum PSA concentration in men with benign prostatic hyperplasia. Results from the North American phase III clinical trial. Urol Clin North Am 1993;20(4):627–36.

64. Lange PH. Is the prostate pill finally here? N Engl J Med 1992;327(17):1234–6.

65. Oesterling JE, Roy J, Agha A, et al. Biologic variability of prostate-specific antigen and its usefulness as a marker for prostate cancer: effects of finasteride. The Finasteride PSA Study Group. Urology 1997;50(1):13–8.

66. Thompson IM, Goodman PJ, Tangen CM, et al. The influence of finasteride on the development of prostate cancer. N Engl J Med 2003;349(3):215–24.

67. Lucia MS, Epstein JI, Goodman PJ, et al. Finasteride and high-grade prostate cancer in the Prostate Cancer Prevention Trial. J Natl Cancer Inst 2007; 99(18):1375–83.

68. Data show Dutasteride reduces prostate cancer diagnosis in men with increased risk, in article number 130, vol. 2009. Available at: www.auanet.org/content/press/press-release/article.cfm.

69. Lepor H, Williford WO, Barry MJ, et al. The efficacy of terazosin, finasteride, or both in benign prostatic hyperplasia. Veterans Affairs Cooperative Studies Benign Prostatic Hyperplasia Study Group. N Engl J Med 1996;335(8):533–9.

70. Bautista OM, Kusek JW, Nyberg LM, et al. Study design of the Medical Therapy of Prostatic Symptoms (MTOPS) trial. Control Clin Trials 2003;24(2): 224–43.

71. McConnell JD, Roehrborn CG, Bautista OM, et al. The long-term effect of doxazosin, finasteride, and combination therapy on the clinical progression of benign prostatic hyperplasia. N Engl J Med 2003;349(25):2387–98.

72. Roehrborn CG, Siami P, Barkin J, et al. The effects of dutasteride, tamsulosin and combination therapy on lower urinary tract symptoms in men with benign prostatic hyperplasia and prostatic enlargement: 2-year results from the CombAT study. J Urol 2008;179(2):616–21 [discussion: 21].

73. Abrams P, Cardozo L, Fall M, et al. The standardisation of terminology of lower urinary tract function: report from the Standardisation Sub-committee of the International Continence Society. Am J Obstet Gynecol 2002;187(1):116–26.

74. Abrams P, Kaplan S, De Koning Gans HJ, et al. Safety and tolerability of tolterodine for the treatment of overactive bladder in men with bladder outlet obstruction. J Urol 2006;175(3 Pt 1): 999–1004 [discussion].

75. Blake-James BT, Rashidian A, Ikeda Y, et al. The role of anticholinergics in men with lower urinary tract symptoms suggestive of benign prostatic hyperplasia: a systematic review and meta-analysis. BJU Int 2007;99(1):85–96.

76. Kaplan SA, Roehrborn CG, Rovner ES, et al. Tolterodine and tamsulosin for treatment of men with lower urinary tract symptoms and overactive bladder: a randomized controlled trial. JAMA 2006;296(19):2319–28.

77. Bales GT, Christiano AP, Kirsh EJ, et al. Phytotherapeutic agents in the treatment of lower urinary tract symptoms: a demographic analysis of awareness and use at the University of Chicago. Urology 1999;54(1):86–9.

78. Lowe FC. Phytotherapy in the management of benign prostatic hyperplasia. Urology 2001; 58(6 Suppl 1):71–6 [discussion: 76–7].

79. Dedhia RC, McVary KT. Phytotherapy for lower urinary tract symptoms secondary to benign prostatic hyperplasia. J Urol 2008;179(6):2119–25.
80. Dreikorn K, Borkowsi A, Braeckman J, et al. Other medical therapies. In: Denis L, Griffiths K, Khoury S, et al, editors. The 4th International Consultation on BPH Plymouth, United Kingdom. Health Publications; 1998. p. 633–59.
81. Buck AC. Is there a scientific basis for the therapeutic effects of Serenoa repens in benign prostatic hyperplasia? Mechanisms of action. J Urol 2004;172(5 Pt 1):1792–9.
82. Weisser H, Tunn S, Behnke B, et al. Effects of the Sabal serrulata extract IDS 89 and its subfractions on 5 alpha-reductase activity in human benign prostatic hyperplasia. Prostate 1996; 28(5):300–6.
83. Hill B, Kyprianou N. Effect of permixon on human prostate cell growth: lack of apoptotic action. Prostate 2004;61(1):73–80.
84. Rhodes L, Primka RL, Berman C, et al. Comparison of finasteride (Proscar), a 5 alpha reductase inhibitor, and various commercial plant extracts in in vitro and in vivo 5 alpha reductase inhibition. Prostate 1993;22(1):43–51.
85. Vela-Navarrete R, Escribano-Burgos M, Farre AL, et al. Serenoa repens treatment modifies bax/bcl-2 index expression and caspase-3 activity in prostatic tissue from patients with benign prostatic hyperplasia. J Urol 2005;173(2):507–10.
86. Goepel M, Hecker U, Krege S, et al. Saw palmetto extracts potently and noncompetitively inhibit human alpha1-adrenoceptors in vitro. Prostate 1999;38(3):208–15.
87. Cao N, Haynes JM, Ventura S. Saw palmetto is an indirectly acting sympathomimetic in the rat-isolated prostate gland. Prostate 2006;66(2):115–23.
88. Goepel M, Dinh L, Mitchell A, et al. Do saw palmetto extracts block human alpha1-adrenoceptor subtypes in vivo? Prostate 2001;46(3):226–32.
89. Boyle P, Robertson C, Lowe F, et al. Updated meta-analysis of clinical trials of Serenoa repens extract in the treatment of symptomatic benign prostatic hyperplasia. BJU Int 2004;93(6):751–6.
90. Wilt TJ, Ishani A, Stark G, et al. Saw palmetto extracts for treatment of benign prostatic hyperplasia: a systematic review. JAMA 1998;280(18):1604–9.
91. Gerber GS, Kuznetsov D, Johnson BC, et al. Randomized, double-blind, placebo-controlled trial of saw palmetto in men with lower urinary tract symptoms. Urology 2001;58(6):960–4 [discussion: 4–5].
92. Bent S, Kane C, Shinohara K, et al. Saw palmetto for benign prostatic hyperplasia. N Engl J Med 2006;354(6):557–66.
93. Willetts KE, Clements MS, Champion S, et al. Serenoa repens extract for benign prostate hyperplasia: a randomized controlled trial. BJU Int 2003;92(3):267–70.
94. Complementary and Alternative Medicine for Urological Symptoms (CAMUS). 2009. Available at: www.clinicaltrial.gov.
95. Boulbes D, Soustelle L, Costa P, et al. Pygeum africanum extract inhibits proliferation of human cultured prostatic fibroblasts and myofibroblasts. BJU Int 2006;98(5):1106–13.
96. Choo MS, Bellamy F, Constantinou CE. Functional evaluation of Tadenan on micturition and experimental prostate growth induced with exogenous dihydrotestosterone. Urology 2000;55(2):292–8.
97. Lawson RK. Role of growth factors in benign prostatic hyperplasia. Eur Urol 1997;32(Suppl 1):22–7.
98. Paubert-Braquet M, Cave A, Hocquemiller R, et al. Effect of Pygeum africanum extract on A23187-stimulated production of lipoxygenase metabolites from human polymorphonuclear cells. J Lipid Mediat Cell Signal 1994;9(3):285–90.
99. Yoshimura Y, Yamaguchi O, Bellamy F, et al. Effect of Pygeum africanum tadenan on micturition and prostate growth of the rat secondary to coadministered treatment and post-treatment with dihydrotestosterone. Urology 2003;61(2):474–8.
100. Levin RM, Riffaud JP, Bellamy F, et al. Effects of tadenan pretreatment on bladder physiology and biochemistry following partial outlet obstruction. J Urol 1996;156(6):2084–8.
101. Ishani A, MacDonald R, Nelson D, et al. Pygeum africanum for the treatment of patients with benign prostatic hyperplasia: a systematic review and quantitative meta-analysis. Am J Med 2000; 109(8):654–64.
102. Melo EA, Bertero EB, Rios LA, et al. Evaluating the efficiency of a combination of Pygeum africanum and stinging nettle (Urtica dioica) extracts in treating benign prostatic hyperplasia (BPH): double-blind, randomized, placebo controlled trial. Int Braz J Urol 2002;28(5):418–25.
103. Lowe FC, Ku JC. Phytotherapy in treatment of benign prostatic hyperplasia: a critical review. Urology 1996;48(1):12–20.
104. Wilt T, Ishani A, MacDonald R, et al. Beta-sitosterols for benign prostatic hyperplasia. Cochrane Database Syst Rev 2000;(2):CD001043.

Electroresection and Open Surgery

David D. Thiel, MD, Steven P. Petrou, MD*

KEYWORDS

- Transurethral resection of prostate • Prostatic hyperplasia
- Prostatectomy • Urinary retention
- Lower urinary tract symptoms • Robotic surgery

Transurethral resection of the prostate (TURP) is the historical gold standard therapy for lower urinary tract symptoms secondary to obstruction from benign prostatic hyperplasia (BPH). Over the last 15 years, medical therapy (alpha blockers and 5-alpha-reductase inhibitors) and the advent of office-based prostatic ablation for BPH have altered the treatment landscape of men suffering from lower urinary tract symptoms. Efficacy and morbidity of newer minimally invasive surgical therapies (MIST) are often compared with traditional TURP data from the 1960s and 1970s. Technologic improvements in lighting, resectoscope design, lens crafting, anesthetic care, and surgical technique have dramatically improved the efficacy, morbidity, and mortality of the modern TURP. This review outlines the indications, technique, and outcome data of the modern TURP and its variant, the saline bipolar TURP. Current indications and outcomes of simple prostatectomy (open, laparoscopic, and robotic) are also reviewed.

CURRENT USE OF TRANSURETHRAL RESECTION OF THE PROSTATE

In the decade of the 1980s, TURP was the most common operation in the Medicare population after cataract surgery.[1] TURP rates decreased in the 1990s from between 229.2 to 268.3 procedures per 100,000 population (1980–1991) to 131.3 per 100,000 in 1994.[1] This 50% decrease in TURP procedures did not likely represent a decreased prevalence of BPH but rather an increased use of medical treatments and MIST

procedures (eg, laser, microwave).[2] Following a 10-year decrease in the number of BPH procedures, the total number of BPH procedures in Medicare patients increased 44% from 88,868 in 1999 to 127,786 in 2005.[3] The number of MIST procedures for BPH increased 529% during this time.[3] In fact, by 2005, TURP represented only 39% of all BPH procedures compared with 81% in 1999. A 2005 survey of a cohort of urologists demonstrated that 59% said they offer both MIST and TURP. Ten percent of urologists polled would offer only MIST while 29% would only offer TURP.[4] Multiple forces, including economic, may have driven this trend toward increased MIST usage over TURP, but there has been no clear evidence that MIST is more efficacious or cost-effective than traditional TURP.

INDICATIONS FOR TRANSURETHRAL RESECTION OF THE PROSTATE

The traditional absolute indications for TURP were acute urinary retention, bladder stones, postrenal azotemia secondary to bladder outlet obstruction, and intractable gross hematuria from an enlarged adenoma.[5] The clinical literature and the Medical Therapy of Prostate Symptoms Study demonstrated the success of alpha blockers and 5-alpha-reductase inhibitors for improving urinary symptoms and preventing clinical progression of BPH.[6] The above medications, microwave therapy, and interstitial laser therapy have all been used successfully in patients with acute urinary retention.[7,8] Hematuria secondary to BPH has been successfully managed with the

Disclosures: Dr Thiel, none; Dr Petrou, Contura Inc, study participant. Financial support: none.
Department of Urology, Mayo Medical School, Mayo Clinic Florida, San Pablo Road, Jacksonville, FL 32224, USA
* Corresponding author.
E-mail address: petrou.Steven@mayo.edu (S.P. Petrou).

Urol Clin N Am 36 (2009) 461–470
doi:10.1016/j.ucl.2009.08.001
0094-0143/09/$ – see front matter © 2009 Elsevier Inc. All rights reserved.

urologic.theclinics.com

5-alpha-reductase inhibitor finasteride.[9] Even acute urinary retention has been managed successfully with alpha blockers.[10] The modern-day indications for TURP have not changed. However, it would seem that the operation is reserved for those indications for which medical therapy has failed. One could even argue that TURP is reserved for cases in which not only has medical therapy failed for the above indications, but at least one attempt at office-based MIST has also failed. A 2004 retrospective case-note analysis of TURP in 1990 compared with TURP in 2000 in the United Kingdom noted an increase in patients undergoing TURP for urinary retention in the 2000 group (33% to 58%).[11] The same study also noted lower urinary tract symptoms as an indication for TURP fell from 65% to 42% in the year 2000. A comprehensive review of 15 international guidelines for the treatment of BPH listed the indications for TURP that ranged from "complicated BPH," "moderate to severe symptoms," International Prostate Symptom Scores of 20 to 35, or any of the "absolute indications" listed above.[12]

PREOPERATIVE EVALUATION OF TRANSURETHRAL RESECTION OF THE PROSTATE

All patients should be suitable candidates for general anesthesia. Particular vigilance should be paid to the patient's cardiac status. A recent analysis of Australian postoperative deaths over a 3-year period demonstrated that the largest number of deaths after surgery was among patients having TURP.[13] Although the death rate was only 0.05% (9 of 17,044 patients), most of the deaths were secondary to acute myocardial infarction.[13] We do not require formal upper tract imaging before standard TURP. A bowel preparation is not used. A single perioperative dose of cephalosporin antibiotic decreases the perioperative TURP infection rate.[14] We typically use antibiotics until the Foley catheter is removed. It is necessary to select an anesthesiologist who is aware of the unique situations TURP can present both intraoperatively and in the perioperative period. Spinal anesthesia is the most frequently employed anesthetic for TURP in the United States.[15] Blood loss is reduced in TURP with regional anesthesia compared with general anesthesia. More importantly, the signs of water intoxication should be more readily recognized and abdominal/shoulder pain may signify inadvertent bladder perforation.[15]

MODERN TRANSURETHRAL RESECTION OF THE PROSTATE TECHNIQUE

The standard TURP technique has not changed. The patient is placed in dorsal lithotomy position with his buttocks near the end of the table. After a sterile preparation, the urethra is dilated with sounds to one size larger than the resectoscope sheath. To prevent false passages from over-zealous dilation, we usually only dilate the anterior urethra and then pass the scope through the prostatic urethra under direct vision. Lack of attention at this initial step may lead to an inadvertent anterior or posterior false passage (**Fig. 1**). The basic resection technique may vary according to the size or configuration of the prostate but should be based on an orderly plan. Some advocate resecting ventral tissue first so that the adenomatous tissue drops down, allowing the surgeon to resect from the top downward rather than from the floor upward. However, some surgeons have suggested resecting the floor tissue initially to improve water flow during the resection (**Fig. 2**).[16] When dissecting around the floor of the prostate, care should be taken not to undermine the bladder neck. If possible, avoid angling the resectoscope downwards to prevent inadvertent undermining of the bladder neck. Resection should continue to the capsule. A trough should be resected that identifies capsule and all other resection planes on that level. No resection should take place distal to the veromontanum and the ureteral orifices should be identified and not violated.

Numerous irrigating fluids are available to the urologist performing TURP. Because of the dangers of using water (absorption leads to hemolysis, shock, and renal failure), most urologists today use nonhemolytic irrigating solutions, such as 1.5% glycine, 3% sorbitol, or 3% mannitol.[16] These solutions are inexpensive and maintain a degree of the transparency of water. It should be noted that these solutions are not isotonic but merely nonhemolytic and can have some deleterious effects if excessive amounts are absorbed.[15]

Transurethral resection syndrome is characterized by hypertension, bradycardia, visual disturbances, mental confusion, and nausea.[17] Untreated transurethral resection syndrome can have serious consequences, such as cerebral or bronchial edema.[17] If capsular perforation is suspected, the procedure should be terminated. Serum sodium measurements should be monitored frequently and corrected as needed. Generous use of furosemide intravenously corrects sodium levels.[16] We routinely give 20 mg intravenous furosemide following large resections or suspected capsular perforation. Infusion of hypertonic sodium chloride may be needed in certain instances but should be used carefully.[16]

Various attempts have been made to improve the modern TURP technique by altering

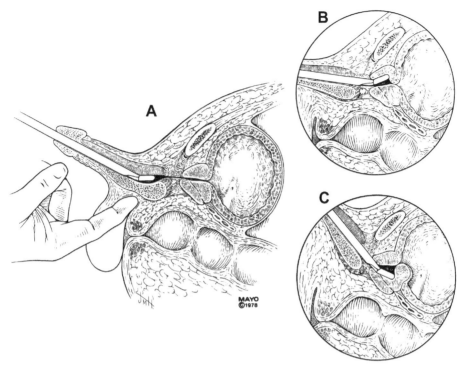

Fig. 1. Passage of resectoscope sheath into the bladder. (*A*) The resectoscope sheath is passed into the urethra. (*B*) At the level of the veromontanum, the scope must take a sharp angle upward to enter the bladder. (*C*) Failure to make the appropriate upward turn can lead to significant false-passage formation. (*From* Mayo Clinic Florida, Jacksonville, Florida; with permission.)

instrumentation. Most changes have focused on improving hemostasis to provide superior intraoperative visualization and thereby safety. Numerous changes in resection loop thickness and shape as well as roller balls with various surface areas have all been used to improve hemostasis and visualization.[18,19] As stated by Issa,[18] irrespective of the shape, thickness, and configuration of TURP loops, hemostasis is determined by the balance of wattage, power, voltage, surface contact, and exposure time to tissue. Excellent results may be achieved with cutting energy of 100 W set to medium "blend" with 30 W of coagulation power. Slowing down the resection through tissue provides longer exposure time and surface contact to improve hemostasis.

It was initially thought that transurethral vaporization of prostate tissue was as effective as TURP while providing the benefit of decreased blood loss that is inherent to techniques that do not actually resect tissue.[20–22] However, despite its introduction in the mid-1990s, there is a dearth of long-term studies with transurethral vaporization of prostate tissue, so its long-term efficacy is not well documented. Most investigators agree that the technique has limited use for intravesical extension of tissue near the apex.[19,20,23]

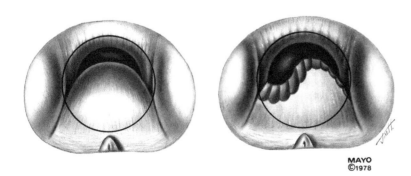

Fig. 2. (*Left*) Before resection. (*Right*) After resection. Transurethral resection of prostate floor. In cases with elevated median lobes, the floor of the prostate is often resected first. This improves water flow during the procedure. Care must be taken not to undermine the bladder neck during this step. (*From* Mayo Clinic Florida, Jacksonville, Florida; with permission.)

EFFICACY OF MODERN TRANSURETHRAL RESECTION OF THE PROSTATE

TURP is the only transurethral procedure for BPH that has durable follow-up in the literature ranging from 8 to 22 years.[24] Wasson and colleagues[25] noted the 5-year reoperation rate after TURP to be approximately 5% in a review of 188,161 Medicare beneficiaries. Nationwide analysis of 20,671 men undergoing TURP in Austria noted the incidence of secondary TURP to be 5.8% at 5 years and 7.4% at 8 years.[26] A study of 577 patients with 10-year follow-up revealed a 6% incidence of re-resection.[27] The studies demonstrate the long-term efficacy of TURP. What is not defined is whether these repeat resections are required because of tissue regrowth or because of inadequate initial resection. What is also not defined is how many patients with recurrent symptoms after TURP forgo repeat operation in favor of adjuvant medical therapy.

Madersbacher and colleagues[28] analyzed 29 randomized controlled trials comparing TURP to less-invasive procedures. The mean decrease in urinary symptom scores after TURP in the 29 studies was 70.6%. Symptom scores decreased by half in 58% of the patients. The same investigators also noted that the mean increase in maximum flow in the TURP groups was 125%. The analysis of the randomized trials also noted that 93% of patients following TURP have a maximum flow greater than 15 mL/s, suggesting an absence of bladder-outlet obstruction in a majority of patients. A United Kingdom urodynamic study from 2005 evaluated 217 patients a mean 13.0 years following TURP. They noted a sustained improvement in a majority of urodynamic parameters over the follow-up period.[29] Long-term symptomatic failure and decreased flow rate were associated with detrusor underactivity as opposed to repeat obstruction. A meta-analysis compared urodynamic efficacy on various forms of bladder-outlet obstruction therapies and found TURP to be better than all modalities except open prostatectomy.[30] It should be noted that most urodynamic measurements improve after surgery but they often do not correlate with lower urinary tract symptoms as measured by symptom scores.[31]

O'Sullivan and colleagues[32] demonstrated that, in addition to improvement in American Urology Association score, patients undergoing TURP had improvement in quality-of-life indices, depression rating scales, and pain indices at 1 month and 3 months postoperatively compared with preoperatively. Although the importance of quality of life and patient satisfaction are acknowledged, long-term data of these measures following bladder-outlet surgery are rare. A 2008 prospective cohort study of 280 consecutive patients following TURP in the years 1993 and 1994 were noted to have consistent and statistically significant improvement in urinary bother and quality of life at 6 months, 6 years, and 12 years of follow-up.[33] At 6 months, 6 years, and 12 years following treatment, 8.4%, 20.8%, and 13.3%, respectively, were truly dissatisfied with their outcome following TURP.

MORBIDITY/MORTALITY OF MODERN TRANSURETHRAL RESECTION OF THE PROSTATE

Improved antibiotics, perioperative care, and instrumentation have greatly improved the mortality/morbidity of the modern TURP. A 2008 prospective evaluation of 10,654 TURPs performed in the years 2002 and 2003 revealed a 0.10% mortality rate, a 2.9% blood transfusion rate, and a 1.4% risk of transurethral resection syndrome.[34] The overall morbidity in the study was 11.1% with urinary retention (5.8%) and urinary tract infection (3.6%) being the most common complications. Mebust and colleagues[35] noted a mortality rate of 0.2% in 3885 patients undergoing TURP. The investigators correlated postoperative morbidity with resection time over 90 minutes, gland size over 45 g, acute urinary retention, and age over 80 years. Both of these studies provide insight into the improved morbidity and mortality rates seen with TURP in the 1960s and 1970s.[36,37] The published mortality rates were 1.3% to 2.5% in those earlier experiences. Myocardial infarction and septic complications were more prevalent in the earlier studies compared with the modern experience listed above. What is also becoming clear is that mortality and morbidity of the modern TURP have improved even though patients currently getting TURP are older and have more medical comorbidities than those in earlier TURP studies.[25]

A comparison of TURP over 17 years at a single center revealed a significant decrease in mortality (0.5% to 0%), transfusion rates (20.3% to 3.8%), and postoperative urinary tract infections (37.1% to 6.2%) in TURPs performed from 1997 to 2004 versus those performed from 1987 to 1997.[38] Examination of 577 patients 10 years following TURP demonstrated reoperation for bladder neck contracture to be 2.4% and for urethral stricture to be 1.9%.[27] The data from most cohort studies do suggest that patient morbidity decreases with increased urologist caseload volume although the most recent studies examining caseload volumes and TURP are not consistent with the definition of high-volume surgeons.[25,39] One study notes improved outcomes with high-volume surgeons (more than 55 cases annually), while the earlier study[25] defines improved outcomes with surgeon volume over 29 cases per year. Incontinence following TURP for benign conditions has a noted incidence in the literature of 1% to 5%.[40] Improved visualization of the modern TURP may limit accidental resection distal to the urethral sphincter and thereby decrease incontinence. Consequently, most surgeons today find urinary incontinence following TURP in the obstructed patient to be a rare event. Obstructed patients undergoing TURP following brachytherapy or radiation are at a much higher risk of urinary incontinence than the general population.[41] Kollmeier and colleagues[41] noted an 18% post-TURP incontinence rate in 38 patients following brachytherapy. The investigators noted that the incontinence rate increased if the procedure was performed more than 2 years following seed implantation.

Systematic reviews note that approximately 75% of patients experience retrograde ejaculation following TURP.[5,16,42,43] Given the current medical-legal environment, it is highly prudent to clearly alert any patient undergoing an outlet procedure, especially TURP, of the high risk of retrograde ejaculation and the consequences for fertility and sexual functioning. Most studies dealing with sexual dysfunction following TURP lack a standard definition of sexual dysfunction. The most recent study examining erectile dysfunction following TURP concluded that the incidence of newly reported erectile dysfunction following TURP was 12% in 629 TURP procedures at 6-month follow-up.[42] The investigators found that diabetes mellitus and observed intraoperative capsular perforation were statistical predictors of postoperative erectile dysfunction. The study is notable for using the validated International Index of Erectile Function Instrument (IEFF-5) to measure erectile dysfunction following TURP. A 2007 study of 1014 patients following TURP in Switzerland between January 2000 and January 2005 noted that 3 of 4 patients undergoing TURP remain sexually active and the surgery itself had no influence on this ratio.[44]

SALINE TRANSURETHRAL RESECTION OF THE PROSTATE

The Achilles heal of the standard monopolar TURP is the requirement of hypotonic irrigating solutions that carry the risk of dilutional hyponatremia and transurethral resection syndrome. Bipolar TURP was developed to allow the operation to be performed in a normal saline environment and theoretically allow for longer and safer resection.[18] The traditional monopolar TURP uses an active electrode loop to transmit energy into tissue and a return electrode at the skin to complete the circuit.[18,45] The energy must travel through the body to complete the circuit. The electrical resistance creates temperatures as high as 400°C.[46] Bipolar technology allows high initializing voltage to establish a voltage gradient in the gap between two electrodes.[45] In essence, the active and return poles are incorporated into the electrode design.[18] This energy converts the conductive medium (saline) into a plasma field of highly ionized particles. This field disrupts the molecular bonds between the tissues. This allows the high-temperature loop to provide rapid vaporization and desiccation of prostate tissue and result in a "cut and seal" effect.[46] Since these charge ions have only a short penetration of 50 to 100 μm, there should be less collateral thermal damage to the surrounding tissue and less tissue char.[45]

Five types of bipolar resection devices appear in the medical literature.[46,47] The PlasmaKinetic system (Gyrus-ACMI, Southborough, Massachusetts) was the first true bipolar TURP system. Karl Storz, Wolf, Olympus, and ACMI all offer similar bipolar resection devices.[47] Depending on the system used, the resectoscope loop can be used with 25F to 27F sheaths.[46,47] Issa[18] performed a meta-analysis on 12 randomized controlled trials of saline TURP compared with traditional TURP. The four outcome parameters of American Urologic Association symptom score, quality-of-life scores, peak urinary flow rate, and postvoid residual urine volume were all evaluated. The meta-analysis showed similar efficacy between monopolar TURP and saline bipolar TURP. The same meta-analysis demonstrated overall adverse events to be lower with bipolar TURP compared with monopolar TURP (28.6% versus 15.5%). Although not statistically significant, there was a lower transfusion rate, less hyponatremia, and lower transurethral resection syndrome in bipolar group. There was a slight decrease in urethral stricture rates in the bipolar group (1.6% versus 2.7%).

Several surgeons note that the sharper, smoother, "cut and seal" mechanism of the bipolar TURP shortens resection times. A prospective randomized trial of bipolar TURP versus monopolar TURP on prostates of similar size (40 mL) demonstrated the mean operative time to be 36 minutes for the bipolar system compared with 57 minutes for the monopolar system ($P<.001$).[48] The saline irrigation used during bipolar TURP has led to a much less significant drop in serum sodium level compared with monopolar TURP.[49] However, there is a randomized controlled trial that does show a significant decrease in postoperative sodium with the bipolar device while the monopolar device had no change.[46,50] The reason for this decrease is unclear but it does call into question the predictions by some that bipolar saline systems may forever solve the problem of dilutional hyponatremia.[51] However, to date no reports have appeared about any case of clinically significant transurethral resection syndrome with saline bipolar TURP.

The average number of TURPs performed by graduating chief residents in the early 1990s was 120.[52] In 2006, graduating chief residents performed a mean of 61.6 TURPs by graduation.[18,53] This decrease in surgical cases performed by graduating residents has raised the question of training proficiency for TURP in the modern urology residency. The bipolar TURP allows for longer resection times without the risk of hyponatremia and transurethral resection syndrome. Issa[18] also proposed that the slower pace of resection is also more comfortable for the resident in training and will only enhance resident training in the future. The advantages of saline TURP has also allowed safe resection of very large glands without the large risk of dilutional hyponatremia and copious bleeding. Finley and colleagues[54] reported on the safe resection of three patients with preoperative gland size over 160 cm^3. The mean resection time was 163 minutes and average resection weight was 80.8 g. The mean change in hemoglobin was 2.1 g/dL and the mean serum sodium change was 3.3 mEq/L. The mean hospital stay was 12 hours. The investigators proposed saline bipolar TURP as a safe alternative to open simple prostatectomy in patients with extremely large adenomas.

OPEN SIMPLE PROSTATECTOMY

Open prostatectomy remains the procedure of choice at most centers for the majority of patients with very large prostates.[16,55] Although it was traditionally thought that glands over 100 g were best managed with open prostatectomy as opposed to TURP, this upper limit is often challenged by some resectionists. Open prostatectomy holds appeal in dealing with large glands with associated pathology and need of correction synchronously (bladder calculi, bladder diverticulum, large intravesical median lobes). Open simple prostatectomy is also potentially more beneficial than TURP in large glands that have associated urethral strictures, ankylosing spondylitis preventing hip flexion, and concurrent inguinal hernia.[56] The choice of whether to perform the operation in a retropubic or suprapubic (transvesical) manner remains controversial and depends on surgeon training or comfort. The suprapubic approach is preferred by most if there is an extremely large median lobe, concomitant bladder stones, or a bladder diverticulum requiring repair.[16] Unfortunately there is a paucity of contemporary Western literature pertaining to open simple prostatectomy. Most references to open simple prostatectomy refer to old Western series or contemporary experience from developing nations lacking access to modern TURP technology.[57]

Our technique for suprapubic prostatectomy consists of placing the patient in the dorsal lithotomy position on a slightly tilted Trendelenburg. A 22F catheter is placed in the bladder and 20 mL of fluid is placed in the balloon. A midline incision is made from below the umbilicus to the pubic bone. The extraperitoneal prevesical space is developed and a retractor placed. The bladder is distended with normal saline through the indwelling catheter and a midline cystotomy is made. The incision is carried down to the bladder neck region but care must be taken not to extend the incision too cephalad so that the bladder can later be retracted easily with the self-retaining retractor. Moist sponges are placed in the dome of the bladder and the self-retaining retractor is configured to hold the bladder open in a method to optimize exposure. Consideration can be given to placing 5F localization stents in the ureteral orifices to accentuate identification and exposure, especially if there is a large intravesical component.

A circular incision is made in the bladder mucosa distal to the trigone region. A plane is created between the adenoma and the prostate capsule at the 6-o'clock position. Blunt dissection is performed to enucleate the adenoma after the surgical plane has been initially developed sharply. The apical prostatic urethra is transected by placing the index finger at the apex of the prostate and retracting the adenoma posteriorly (**Fig. 3**). To avoid injuring the sphincter complex, care is taken not to apply excessive retraction on the apex. The adenoma is removed and hemostasis secured. If notable bleeding is encountered from the floor of the capsule, absorbable suture ligatures may be applied in a step-wise fashion. Use 2-0 Vicryl sutures to advance the bladder mucosa to the prostatic urethra at the 5- and 7-o'clock position and thus retrigonalize the bladder neck. A 22F three-channel irrigation catheter is placed in the urethra and a 24F suprapubic tube is passed through the lateral aspect of the dome of bladder.

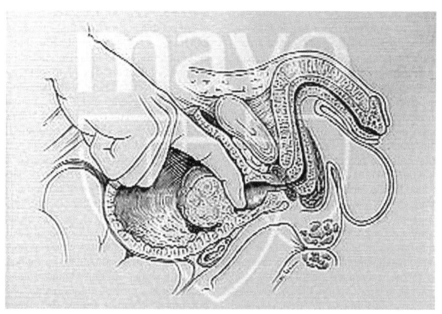

Fig. 3. Apical dissection during suprapubic prostatectomy. The apex of the prostate is dissected during suprapubic prostatectomy by placing the index finger at the apex of the prostate and retracting the adenoma posteriorly. This will expose the apex of prostate to be cut sharply. (*From* Mayo Clinic Florida, Jacksonville, Florida; with permission.)

The cystotomy is closed in two or three separate layers using absorbable sutures. The completed repair is tested with fluid to confirm a watertight closure. Though some would debate the need for the suprapubic tube, the authors have found it useful because continuous bladder irrigation may be accommodated by one catheter with drainage through the second. The suprapubic tube is removed in 3 days with the urethral catheter removed in 7 days.

Some steps used with prostates of impressive proportions have included placing a silk stitch through the eye of the initial catheter after completing the opening cystotomy. After the enucleation is completed and the initial catheter is withdrawn, the silk suture may be applied to the final catheter to ensure an effortless passage into the bladder through a potentially cavernous space. In addition, if worrisome apical bleeding is encountered after the enucleation is completed, a gel foam pack may be created by folding the material on itself numerous times and passing the catheter through an iatrogenic hole in the gel foam and then expanding the balloon and applying traction to the catheter. The pack will now rest nicely in the deep, difficult-to-visualize space with the gel foam resting in an occlusive and hemostatic position. In many cases, the catheter balloon may be inflated to up to 100 mL to increase

hemostatic occlusion when traction is applied. However, care should be taken to deflate the balloon somewhat the next morning.

The Sicilian-Calabrian Society of Urology reviewed 1804 open simple prostatectomies performed for BPH in 1997 and 1998.[57] This large contemporary series noted that only 11.2 % of cases were performed in a retropubic manner. There was 1 death noted (0.05%). Investigators found that 8.2% of patients required blood transfusion and 1.1% of patients required surgical reintervention (usually for clot retention). Also, 2.1% of patients had a postoperative bladder neck contracture, 1.2 % had significant urinary incontinence postoperatively, and 3.6% of patients required a second BPH intervention at some point postoperatively. This large review provides excellent insight into the expected morbidity associated with open simple prostatectomy performed in a contemporary setting.

LAPAROSCOPIC AND ROBOTIC SIMPLE PROSTATECTOMY

Most traditional urologic procedures can now be performed laparoscopically. Mariano[58] described the first laparoscopic simple prostatectomy in 2002. Numerous reports have described laparoscopic simple prostatectomy performed both in an intraperitoneal and extraperitoneal fashion.[56,59–63] McCullough and colleagues[56] compared 96 extraperitoneal laparoscopic prostatectomies performed with a transcapsular incision to 184 open transvesical open simple prostatectomies. The operating time was significantly longer in the laparoscopic group (95.1 ± 32.9 minutes) than the open group (54.7 ± 19.7 minutes). The laparoscopic group required fewer hospital days and less total catheter time. However, there was no difference between the groups with regards to estimated blood loss and continuous bladder irrigation time. Only 1 patient in the laparoscopy group developed a postoperative urinary tract infection compared with 18 (9.8%) in the open group despite using similar perioperative antibiotic regimens. The investigators attributed this low rate of infection to the decreased hospital time and catheter time in the laparoscopic group. A similar comparison was performed by Baumert and colleagues[59] in 2006 (30 laparoscopic simple prostatectomies versus 30 open simple prostatectomies), which also noted a statistically significant decrease in catheter time and hospital stay in the laparoscopic group at the expense of longer operative times and no difference in blood loss.

Investigators of laparoscopic simple prostatectomy series comment on the advanced nature of the procedure and the requirement of expert-level laparoscopic skills. Investigators have noted that approaching the prostate via a transverse cystotomy just proximal to the junction of the bladder and prostate leads to less blood loss than an approach involving a vertical incision over the prostate.[56,59,60] McCullough and colleagues[56] now place an index finger through the 12-mm umbilical port to complete much of the adenomectomy manually in a hybrid fashion (ie, "finger assisted"). They note that this may offset some of the disadvantages of the lack of tactile dissection associated with laparoscopic simple prostatectomy. Sotelo and colleagues[60] believe the most significant advantage of laparoscopic simple prostatectomy is the ability to precisely transect the adenoma at the apex while maintaining the integrity of the sphincter at the membranous urethra.

In 2008, the Cleveland Clinic group reported their initial experience with single-port transvesical simple prostatectomy.[64] A single-port access device was placed intravesically and the bladder inflated with carbon dioxide. The entire dissection was completed intravesically. Three surgeries were completed with a gradual reduction in operating room time from 6 hours to 1.5 hours noted with increasing experience. There was one inadvertent enterotomy reported. Blood loss and outcomes were not reported. The one possible benefit of this approach is that intravesical insufflation may provide a tamponade that decreases intraoperative blood loss. Robotic simple prostatectomy has been described with a technique similar to that used in laparoscopic simple prostatectomy.[65] Seven cases were completed with mean estimated blood loss of 382 mL and hospital stay of 1.33 days. The mean operating room time was 195 minutes. No outcome data was reported. What is absent from an abundance of the laparoscopic simple prostatectomy literature is a comparison of functional outcomes (eg, continence, flow) to those after standard open prostatectomy. It is clear that the use of laparoscopic and robotic technology for patients with BPH and large glands is on the rise. Good comparative trials are needed to ensure that the marked increase cost and longer operative times required for these procedures provide equivalent or improved outcomes to open simple prostatectomy with a demonstrated benefit in convalescence and no deleterious consequences.

SUMMARY

Improvements in instrumentation, surgical technique, irrigation fluids, antibiotics, and anesthesia have made the modern TURP a safe and efficacious operation. Newer MIST procedure data need to be compared with modern TURP data with regards to efficacy and morbidity. Simple prostatectomy still has a role in certain instances and also appears to be safe and efficacious in modern settings. It remains to be seen if laparoscopy and robot-assisted applications will provide a benefit in simple prostatectomy.

REFERENCES

1. Wei JT, Calhoun E, Jacobsen SJ. Urologic diseases in America project: benign prostatic hyperplasia. J Urol 2005;173:1256–61.
2. Xia Z, Roberts RO, Schottenfeld D, et al. Trends in prostatectomy for benign prostatic hyperplasia among black and white men in the United States: 1980 to 1994. Urology 1999;53:1154–9.
3. Yu X, Elliott SP, Wilt TJ, et al. Practice patterns in benign prostatic hyperplasia surgical therapy: the dramatic increase in minimally invasive technologies. J Urol 2008;180:241–5.
4. Ercole B, Lee C, Best S, et al. Minimally invasive therapy of benign prostatic hyperplasia: practice patterns in Minnesota. J Endourol 2005;19(2): 159–62.

5. Nudell DM, Cattolica EV. Transurethral prostatectomy: an update. AUA update series. 2000; Lesson 5 vol. XIX.

6. McConnell JD, Roehrborn CG, Buatista OM, et al. The long-term effect of doxazosin, finasteride, and combination therapy on the clinical progression of benign prostatic hyperplasia. N Engl J Med 2003; 349:2387–98.

7. Berger AP, Niescher M, Spranger M, et al. Transurethral microwave therapy (TUMT) with the Targis System: a single-centre study on 78 patients with acute urinary retention and poor general health. Eur Urol 2003;42(2):176–80.

8. Nishizawa K, Kobayashi T, Wantanabe J, et al. Iterstitial laser therapy of the prostate for management of acute urinary retention. J Urol 2003;170(3):879–82.

9. Donohue JF, Hayne D, Kornik U, et al. Randomized, placebo-controlled trial showing that finasteride reduces prostatic vascularity rapidly within 2 weeks. BJU Int 2005;96(9):1319–22.

10. Lucas MG, Stephenson TP, Narqund V. Tamsulosin in the management of patients in acute urinary retention from benign prostatic hyperplasia. BJU Int 2005;95(3):354–7.

11. Wilson JR, Urwin GH, Stower MJ. The changing practice of transurethral prostatectomy: a comparison of cases performed in 1990 and 2000. Ann R Coll Surg Engl 2004;86:428–31.

12. Roehrborn CG, Bartsch G, Kirby R, et al. Guidelines for the diagnosis and treatment of benign prostatic hyperplasia: a comparative, international overview. Urology 2001;58:642–50.

13. Gyomber D, Lawrentschuk N, Ranson DL, et al. An analysis of deaths related to urologic surgery, reviewed by the state coroner: a case for cardiac vigilance before transurethral prostatectomy. BJU Int 2006;97:758–61.

14. Nielsen OS, Maigaard S, Frimodt-Moller N, et al. Prophylactic antibiotics in transurethral prostatectomy. J Urol 1981;126(1):60–2.

15. Malhotra V. Transurethral resection of the prostate. Anesthesiol Clin North America 2000;18(4):883–97.

16. Fitzpatrick JM. Minimally invasive and endoscopic management of benign prostatic hyperplasia. In: Wein AJ, Kavoussi LR, Nocick AC, editors. Campbell-Walsh urology. 9th edition. Philadelphia: Saunders Elsevier; 2007. Chapter 88.

17. Rassweiler J, Teber D, Kuntz R, et al. Complications of transurethral resection of the prostate (TURP)—incidence, management, and prevention. Eur Urol 2006;50:969–80.

18. Issa MM. Technological advances in transurethral resection of the prostate: bipolar versus monopolar TURP. J Endourol 2008;22(8):1587–95.

19. Barba M, Leyh H, Hartung R. New technologies in transurethral resection of the prostate. Curr Opin Urol 2000;10:9–14.

20. Gallucci M, Puppo P, Perachino M, et al. Transurethral electrovaporization of the prostate vs. transurethral resection—results of a mulitcentre, randomized clinical study on 150 patients. Eur Urol 1998;33:359–64.

21. Cetinkaya M, Ulusoy E, Adsan O, et al. Comparative early results of transurethral electoresection and transurethral electrovaporization in benign hyperplasia. Br J Urol 1996;78:901–3.

22. Hammadeh MY, Madann S, Singh M, et al. Two-year follow-up of a prospective randomized trial of electrovaporization versus resection of prostate. Eur Urol 1998;34:188–92.

23. Weiner DM, Kaplan SA. Electrosurgery: VaporTrode. Eur Urol 1999;35:166–72.

24. Reich O, Gratzke C, Stief CG. Techniques and long-term results of surgical procedures for BPH. Eur Urol 2006;49:970–8.

25. Wasson JH, Bubolz TA, Lu-Yao GL, et al. Transurethral resection of the prostate among Medicare beneficiaries: 1984 to 1997. J Urol 2000;164: 1212–5.

26. Madersbacher S, Lackner J, Brossner C, et al. Reoperation, myocardial infarction and mortality after transurethral and open prostatectomy: a nationwide, long-term analysis of 23,123 cases. Eur Urol 2005;47:499–504.

27. Varkarakis J, Bartsch G, Horninger W. Long-term morbidity and mortality of transurethral prostatectomy: a 10-year follow-up. Prostate 2004;58:248–51.

28. Madersbacher S, Marberger M. Is transurethral resection of the prostate still justified? BJU Int 1999;83:227–37.

29. Thomas AW, Cannon A, Bartlett E, et al. The natural history of lower urinary tract dysfunction in men: minimum 10-year urodynamic followup of transurethral resection of prostate for bladder outlet obstruction. J Urol 2005;174:1887–91.

30. Bosch JLHR. Urodynamic effects of various treatment modalities for benign prostatic hyperplasia. J Urol 1997;158:2034–44.

31. Hakenberg OW, Pinnock CB, Marshall VR. Preoperative urodynamic and symptom evaluation of patients undergoing transurethral prostatectomy: analysis of variables relevant for outcome. BJU Int 2003;91:375–9.

32. O'Sullivan MJ, Murphy C, Deasy C, et al. Effects of transurethral resection of prostate on the quality of life of patients with benign prostatic hyperplasia. J Am Coll Surg 2004;198:394–403.

33. Mishriki SF, Grimsley SJS, Nabi G, et al. Improved quality of life and enhanced satisfaction after TURP: prospective 12-year follow-up study. Urology 2008;72:322–8.

34. Reich O, Gratzke C, Bachman A, et al. Morbidity, mortality and early outcome of transurethral resection of the prostate: a prospective multicenter evaluation of 10,654 patients. J Urol 2008;180:246–9.

35. Mebust WK, Holtgrewe HL, Cockett ATK, et al. Writing Committee. Transurethral prostatectomy: immediate and postoperative complications cooperative study of 13 participating institutions evaluating 3,885 patients. J Urol 1989;141:243–7.

36. Holtgrewe HL, Valk WL. Factors influencing the mortality and morbidity of transurethral prostatectomy: a study of 2,015 cases. J Urol 1962;87: 450–9.

37. Melchior J, Valk W, Foret JD, et al. Transurethral prostatectomy: computerized analysis of 2,223 consecutive cases. J Urol 1974;112:634–42.

38. Wendt-Nordahl G, Bucher B, Hacker A, et al. Improvement in mortality and morbidity in transurethral resection of the prostate over 17 years in a single center. J Endourol 2007;21(9):1081–7.

39. Chen YK, Lin HC. Association between urologists' caseload volume and in-hospital mortality for transurethral resection of prostate: a nationwide population-based study. Urology 2008;72:329–35.

40. Foote J, Yun S, Leach GE. Postprostatectomy incontinence. Pathophysiology, evaluation, and management. Urol Clin North Am 1991;18:229–41.

41. Kollmeier MA, Stock RG, Cesaretti J, et al. Urinary morbidity and incontinence following transurethral resection of the prostate after brachytherapy. J Urol 2005;173:808–12.

42. Poulakis V, Ferakis N, Witzsch U, et al. Erectile dysfunction after transurethral prostatectomy for lower urinary tract symptoms: results from a center with over 500 patients. Asian J Androl 2006;8(1): 69–74.

43. US Department of Health and Human Services. Benign prostatic hyperplasia: diagnosis and treatment. Bethesda (MD): Agency for Health Care Policy and Research; 1994.

44. Muntener M, Aellig S, Kuettel R, et al. Sexual function after transurethral resection of the prostate (TURP): results of an independent prospective multicentre assessment of outcome. Eur Urol 2007;52: 510–6.

45. Smith D, Khoubehi B, Patel A. Bipolar electrosurgery for benign prostatic hyperplasia: transurethral electrovaporization and resection of the prostate. Curr Opin Urol 2005;15:95–100.

46. Ho HSS, Cheng CWS. Bipolar transurethral resection of prostate: a new reference standard? Curr Opin Urol 2008;18:50–5.

47. Rassweiller J, Schlze M, Stock C, et al. Bipolar transurethral resection of the prostate—technical modifications and early clinical experience. Minim Invasive Ther Allied Technol 2007;16:11–21.

48. Erturhan S, Erbagci A, Seckiner L, et al. Plasmakinetic resection of the prostate versus standard transurethral resection of the prostate: a prospective randomized trial with a 1 year follow-up. Prostate Cancer Prostatic Dis 2007;10:97–100.

49. Singh H, Desai MR, Shrivastav P, et al. Bipolar versus monopolar transurethral resection of prostate: randomized controlled study. J Endourol 2005;19:333–8.

50. Yang S, Lin WC, Chang HK, et al. Gyrus Plasmasect: is it better than monopolar transurethral resection of the prostate? Urol Int 2004;73:258–61.

51. Issa MM, Young MR, Bullock AR, et al. Dilutional hyponatremia of TURP syndrome: a historical event in the 21st century. Urology 2004;64:298–301.

52. Accreditation Council for Graduate Medical Education. Urology residency case log report. Chicago: ACGME; 2004.

53. Resident National Data Summary Report 2005–2006. Residency Review Committee for Urology, American Board of Urology. ANA Residency Review Committee; 2005–2006

54. Finley DS, Beck S, Szabo RJ. Bipolar saline TURP for large prostate glands. ScientificWorldJournal 2007;7:1558–62.

55. AUA Practice Guidelines Committee. AUA guideline on management of benign prostatic hyperplasia (2003). Chapter 1: diagnosis and treatment recommendations. J Urol 2003;170:530–47.

56. McCullough TC, Heldwein FL, Soon SJ, et al. Laparoscopic versus open simple prostatectomy: an evaluation of morbidity. J Endourol 2009;23(1):129–33.

57. Serretta V, Morgia G, Fondacaro L, et al. Open prostatectomy for benign prostatic enlargement in southern Europe in the late 1990s: a contemporary series of 1800 interventions. Urology 2002;60:623–7.

58. Mariano MB, Graziottin TM, Tefilli MV. Laparoscopic prostatectomy with vascular control for benign prostatic hyperplasia. J Urol 2002;167:2528–9.

59. Baumert H, Ballaro A, Dugardin F, et al. Laparoscopic versus open simple prostatectomy: a comparative study. J Urol 2006;175:1691–4.

60. Sotelo R, Spaliviero M, Garcia-Segui A, et al. Laparoscopic retropubic simple prostatectomy. J Urol 2005;173:757–60.

61. Nadler RB, Blunt LW, User HM, et al. Preperitoneal laparoscopic simple prostatectomy. Urology 2004; 63:778–9.

62. Porpiglia F, Terrone C, Renard J, et al. Transcapsular adenomectomy (Millin): a comparative study, extraperitoneal laparoscopy versus open surgery. Eur Urol 2006;49:120–6.

63. Rehman J, Khan SA, Sukkarieh T, et al. Extraperitoneal laparoscopic prostatectomy (adenomectomy) for obstructing benign prosatatic hyperplasia transvesical and transcapsular (Millin) techniques. J Endourol 2005;19:491–6.

64. Desai MM, Aron M, Canes D, et al. Single-port transvesical simple prostatectomy: initial clinical report. Urology 2008;72:960–5.

65. Sotelo R, Clavijo R, Carmona O, et al. Robotic simple prostatectomy. J Urol 2008;179:513–5.

KTP/LBO Laser Vaporization of the Prostate

Matthew S. Wosnitzer, MD, Matthew P. Rutman, MD*

KEYWORDS

- BPH • GreenLight laser
- KTP laser • Vaporization • Minimally invasive

Laser-based treatments have been developed in the past 15 years as an alternative to transurethral resection of the prostate (TURP) for treatment of symptomatic benign prostatic hyperplasia (BPH). Increasing demand for a minimally invasive procedure to alleviate lower urinary tract symptoms (LUTS) with greater efficacy and fewer side effects has led to the introduction of various lasers, including photoselective vaporization of the prostate (PVP) using "GreenLight PV" KTP (potassium-titanyl-phosphate) laser, or most recently, the "GreenLight High Performance System (HPS)" LBO (lithium triborate) laser. Laser prostatectomies may be performed with coagulative lasers such as neodymium:yttrium-aluminium-garnet (Nd:YAG) and diode lasers, cutting lasers such as holmium:YAG, (Ho:YAG) and thulium:YAG (Tm:YAG), or vaporization lasers such as Nd:YAG, Ho:YAG, diode, KTP, and lithium triborate (LBO) lasers. The search for an ideal minimally invasive treatment option for BPH to reduce morbidity and expense is constantly evolving. Many earlier modalities using various delivery systems did not result in consistent and durable outcomes compared with the reference standard, TURP. Since its introduction in 1998 by Malek and colleagues, the excellent clinical outcomes, low morbidity, technical simplicity, and cost-effectiveness of GreenLight laser photoselective vaporization (American Medical Systems, Minnetonka, MN) have made this technology a valid and efficacious clinical alternative to TURP.

Most early data on laser treatment of BPH were based on an Nd:YAG laser using visual laser ablation of the prostate (VLAP), as initially introduced by Costello and colleagues.[1] Limitations included prolonged operative time because of the lack of a continuously emitting laser beam, significant dysuria, and extended postoperative catheterization time secondary to massive sloughing of necrotic tissue.[2] The key determinant of efficacy with laser vaporization is based on the interaction between the laser beam and target tissue. The laser energy (collimated coherent light emitted from an energized source at a single wavelength) can produce either coagulation, when tissue is heated to below the boiling/vaporization temperature but above that required to denature protein, or vaporization, in which the tissue is evaporated by being heated to above the vaporization/boiling temperature. The wavelength of Nd:YAG (1064 nm) is double the wavelength (532 nm) and half of the frequency of KTP or LBO lasers. The KTP and LBO lasers produce the same 532-nm light beam within the visible green region of the electromagnetic spectrum with different maximal average power (80 W vs 120 W, respectively).[3,4] Unlike the 1064 nm wavelength of the Nd:YAG laser, which is found within the infrared portion of the electromagnetic spectrum, the KTP or LBO lasers are selectively absorbed by hemoglobin within prostatic tissue, thus permitting photoselective vaporization and removal of prostatic tissue by rapid photothermal vaporization of heated intracellular water.[5] With a short optical penetration of 0.8 mm because of the shorter wavelength and absorption by hemoglobin, the resulting coagulation zone is limited to 1 to 2 mm, which leads to

Department of Urology, Columbia University College of Physicians and Surgeons, New York, NY 10032, USA
* Corresponding author.
E-mail address: mr2423@columbia.edu (M.P. Rutman).

Urol Clin N Am 36 (2009) 471–483
doi:10.1016/j.ucl.2009.08.004
0094-0143/09/$ – see front matter © 2009 Elsevier Inc. All rights reserved.

urologic.theclinics.com

a more focused and effective vaporization when compared with the 4 to 7 mm coagulation zone of Nd:YAG.[6] Unlike KTP or LBO lasers, Nd:YAG laser treatment often leads to severe postoperative dysuria and delayed sloughing, resulting in prolonged obstruction.[7]

The GreenLight HPS (120-W LBO laser), which is currently used at our institution, permits more rapid and effective tissue vaporization, greater maximum average power, and improved collimation of the laser beam than the older GreenLight PV (KTP laser) system (**Fig. 1**). For these reasons, the GreenLight HPS laser can be used to treat larger prostate glands with up to 3-mm working distance between the laser fiber and the tissue compared with the required "near contact" of tissue (0.5 mm distance) for vaporization with the older GreenLight PV system (**Fig. 2**). Increased working distance with the older PV system results in coagulation rather than vaporization. By contrast, the GreenLight HPS uses separate footswitches for vaporization and coagulation (default 20 W) (**Figs. 3** and **4**). With either system, hemostasis is gained by the inherent superficial coagulative effect of the KTP or LBO laser beam,

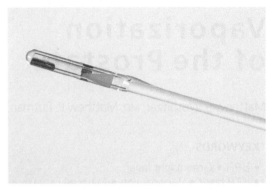

Fig. 2. GreenLight HPS laser fiber (532 nm).

which permits a nearly bloodless procedure. In the first study of pure KTP, bleeding hemostasis was successfully obtained by defocusing the laser beam (3–4 mm) without the need to switch to Nd:YAG laser for coagulation.[8] Specific studies establishing the efficacy of GreenLight PV and GreenLight HPS laser are discussed later in this review.

Preoperative evaluation may include accurate transrectal ultrasound (TRUS) prostate volume assessment to properly gauge required vaporization energy and operative time. Preoperative evaluation is surgeon-dependent and may include uroflowmetry, postvoid residual (PVR) measurement, cystoscopy, and urodynamic evaluation. In contrast to TURP, no tissue specimen is provided by photovaporization of the prostate (PVP). Therefore histopathologic abnormalities, including high-grade prostatic intraepithelial neoplasia (HGPIN), atypical small cell acinar proliferation (ASAP), and cancer cannot be diagnosed. With preoperative elevated prostate-specific antigen (PSA) or suspicious digital rectal examination (DRE), a TRUS-guided biopsy should be performed. The clinical significance of cancers not identified preoperatively as a result of normal PSA and DRE is not clear. Patients may in the future develop prostate cancer, and should be followed postoperatively by DRE and PSA surveillance in specific circumstances when a proactive follow-up is agreed on by urologist and patient. The procedure may be performed on patients taking 5α-reductase inhibitors for more than 6 months without compromising efficiency or efficacy as described by Araki and colleagues[9] in a prospective nonrandomized trial. GreenLight laser photovaporization has a high absorption affinity for hemoglobin, making prostate tissue a good candidate target tissue. Because 5α-reductase inhibitors reduce angiogenesis and blood vessel formation in prostate tissue, it had

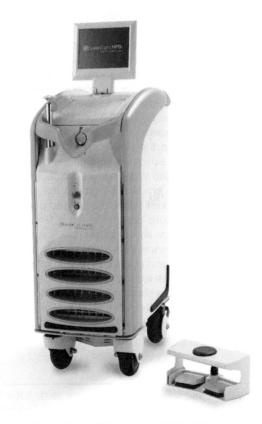

Fig. 1. GreenLight HPS system (AMS, Minnetonka, MN).

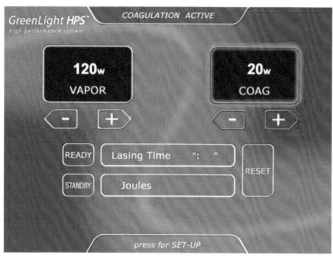

Fig. 3. GreenLight HPS coagulation screen.

been hypothesized that BPH patients treated chronically with 5α-reductase inhibitors would have less significant responses with GreenLight laser photovaporization of the prostate, but this has not been demonstrated. Anesthetic options during the procedure include general and regional anesthesia. Regional anesthesia is effective, but does delay immediate catheter removal.[10] In the outpatient setting, local anesthesia with sedation, oral analgesics, and nonsteroidal anti-inflammatory medications have all been used with excellent safety and recovery profiles, and equivalent outcomes at 2-year follow-up.[11] The efficacy of local anesthetic, periprostatic and pudendal nerve blocks using lidocaine, bupivacaine, or ropivacaine remain controversial. Perioperative antibiotics are given based on urine culture results, and follow-up antibiotics for 3 days are prescribed on an outpatient basis.

SURGICAL TECHNIQUE

The GreenLight HPS laser procedure begins with careful introduction of a continuous-flow cystoscope with a visual obturator. Blind insertion of the cystoscope without the visual obturator can result in urethral trauma and unnecessary bleeding. Prostate size, prostatic urethral length, ureteral orifice position, and bladder neck are evaluated. If the prostate is too large or friable to inspect without causing bleeding, flexible cystoscopy can be performed initially, although this is rarely necessary. A camera filter insert is placed between the telescope and the videocamera to protect the charge-coupled device chip in the camera from being damaged by the laser light. The laser fiber is inserted into a special laser

cystoscope with separation for the fiber and irrigant solution. The authors use a 30 degree cystoscopic lens, as it allows for good visualization of the prostatic urethra and inspection of the ureteral orifices. Alternatively, a 12 degree cystoscopic lens can be used. The KTP or LBO laser generators deliver a continuously emitted beam using a 21 to 23 French continuous-flow cystoscope with a 70-degree side-firing fiber. The continuous nature of the laser beam permits efficient vaporization of gland tissue to the level of the hypovascular prostatic capsule. The routine irrigant is normal saline, although sterile water may also be used without compromising visualization as described by Barber and colleagues[12] in their study of expired breath ethanol measurements during PVP. The goal is to maintain a filled but not over-distended bladder during surgery. Because the electrosurgical resection instruments

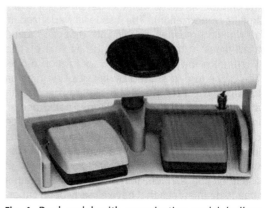

Fig. 4. Dual pedal with vaporization pedal (*yellow, left*) and coagulation pedal (*blue, right*).

required for TURP are not used, glycine is not required during photovaporization. This eliminates the possibility of transurethral resection (TUR) syndrome including hypertension, hyponatremia, glycine toxicity, disorientation, and tachycardia, which was traditionally a possible complication during TURP.

The laser fiber has several key markings, including a blue triangle on the quartz cap of the fiber, which is located opposite to where the laser beam fires (see **Fig. 2**). This blue triangle should be visible at all times to avoid damaging the cystoscopic sheath. There is a red stop sign on the opposite side (relative to the blue triangle) of the fiber. This is aligned with the aiming beam of the fiber. The red aiming beam is aligned in the same direction as the laser beam itself and should be directed toward the targeted tissue. The laser beam should not be fired under any circumstance until the aiming beam is visible on the targeted tissue. The laser beam itself exits at a 70-degree forward deflection angle to the fiber axis. The foot pedal has a standby/ready mode pedal in addition to a left vaporization and right coagulation pedal. Default settings on the HPS system include 80 W for vaporization and 20 W for coagulation. The laser can be adjusted accordingly in 10-W increments. The authors routinely start at 60 W and evaluate the effect of the laser on tissue before titrating the power to a higher setting.

The creation of a working space at the start of the procedure is essential; this avoids contact with tissue and consequent fiber degeneration. This working space is formed by enlarging the urethral lumen by strategic removal of prostatic tissue that may limit maneuverability of the laser fiber and cause full contact with the prostatic tissue. The working space facilitates near-contact vaporization and subsequent optimal irrigation and visualization during lasing, defining the bladder neck (proximal limit of vaporization) and the urethral sphincter at the verumontanum (distal limit of vaporization). The tissue is vaporized in a sweeping manner, keeping the fiber in motion at all times at the ideal working distance of 1 to 3 mm from the tissue during vaporization mode. The procedure is started by lasering the median lobe (when present) and the bladder neck. Initiating the procedure at the bladder neck/median lobe ensures sufficient irrigation and visualization during the remainder of the procedure. The lateral lobes are then vaporized in a symmetric manner, with the laser fired selectively against peaks of tissue on the surface, flattening them out rather than targeting areas that have already been vaporized. A smooth surface permits easier control of any bleeding that may occur than if the surface

were irregular. Next, lasering of the apex is performed, and this must be precise without lasering distal to the verumontanum to avoid damage to the urethral sphincter. Anterior vaporization may be performed without scope rotation if the fiber is maintained far from the cystoscope. At the end of the procedure, the bladder neck and middle lobe can be further assessed to ensure prior vaporization was complete, because it is sometimes technically simpler to complete the middle lobe after the lateral lobes have been vaporized. If the bladder neck remains elevated after vaporization of the middle lobe, bladder neck incision at 5 and 7 o'clock (or 6 o'clock) may be performed. Tissue should be vaporized down to the prostatic capsule until an unobstructed view of the trigone and a TURP-like defect are obtained. At the completion of the procedure, the bladder should be emptied, bleeders should be identified and coagulated, and the contour should be smooth without significant irregular peaks of tissue.

Throughout the procedure, the laser fiber is moved slowly and constantly with a "paint brush motion" to avoid drilling holes in the prostate tissue; spreading the energy in this way promotes a smooth surface. The rotation speed of the fiber must be adapted to efficiency of vaporization. For example, if vaporization is efficient, rotation speed can be increased, whereas if vaporization is less efficient, rotation speed should be decreased. The rotation angle of the fiber must be limited (eg, from 5 to 7 o'clock) to maintain the angle of incidence of the beam perpendicular to the tissue. Bubble formation is representative of effective vaporization. Direct contact with the tissue should be avoided because excessive heat reflection damages the fiber. If tissue build-up occurs on the fiber at any time, it should be immediately cleaned by 1 of 2 techniques. Gently advancing the fiber against the prostatic tissue and then pulling back the fiber towards the cystoscope may remove the excess tissue most efficiently. This may be repeated several times to remove all tissue. If this is not successful, the laser generator should be put in standby mode, and the laser fiber should be gently removed from the cystoscope and cleaned with a clean sterile towel moving from the tip of the fiber toward the fiber control knob and surgeon. It is critical to maintain a clean fiber to allow for efficient vaporization throughout the procedure and maximal use of the fiber (energy limit is 275,000 J).

Bleeding vessels, although rare, may occur during photovaporization of the prostate. With the HPS laser, the coagulation footswitch is used to cauterize bleeding using 20 W. Power can be increased if needed at the discretion of the surgeon. On the older system without individual foot pedals for vaporization and coagulation, the laser power had to be adjusted on the machine to 20 W, and the tissue distance of 0.5 mm was maintained during coagulation. Alternatively with the older GreenLight PV system, the beam can be defocused by increasing the distance between the fiber and tissue. Bleeding during PVP can be classified as venous, from congested mucosa, or prostate tissue, and can negatively affect visibility. Gentle movement of the cystoscope along the urethral path can reduce such bleeding. Maintaining a sweeping motion with the laser fiber can prevent crater development, which can hinder the ability to obtain hemostasis. The surgeon should be especially careful at the bladder neck, median lobe, and verumontanum, where bleeding is most likely to occur. The authors recommend continuing laser vaporization if bleeding is not severe, as further vaporization of the periurethral tissue can cause bleeding to cease. Arterial bleeding is also possible, and may be noted as pulsatile flow. Smooth rotation of the laser fiber and avoidance of crater formation usually prevents this type of bleeding. An irrigation pump may be used to improve visibility, and coagulation (with reduced power to 20 W) should be obtained by coagulating around the bleed, but not directly on it. With venous or arterial bleeding, the laser should be used to paint circumferentially around the bleeding region. If this is not successful, the Bugbee electrocautery (passed through the laser port) can be used to cauterize the bleeder after irrigation is switched from saline to water. Traditional electrocautery resection can be used if other methods are not effective, although this is rarely necessary.

Gentle movement of the laser fiber and cystoscope are recommended, and, overall, GreenLight laser PVP is a more static approach than the movements used with TURP. One may choose to move the fiber in association with the cystoscope when active, or the cystoscope can remain fixed in position while the fiber is moved. The learning curve for the PVP technique is significantly shorter compared with other modalities such as holmium laser enucleation of the prostate (HoLEP),[13] and outcomes such as blood loss, Q_{max}, PVR, and quality of life were not affected when compared early versus later in the learning curve of a surgeon.[14] Overall, good treatment efficacy occurs early in the learning curve of a surgeon. KTP laser vaporization is also considered to be easier to learn and perform than TURP. Competence occurs following 5 to 20 procedures, with larger glands requiring more training. Nonetheless, a mentorship is essential before performing PVP.

With the GreenLight PV 80-W KTP laser and the GreenLight HPS 120-W laser, patients with normal preoperative urodynamics and no history of urinary retention undergo Foley catheter removal 1 hour postoperatively or 1 hour following resolution of spinal anesthetic in the recovery room, before same-day discharge. Patients who have poor compliance, poor detrusor activity, or elevated PVR on preoperative urodynamics, or history of urinary retention have the Foley catheter removed 2 days following discharge. In a recent study by Spaliviero and colleagues,[15] 70% of patients undergoing GreenLight laser PVP were discharged catheter-free on the day of surgery, and the remaining 30% had their catheter removed on postoperative day 1. Two of 21 patients having the catheter removed on postoperative day 1 required reinsertion 3 weeks post surgery for urinary retention, with successful trial of void 1 day later. Other studies have also shown that catheter removal following the operation or on postoperative day 1 is feasible.[16] All patients at our center are discharged with oral pain medication (oxycodone/acetaminophen), oral stool softener (docusate sodium), oral antibiotic for 3 to 5 days, and urinary tract analgesic (phenazopyridine, hyoscyamine).

The evolution of the GreenLight laser system includes an initial hybrid system, followed by stand-alone GreenLight laser with gradually increasing power as studies proved efficacy and safety. KTP lasers with 532-nm wavelength were initially introduced in BPH treatment as part of a hybrid technique with Nd:YAG laser. KTP laser allowed effective vaporization and excision of prostate tissue, whereas Nd:YAG allowed for excellent coagulation and hemostasis. In the first description of KTP laser prostatectomy, Watson[17] described the 30-W KTP laser used in this hybrid technique, followed by Nd:YAG laser coagulation. The hybrid group (using 30-W KTP laser) was identified to have lower recatheterization rates (33% vs 70.5%) compared with 40-W Nd:YAG alone.[18] During brief follow-up, there was significant postoperative retention and delayed onset of therapeutic benefit.[19] At 2.5-year follow-up, higher power 40-W KTP laser was identified to promote more rapid improvement in symptoms than 20-W KTP laser when either was part of the hybrid technique.[20]

Compared with TURP, the randomized controlled trial by Carter and colleagues[16] demonstrated that a hybrid technique (using 30-W KTP laser) gave similar rates of dysuria and median duration of postoperative catheterization. Results after 1 year showed a higher urethral stricture rate in the TURP arm (10% vs 2%) attributed to the larger scope diameter used in TURP. Postoperative urosepsis was more common in the hybrid group, likely secondary to sloughing necrotic tissue following completion of the procedure. Re-operation rate was similar between the 2 groups (2 patients in the hybrid group vs 1 patient in the TURP group). Improvements in international prostatic symptom score (IPSS), Q_{max}, PVR, and LUTS were similar in both groups at 1.5 years. Another study comparing the hybrid technique to TURP in 100 patients showed equivalent improvements in flow rate and symptoms at 3-year follow-up.[21] Retreatment rates were low with no re-operations required in the TURP arm versus 6% in the hybrid group.

Eventually the hybrid technique, which had prolonged operative time and limited tissue ablation, was replaced by pure KTP laser vaporization as laser power capabilities increased. Successful pure KTP laser vaporization (38 and 60 W) using the canine prostate model and human cadaver model has been described[7,22] The technique was described as technically easy, safe, and rapid for the hemostatic removal of prostate tissue with a 2-mm-thick rim of coagulation. In 1998, the first clinical trial of pure KTP laser vaporization described 10 patients with prostate glands up to 60 g undergoing successful treatment.[8] Hemostasis was excellent, and catheters were removed less than 24 hours postoperatively with dramatic Q_{max} improvement rate of 142% without recatheterization required. At 3-month follow-up, this study revealed a mean peak flow rate increase of 166%, mean PVR volume decrease of 82%, and mean American Urological Association (AUA) symptom score reduction of 77%. In 2000, 2-year follow-up results of 55 well-selected patients (without history of urinary retention, urethral strictures, previous prostatic surgery, prostate cancer, or neurogenic bladder) showed a statistically significant improvement in postoperative Q_{max} (mean 29.1 mL/s, 278% improvement), PVR (27 mL, 75% improvement), and AUA symptom score (mean 14, 82% improvement).[23] Data from this group showed that recatheterization was still not required, although 4% of patients had postoperative delayed gross hematuria (6–8 weeks) following strenuous physical activity, and 9% of patients had retrograde ejaculation.

Although the first pure KTP laser vaporization studies reported impressive results, the power of the 60-W KTP laser was not adequate to treat prostate glands larger than 60 g in a reasonable time period. To improve the vaporization speed, the GreenLight PV (80-W KTP) laser system was introduced. Total energy delivery is approximately 200,000 J in 1 hour for a prostate of 80 g. The 80-W

KTP laser has been shown to be effective with prompt improvement in maximum urinary flow rate and symptom scores in multiple studies with prostate volume reduction ranging between 30% and 44%, and PSA reduction ranging between 30% and 42% (**Table 1**).[24] Outcomes for the 80-W KTP laser in the study of Hai and colleagues[25] describe reduction in prostate volume of 27% in 10 patients at 1-year follow-up. In several uncontrolled clinical trials, 759 men with prostate weight ranging from 15 to 250 g (mean 49.6 g) were treated in a mean operative time of 53.7 minutes, with reduction in prostate volume of 37% to 53%.[4,10,26–28] No significant bleeding was recorded, and the mean improvement from preoperative Q_{max} was 13.6 mL/s; the mean decrease in IPSS was 14 points.[4] Twelve-month outcome was reported by Te and colleagues[28] from a multicenter prospective study including 145 patients. AUA symptom index (SI), Q_{max}, and PVR were found to be significantly improved as early as 1 month postoperatively. At 12 months, the mean AUA-SI score decreased from 23.9 to 4.3, whereas the mean Q_{max} increased from 7.8 to 22.6 mL/s ($P<.0001$). PVR decreased from 114.3 to 24.8 mL and the mean prostate volume was reduced from 54.6 mL to 34.4 mL (37%) ($P<.0001$). Twelve-month follow-up was also described in 78 patients from Japan by Seki and colleagues[29] with durable improvement in urinary flow with no effect on serum sodium or hemoglobin levels.

Twelve-month follow-up of 45 patients from Germany has been described by Hamann and colleagues[30] with characteristic urodynamic functional improvement. Three-year follow-up from a multicenter study of 139 men confirmed the overall efficacy of the PVP procedure.[31] Results from the study with extensive follow-up (5 years) cannot be extrapolated directly because only 15 of the 94 patients received treatment with the 80-W KTP laser, and only 14 of 94 patients were evaluated at 5 years.[32] Seventy-nine percent of patients at 5 years had 100% improvement in Q_{max} from baseline, whereas all patients had at least a 50% decline in mean IPSS score.[32] The complications in these early uncontrolled studies included urinary retention (1% to 15.4%), dysuria (6.2% to 30%), minor hematuria (<18%), and retrograde ejaculation (36% to 55% in previously potent men).[4]

Unlike candidates for conventional TURP, candidates for PVP include patients who are high risk and on anticoagulation. The nearly bloodless tissue ablation procedure can be applied to men with elevated American Society of Anesthesiologists (ASA) scores of 3 or greater.[33,34] In 1 of the first studies of the 80-W KTP laser, Reich and colleagues[33] described 66 patients who did not require blood transfusions; there was an 11% need for recatheterization with dramatic 222% improvement (6.7 to 21.6 mL/s) in Q_{max} from baseline and 14 point reduction (20.2 to 6.5) in mean IPSS at 1-year follow-up. Overall, there were no major perioperative complications, with 2 patients requiring re-operation secondary to persistent obstructive voiding. Patients on anticoagulation are typically required to discontinue aspirin or clopidogrel several days before TURP, and to convert from warfarin to low molecular weight heparin (LMWH). Despite these measures, there is increased catheterization time and an elevated transfusion rate of 20%.[35] In a study by Ruszat and colleagues,[36] the safety of 114 men on oral anticoagulation (including 36 on warfarin, 71 on aspirin, and 9 on clopidogrel) was compared with a control group without anticoagulation undergoing PVP. There was similar efficacy with improved voiding parameters at 24 months, and no bleeding complications, blood transfusions, or clot retention occurred. There was a slightly elevated incidence of postoperative irrigation during the first 24 hours (17% vs 5%), which resulted in longer catheterization time. Equivalent PSA decline of 40% at 2 years was observed, reflecting similar volumes of prostate tissue removed in each group. Similar results were reported by Sandhu and colleagues[37] in their study of 24 patients receiving 80-W KTP laser PVP treatment, including 14 men on aspirin, 8 on warfarin, and 2 on clopidogrel (warfarin was discontinued and coagulation normalized before PVP performance). Mean IPSS declined from 18.7 to 9.5 (49.2%) at 1 year, mean Q_{max} increased from 9 to 20.1 mL/s (123%) at 1 year, and mean PVR decreased from 134 to 69 mL (48.5%) at 1-month follow-up. There was no reported occurrence of clot retention or other significant complications.

Patients with larger prostates (>60 g, mean 101.3 g) were evaluated by Sandhu and colleagues[38] with the 80-W KTP (GreenLight PV) laser in 64 patients. Twenty-eight percent of men were had urinary retention preoperatively, the mean prostate volume was 100 g, and the mean operative time was 123 minutes. Ninety-five percent of patients had catheters removed within 23 hours, and 3 patients required recatheterization; the re-operation rate at 1 year was 5%. Q_{max} improved from 7.9 mL/s to 18.9 mL/s (139.2%), whereas mean IPSS decreased from 18.4 to 6.7 (63.6%), and PVR decreased from 189 to 109 mL (42.3%). Complications were minimal with a 4.7% re-operation rate, and no blood transfusions were required. A prospective

randomized controlled trial by Skolarikos and colleagues[39] compared 65 men undergoing 80-W KTP (GreenLight PV laser) to 60 men undergoing open prostatectomy for surgical treatment of prostates greater than 80 g. There were no differences in urodynamic parameters (Q_{max}, PVR) or erectile function by questionnaire at 18-month follow-up. There was no difference in IPSS 18 months postoperatively, but IPSS quality-of-life score was significantly improved in the open prostatectomy group. Prostate volume was significantly lower starting at 3 months postoperatively. Overall, the PVP was established as a reasonable alternative for the surgical management of BPH.

Patients who present with preoperative urinary retention typically have higher complication rates and less benefit reflected in postoperative voiding parameters.[40] Ruszat and colleagues[40] compared 70 patients with preoperative refractory urinary retention to 113 patients with BPH without retention undergoing KTP laser prostate vaporization. The postoperative retention rate was comparable between groups (12.9% vs 10.6%). No statistically significant differences in Q_{max}, IPSS mean decline, or PVR were noted between the 2 groups. In a study of the 80-W KTP laser in 54 men with prostates larger than 100 g, Rajbabu and colleagues[41] described excellent urodynamic outcomes at 24-month follow-up: mean IPSS declined 75.1% (22.9 to 5.7), Q_{max} increased from 8 to 17.9 mL/s (123.8%), and PVR reduced from 134 to 48 mL (64.2%). Complications were minimal, and no blood transfusions were required. At a follow-up of 2 years, Tasci and colleagues[42] identified improved urodynamic outcomes and IPSS scores in 40 patients with large prostates (70–150 g) having 80-W KTP laser PVP compared with TURP. One of the most comprehensive studies with regard to patient cohort and duration of follow-up was the study by Ruszat and colleagues[43] of 500 patients undergoing 80-W KTP laser PVP (including 225 patients on anticoagulation and 80 patients with prostates larger than 80 g). Here, a characteristic sustained voiding parameter improvement was identified without severe intraoperative complications at mean follow-up of 30.6 months. There was no relationship between prostate volume and functional outcome, and late complication rates were comparable to TURP.

Although morbidity is generally low with the 80-W KTP laser, low rates of incontinence (0–1.4%), urethral stricture (0%–4%), bladder neck contracture (0%–3.5%), and urinary tract infection (UTI) (0%–6%), have been reported.[15,27,28,32,33,38,44] Retrograde ejaculation has been reported in

Table 1
Comparison of complications associated with 80-W KTP laser and 120-W LBO laser

Complications of TURP, 80-W KTP (GreenLight PV), and 120-W LBO (GreenLight HPS)

Surgical method	TURP	80 W	80 W	60/80 W	80 W
Authors	Multiple[45–51]	Te et al[28]	Sulser et al[44]	Malek et al[32]	Bachmann et al[27]
Subjects	>20,000[45–51]	139	65	94	108
Follow-up (months)	≤96[50]	12	3	60	12
Hematuria (requiring clot evacuation)	1.3%[45]	0	0	0	NA
Intraoperative bleeding	0.4%[45]–21%[50]	0	0	NA	1 (0.9%)
Dysuria	NA	13 (9.4%)	4 (6.2%)	6 (6%)	7 (6%)
UTI	2.1%–4%[45]	4 (2.2%)	5 (7.7%)	0	5 (5%)
Recatheterization	7.1%[45]–11.4%[50]	7 (5%)	10 (15.4%)	1 (1%)	12 (11%)
Incontinence	1.7%[48]–3.2[49]	2 (1.4%)	NA	0	2 (1.9%)
Re-operation	2.5%[45]–14.7%[50]	0	0	0	0
Bladder neck contracture	2.1%[45]–3.7%[49]	2 (1.4%)	0	2 (2%)	1 (0.9%)
Urethral stricture	1%[45]–3.7%[49]	1 (0.7%)	0	0	4 (4%)
Erectile dysfunction	2.1%[45]–6.3%[46]	0	NA	0	0
Retrograde ejaculation	53%–75%[51]	27 (36%)	NA	≤26%	NA

Surgical method	80 W	80 W	80 W
Authors	Sarica et al[10]	Rajbabu et al[41]	Tasci et al[42]
Subjects	240	54	40
Follow-up (months)	12	24	24
Hematuria (requiring clot evacuation)	0	1 (1.8%)	1 (2.5%)
Intraoperative bleeding	0	0	4 (10%)
Dysuria	26 (10.8%)	3 (5.5%)	7 (17.5%)
UTI	0	5 (9.2%)	3 (7.5%)
Recatheterization	13 (5.4%)	6 (11.1%)	5 (12.5%)
Incontinence	8 (3.3%)	3 (6%)	2 (5%)
Re-operation	0	4 (7%)	3 (7.5%)
Bladder neck contracture	0	0	0
Urethral stricture	2 (0.8%)	2 (3.7%)	0
Erectile dysfunction	0	NA	NA
Retrograde ejaculation	96 (52%)	NA	NA

Surgical method	120 W	120 W	120 W
Authors	Woo et al[53]	Spaliviero et al[15]	Ruszat et al[55]
Subjects	305	70	62
Follow-up (months)	4.2	12	6
Hematuria (requiring clot evacuation)	0	1 (1.4%)	NA
Intraoperative bleeding	8 (2.6%)	1 (1.4%)	8 (13%)
Dysuria	8 (2.6%)	0	11 (18%)
UTI	13 (4.3%)	3 (4.3%)	9 (15%)
Recatheterization	14 (4.6%)	2 (2.9%)	5 (8%)
Incontinence	2 (0.7%)	0	0
Re-operation	2 (0.7%)	0	1 (1.6%)

(continued on next page)

Table 1			
(continued)			
Complications of TURP, 80-W KTP (GreenLight PV), and 120-W LBO (GreenLight HPS)			
Bladder neck contracture	1 (0.3%)	0	1 (1.6%)
Urethral stricture	1 (0.3%)	0	0
Erectile dysfunction	0	NA	NA
Retrograde ejaculation	NA	10 (14.3%)	NA

Abbreviation: NA, data not included in study.

approximately 33% of patients, and erectile dysfunction occurs in usually less than 1% of patients. Recatheterization rates range from 5% to 15%, but these rates are consistent with other surgical interventions. Transfusion is rarely required, and re-operation rate was reported in the range of 0% to 7% at 5-year follow-up. **Table 1** compares the complication rates among studies of the 80-W KTP laser with TURP (individual studies and meta-analysis data).[45–52] Several large studies of TURP published since 1995, including long-term data on 20,671 men,[50] describe transfusion rates between 0.4% and 7.1%,[45,47] TUR syndrome in 2%, incidence of re-operation at 1-, 5- and 8-year follow-up of 5.8%, 12.3%, and 14.7%, respectively (compared with 3.8%, 8.5%, 9.5% for open prostatectomy),[50] urethral stricture rate 1.7% to 9.8%,[49,51] bladder neck contracture rates between 1.7% and 3.7%,[49] erectile dysfunction in 6.3%,[46] and retrograde ejaculation in 50% to 75%.[52]

Other complications include dysuria, which is primarily caused by coagulation rather than vaporization of tissue. The volume of coagulated tissue correlates with the severity of dysuria. Patients with large median lobes, those treated with increased energy because of dense tissue, or patients with prostatitis, fibrosis, or calcifications have an increased risk of dysuria. Antibiotic treatment beyond the standard course given for 5 days postoperatively should not be initiated unless dysuria persists and a positive urine culture is identified. If dysuria without positive urine culture persists, a urinary tract analgesic such as hyoscyamine or phenazopyridine may be prescribed. Bladder neck contracture may result from excessive coagulation of tissue, and/or trauma at the bladder neck. Based on our experience, inward and outward movement of the cystoscope should be minimized at the bladder neck and in the urethra to prevent bladder neck contractures and urethral strictures. Sweeping motion of the laser fiber must be used to avoid capsular perforation. Unlike electrocautery, the GreenLight laser system does not affect the deeper tissue layer of the external sphincter. Creation of an adequate

working channel and avoidance of vaporizing anterior tissue near the verumontanum prevent iatrogenic incontinence. Retrograde ejaculation may occur if the bladder neck is deliberately widened. Anejaculation may occur as a result of disruption of ejaculatory ducts posterolateral to the verumontanum and posterior to the urethra if deep near the seminal vesicles.

In addition, urethral injury with subsequent TUR syndrome has been reported following intravascular absorption of sterile water during KTP laser vaporization. This case report described initial injury to the prostatic urethra after insertion of the cystoscope without the visual obturator. In our judgment, the visual obturator should always be used when any difficulty is encountered with cystoscopic entry. The use of normal saline would have likely prevented the TUR syndrome caused by hypotonic sterile water in this case.[53]

When 80-W KTP laser photoselective vaporization of the prostate was compared with TURP, a nonrandomized controlled prospective study identified PVP as superior to TURP in catheter duration (1.8 vs 3 days) and hospital stay (5.5 vs 7.1 days), whereas the length of surgery was greater with the PVP procedure (59.6 vs 49.4 minutes).[54] Intraoperative bleeding was encountered in 10.8% (4 of 37 patients) of TURP cases but not in PVP. Similar results in voiding parameter improvement occurred at 6 months. Prostate volume reduction was significantly greater in the TURP group, but longer follow-up is required to draw definitive conclusions. The first randomized study of 76 patients treated with either PVP or TURP and followed for at least 6 weeks showed similar improvement rates in IPSS (49.8% vs 50.2% reduction, decreased IPSS 14 vs 12.9), Q_{max} (167% vs 149% increase, 11.96 vs 8.56 mL/s improvement in flow), and PVR (decreased by 125 vs 86 mL) at 12 months (with 44 patients evaluated), with PVP promoting earlier catheter removal (12.2 vs 44.52 hours), shorter hospital stay (1.08 vs 3.39 days), and lower early complication rate including blood loss (0.45 vs 1.46 g/dL decrease in hemoglobin).[55] Follow-up is still in progress, but larger prostates (>85 g) were excluded, the study cohort was limited in size, and the surgeon was early in the learning curve. A more recent nonrandomized prospective study compared 249 patients undergoing 80-W KTP laser (GreenLight PV) with 129 patients undergoing TURP.[56] PVP required significantly longer operative time (73 minutes vs 53 minutes), although patients undergoing PVP were older (72 years vs 68 years) and had larger prostates (62 vs 48 g). KTP laser vaporization had an improved safety profile and earlier hospital discharge than TURP; both had similar IPSS mean decline. There was greater improvement in Q_{max} in the TURP group for any age category. After 12 months, there was a 63% reduction in prostate size in the TURP group versus 44% in the PVP group. At up to 2 years follow-up, there was greater re-operation rate in the PVP group (6.7% versus 3.9%), but this was not statistically significant. The historical re-operation rate for TURP ranges from 2.5% to 14.7% (see **Table 1**).

The evolution of photoselective laser vaporization of the prostate has included increased power, improved accuracy of the laser beam, and overall improved performance. The GreenLight HPS was introduced in 2006, including the 532-nm laser with power settings of 20 to 120 W, which can potentially lead to increased vaporization efficacy as described in bovine, canine, and human studies.[57–60] The HPS system uses a lithium triborate (LBO) crystal rather than the KTP crystal used in the 80-W KTP laser and previous KTP laser systems. The 120-W LBO laser beam is far more collimated than the 80-W KTP laser, allowing maximum focus to be maintained even within 3 mm from the fiber, allowing consistent vaporization, despite changes in the distance between fiber and tissue target. Although there is a theoretic risk of increased morbidity associated with this higher power and more efficient penetrating beam, the fiber is covered with a highly reflective coating to reduce back-scatter effect and inadvertent tissue ablation. The HPS system also has dual-power mode function, as described earlier in this review.

The GreenLight HPS 120-W laser, similar to the 80-W KTP laser,[37,38] has been shown to be safe and effective in men with urinary retention with large prostate glands ($\geq$80 g), and in men on anticoagulant therapy (most patients continued medication during the procedure, "except in outpatient setting" with the actual number not described) (see **Table 1**).[15,61] Although follow-up was short (4.2 months) in the Woo and colleagues[61] cohort of 63 patients with urinary retention, 70 patients on anticoagulant therapy (35 aspirin, 22 warfarin, 13 clopidogrel), and 52 patients with prostate

volume $\geq$80 mL, this study provided initial information regarding the safety and efficacy profile of the 120-W laser. Significant improvements in IPSS, Q_{max} and PVR were similar to the results of the 80-W KTP laser studies[36–38,40,41] The incidence of complications was similar across all groups, with transient urinary retention requiring catheterization occurring most frequently. Blood transfusions were not required, and overall complication rates were lower than the Ruszat and colleagues[36] series using the 80-W KTP laser. In the Spaliviero and colleagues[15] cohort of 70 patients undergoing GreenLight HPS 120-W laser PVP, prostate volume reduction was 53% (P<.001) 12 weeks postoperatively, whereas PSA values decreased 34% (P<.001). Complications included UTI (4.3%), transient urinary retention (2.8%), and retrograde ejaculation (21.4%). No bladder neck contractures or urethral strictures were noted in this study. Limitations also included limited follow-up duration with only 31% of patients evaluated at the 12-month follow-up interval. In addition, perforation of the anterior prostatic capsule has been reported in a single case with the GreenLight HPS system. The patient in this report presented 3 weeks postoperatively with suprapubic pain, and was found to have osteomyelitis of the pubic symphysis and was treated with intravenous antibiotics and suprapubic tube drainage leading to eventual resolution.[62] Comparison of the GreenLight HPS with other modalities is underway, including the high-intensity diode (HiDi) laser system. Equivalence in ablative efficacy, decreased visual acuity and increased bleeding in the HPS group have been reported. Increased postoperative dysuria, transient urge incontinence, stress incontinence, and bladder neck stricture occurred in the HiDi group.[63] Although the HiDi laser seems more favorable for hemostasis, the greater penetration depth results in greater coagulation necrosis and postoperative side effects.

The GreenLight HPS system is cost-effective and versatile. The expected cost per patient at 6 to 24 months postoperatively is significantly less for GreenLight photoselective vaporization ($3020, $3589) than TURP ($4030, $4927). The cost benefit results from decreased rates of adverse outcomes such as retreatment.[64] The GreenLight HPS system may also be used to treat urethral strictures; the 80-W KTP laser has similar success rates with circumferential ablation to cold-knife urethrotomy with success rate of 68% to 80% at mean follow-up of 9.7 months.[65,66] The 80-W KTP laser has been shown to be effective in relieving voiding difficulties in 40 women with anatomic or functional primary bladder neck obstruction.[67] All patients had improvement in voiding symptoms, and urodynamic studies revealed improved parameters.

The evolution of photoselective vaporization laser therapy, including enhanced coagulation and vaporization, has enabled surgeons to perform minimally invasive treatment of BPH with excellent clinical outcomes and reduced morbidity. The GreenLight HPS 120-W system represents the most recent evolution of the Green-Light PVP laser, which has proven, in human studies, to have therapeutic efficacy and efficiency compared with the GreenLight PV 80-W KTP laser. This is especially the case in patients with prostates larger than 80 g and in those patients taking oral anticoagulation.[67] Overall, the functional results for the 80-W KTP laser compare well with TURP results, but with an improved complication profile. Recent studies are comparing the Green-Light HPS to TURP, HiDi, and other modalities, but the long-term results and re-operation rates must be further examined in future, randomized, controlled studies.[63] In the AUA and European Association of Urology guidelines on BPH, laser prostatectomy is recommended for patients receiving anticoagulation, patients unfit for TURP, or patients desiring to maintain ejaculation because electrocautery damage to ejaculatory ducts (when working near verumontanum) is avoided with laser vaporization. The GreenLight HPS must be compared with other laser types and future technologies that arise. Further studies will elucidate whether the GreenLight HPS laser vaporization can surpass TURP as the gold standard therapy for minimally invasive treatment options for BPH.

REFERENCES

1. Costello AJ, Johnson DE, Bolton DM. Nd:YAG laser ablation of the prostate as a treatment for benign prostatic hypertrophy. Lasers Surg Med 1992; 12(2):121–4.
2. Hoffman RM, MacDonald R, Slaton JW, et al. Laser prostatectomy versus transurethral resection for treating benign prostatic obstruction: a systematic review. J Urol 2003;169(1):210–5.
3. Park DS, Cho TW, Lee YK, et al. Evaluation of short term clinical effects and presumptive mechanism of botulinum toxin type A as a treatment modality of benign prostatic hyperplasia. Yonsei Med J 2006;47(5):706–14.
4. Sountoulides P, Tsakiris P. The evolution of KTP laser vaporization of the prostate. Yonsei Med J 2008; 49(2):189–99.
5. Lee R, Gonzalez RR, Te AE. The evolution of photoselective vaporization prostatectomy (PVP): advancing the surgical treatment of benign prostatic hyperplasia. World J Urol 2006;24(4):405–9.
6. Te AE. The next generation in laser treatments and the role of the GreenLight high-performance system laser. Rev Urol 2006;8(Suppl 3):S24–30.
7. Kuntzman RS, Malek RS, Barrett DM, et al. High-power (60-watt) potassium-titanyl-phosphate laser vaporization prostatectomy in living canines and in human and canine cadavers. Urology 1997;49(5): 703–8.
8. Malek RS, Barrett DM, Kuntzman RS. High-power potassium-titanyl-phosphate (KTP/532) laser vaporization prostatectomy: 24 hours later. Urology 1998; 51(2):254–6.
9. Araki M, Lam PN, Culkin DJ, et al. Decreased efficiency of potassium-titanyl-phosphate laser photoselective vaporization prostatectomy with long-term 5 alpha-reductase inhibition therapy: is it true? Urology 2007;70(5):927–30.
10. Sarica K, Alkan E, Luleci H, et al. Photoselective vaporization of the enlarged prostate with KTP laser: long-term results in 240 patients. J Endourol 2005; 19(10):1199–202.
11. Pedersen JM, Romundstad PR, Mjones JG, et al. 2-year followup pressure flow studies of prostate photoselective vaporization using local anesthesia with sedation. J Urol 2009;181(4):1794–9.
12. Barber NJ, Zhu G, Donohue JF, et al. Use of expired breath ethanol measurements in evaluation of irrigant absorption during high-power potassium titanyl phosphate laser vaporization of prostate. Urology 2006;67(1):80–3.
13. de la Rosette J, Alivizatos G. Lasers for the treatment of bladder outlet obstruction: are they challenging conventional treatment modalities? Eur Urol 2006;50(3):418–20.
14. Seki N, Nomura H, Yamaguchi A, et al. Evaluation of the learning curve for photoselective vaporization of the prostate over the course of 74 cases. J Endourol 2008;22(8):1731–5.
15. Spaliviero M, Araki M, Culkin DJ, et al. Incidence, management, and prevention of perioperative complications of GreenLight HPS laser photoselective vaporization prostatectomy: experience in the first 70 patients. J Endourol 2009;23(3):495–502.
16. Carter A, Sells H, Speakman M, et al. A prospective randomized controlled trial of hybrid laser treatment or transurethral resection of the prostate, with a 1-year follow-up. BJU Int 1999;83(3):254–9.
17. Watson G. Contact laser prostatectomy. World J Urol 1995;13(2):115–8.
18. Kollmorgen TA, Malek RS, Barrett DM. Laser prostatectomy: two and a half years' experience with aggressive multifocal therapy. Urology 1996;48(2): 217–22.
19. Miki T, Kojima Y, Nonomura N, et al. Transurethral visual laser ablation of the prostate for benign

prostatic hyperplasia using a KTP/YAG laser. Int J Urol 1997;4(6):576–9.

20. Shingleton WB, Terrell F, Renfroe L, et al. Low-power v high-power KTP laser: improved method of laser ablation of prostate. J Endourol 1999;13(1):49–52.

21. Shingleton WB, Farabaugh P, May W. Three-year follow-up of laser prostatectomy versus transurethral resection of the prostate in men with benign prostatic hyperplasia. Urology 2002;60(2):305–8.

22. Kuntzman RS, Malek RS, Barrett DM, et al. Potassium-titanyl-phosphate laser vaporization of the prostate: a comparative functional and pathologic study in canines. Urology 1996;48(4):575–83.

23. Malek RS, Kuntzman RS, Barrett DM. High power potassium-titanyl-phosphate laser vaporization prostatectomy. J Urol 2000;163(6):1730–3.

24. Bachmann A, Ruszat R. The KTP-(GreenLight-) laser – principles and experiences. Minim Invasive Ther Allied Technol 2007;16(1):5–10.

25. Hai MA, Malek RS. Photoselective vaporization of the prostate: initial experience with a new 80 W KTP laser for the treatment of benign prostatic hyperplasia. J Endourol 2003;17(2):93–6.

26. Dincel C, Samli MM, Guler C, et al. Plasma kinetic vaporization of the prostate: clinical evaluation of a new technique. J Endourol 2004;18(3):293–8.

27. Bachmann A, Ruszat R, Wyler S, et al. Photoselective vaporization of the prostate: the basel experience after 108 procedures. Eur Urol 2005;47(6):798–804.

28. Te AE, Malloy TR, Stein BS, et al. Photoselective vaporization of the prostate for the treatment of benign prostatic hyperplasia: 12-month results from the first United States multicenter prospective trial. J Urol 2004;172(4 Pt 1):1404–8.

29. Seki N, Nomura H, Yamaguchi A, et al. Effects of photoselective vaporization of the prostate on urodynamics in patients with benign prostatic hyperplasia. J Urol 2008;180(3):1024–8 [discussion: 1028–29].

30. Hamann MF, Naumann CM, Seif C, et al. Functional outcome following photoselective vaporisation of the prostate (PVP): urodynamic findings within 12 months follow-up. Eur Urol 2008;54(4):902–7.

31. Te AE, Malloy TR, Stein BS, et al. Impact of prostate-specific antigen level and prostate volume as predictors of efficacy in photoselective vaporization prostatectomy: analysis and results of an ongoing prospective multicentre study at 3 years. BJU Int 2006;97(6):1229–33.

32. Malek RS, Kuntzman RS, Barrett DM. Photoselective potassium-titanyl-phosphate laser vaporization of the benign obstructive prostate: observations on long-term outcomes. J Urol 2005;174(4 Pt 1):1344–8.

33. Reich O, Bachmann A, Siebels M, et al. High power (80 W) potassium-titanyl-phosphate laser vaporization of the prostate in 66 high risk patients. J Urol 2005;173(1):158–60.

34. Fu WJ, Hong BF, Wang XX, et al. Evaluation of GreenLight photoselective vaporization of the prostate for the treatment of high-risk patients with benign prostatic hyperplasia. Asian J Androl 2006;8(3):367–71.

35. Dotan ZA, Mor Y, Leibovitch I, et al. The efficacy and safety of perioperative low molecular weight heparin substitution in patients on chronic oral anticoagulant therapy undergoing transurethral prostatectomy for bladder outlet obstruction. J Urol 2002;168(2):610–3 [discussion: 614].

36. Ruszat R, Wyler S, Forster T, et al. Safety and effectiveness of photoselective vaporization of the prostate (PVP) in patients on ongoing oral anticoagulation. Eur Urol 2007;51(4):1031–8 [discussion: 1038–41].

37. Sandhu JS, Ng CK, Gonzalez RR, et al. Photoselective laser vaporization prostatectomy in men receiving anticoagulants. J Endourol 2005;19(10):1196–8.

38. Sandhu JS, Ng C, Vanderbrink BA, et al. High-power potassium-titanyl-phosphate photoselective laser vaporization of prostate for treatment of benign prostatic hyperplasia in men with large prostates. Urology 2004;64(6):1155–9.

39. Skolarikos A, Papachristou C, Athanasiadis G, et al. Eighteen-month results of a randomized prospective study comparing transurethral photoselective vaporization with transvesical open enucleation for prostatic adenomas greater than 80 cc. J Endourol 2008;22(10):2333–40.

40. Ruszat R, Wyler S, Seifert HH, et al. Photoselective vaporization of the prostate: subgroup analysis of men with refractory urinary retention. Eur Urol 2006;50(5):1040–9 [discussion: 1049].

41. Rajbabu K, Chandrasekara SK, Barber NJ, et al. Photoselective vaporization of the prostate with the potassium-titanyl-phosphate laser in men with prostates of >100 mL. BJU Int 2007;100(3):593–8 [discussion: 598].

42. Tasci AI, Tugcu V, Sahin S, et al. Rapid communication: photoselective vaporization of the prostate versus transurethral resection of the prostate for the large prostate: a prospective nonrandomized bi-center trial with 2-year follow-up. J Endourol 2008;22(2):347–53.

43. Ruszat R, Seitz M, Wyler SF, et al. GreenLight laser vaporization of the prostate: single-center experience and long-term results after 500 procedures. Eur Urol 2008;54(4):893–901.

44. Sulser T, Reich O, Wyler S, et al. Photoselective KTP laser vaporization of the prostate: first experiences with 65 procedures. J Endourol 2004;18(10):976–81.

45. Borboroglu PG, Kane CJ, Ward JF, et al. Immediate and postoperative complications of transurethral

prostatectomy in the 1990s. J Urol 1999;162(4): 1307–10.

46. Muntener M, Aellig S, Kuettel R, et al. Sexual function after transurethral resection of the prostate (TURP): results of an independent prospective multi-centre assessment of outcome. Eur Urol 2007;52(2): 510–5.

47. Muzzonigro G, Milanese G, Minardi D, et al. Safety and efficacy of transurethral resection of prostate glands up to 150 ml: a prospective comparative study with 1 year of followup. J Urol 2004;172(2): 611–5.

48. Wasson JH, Reda DJ, Bruskewitz RC, et al. A comparison of transurethral surgery with watchful waiting for moderate symptoms of benign prostatic hyperplasia. The Veterans Affairs Cooperative Study Group on Transurethral Resection of the Prostate. N Engl J Med 1995;332(2):75–9.

49. Zwergel U, Wullich B, Lindenmeir U, et al. Long-term results following transurethral resection of the prostate. Eur Urol 1998;33(5):476–80.

50. Madersbacher S, Lackner J, Brossner C, et al. Re-operation, myocardial infarction and mortality after transurethral and open prostatectomy: a nation-wide, long-term analysis of 23,123 cases. Eur Urol 2005;47(4):499–504.

51. Gilling PJ, Mackey M, Cresswell M, et al. Holmium laser versus transurethral resection of the prostate: a randomized prospective trial with 1-year followup. J Urol 1999;162(5):1640–4.

52. Rassweiler J, Teber D, Kuntz R, et al. Complications of transurethral resection of the prostate (TURP) – incidence, management, and prevention. Eur Urol 2006;50(5):969–79 [discussion: 980].

53. Dilger JA, Walsh MT, Warner ME, et al. Urethral injury during potassium-titanyl-phosphate laser prostatectomy complicated by transurethral resection syndrome. Anesth Analg 2008;107(4):1438–40.

54. Bachmann A, Schurch L, Ruszat R, et al. Photoselective vaporization (PVP) versus transurethral resection of the prostate (TURP): a prospective bi-centre study of perioperative morbidity and early functional outcome. Eur Urol 2005;48(6):965–71 [discussion: 972].

55. Bouchier-Hayes DM, Anderson P, Van Appledorn S, et al. KTP laser versus transurethral resection: early results of a randomized trial. J Endourol 2006;20(8): 580–5.

56. Ruszat R, Wyler SF, Seitz M, et al. Comparison of potassium-titanyl-phosphate laser vaporization of the prostate and transurethral resection of the prostate: update of a prospective non-randomized two-centre study. BJU Int 2008;102(10):1432–8 [discussion: 1438–9].

57. Kang HW, Jebens D, Malek RS, et al. Laser vaporization of bovine prostate: a quantitative comparison of potassium-titanyl-phosphate and lithium triborate lasers. J Urol 2008;180(6):2675–80.

58. Lee R, Saini R, Zoltan E, et al. Photoselective vaporization of the prostate using a laser high performance system in the canine model. J Urol 2008; 180(4):1551–3.

59. Schwartz MJ, Wysock JS, Wang GJ, et al. Comparison of vaporization efficiency of the 80W potassium-titanyl-phosphate (KTP) GreenLight laser and the 120W GreenLight high performance system (HPS) laser for photoselective vaporization of the prostate [abstract]. AUA Annual Meeting. Orlando, Florida, 2008.

60. Zoltan E, Lee RK, Saini R, et al. Comparative evaluation of high power 532nm laser systems, 120 watt (HPS) vs. 80 watt (KTP), for photoselective vaporization of the prostate (PVP) of large glands with vaporization incision technique (VIT) [abstract]. AUA Annual Meeting. Orlando, Florida, 2008.

61. Woo H, Reich O, Bachmann A, et al. Outcome of GreenLight HPS 120-W laser therapy in specific patient populations: those in retention on anticoagulants, and with large prostates (≥80 ml). Eur Urol 2008;7(4):378–83.

62. Kaplon DM, Iannotti H. Prostatic capsular perforation with extravasation resulting in pubic osteomyelitis: a rare complication of KTP laser prostatectomy. J Endourol 2008;22(12):2705–6.

63. Ruszat R, Seitz M, Wyler SF, et al. Prospective single-centre comparison of 120-W diode-pumped solid-state high-intensity system laser vaporization of the prostate and 200-W high-intensive diode-laser ablation of the prostate for treating benign prostatic hyperplasia. BJU Int 2009;104(6):820–5.

64. Stovsky MD, Griffiths RI, Duff SB. A clinical outcomes and cost analysis comparing photoselective vaporization of the prostate to alternative minimally invasive therapies and transurethral prostate resection for the treatment of benign prostatic hyperplasia. J Urol 2006;176(4 Pt 1):1500–6.

65. Turek PJ, Malloy TR, Cendron M, et al. KTP-532 laser ablation of urethral strictures. Urology 1992;40(4):330–4.

66. Shanberg A, Baghdassarian R, Tansey L, et al. 532 laser in treatment of urethral strictures. Urology 1988;32(6):517–20.

67. Fu Q, Xu YM. Transurethral incision of the bladder neck using KTP in the treatment of bladder neck obstruction in women. Urol Int 2009;82(1):61–4.

Holmium Laser Applications of the Prostate

Lori B. Lerner, MD[a,b,*], Mark D. Tyson, BS[c]

KEYWORDS

- Holmium laser enucleation of the prostate • Holmium
- Laser • Prostate • Surgery • Laser physics

Over the past decade, urologists have witnessed an expansion in the number of various techniques used for the treatment of benign prostatic hyperplasia, especially in the arena of laser surgery. The use of neodymium: yttrium aluminium garnet (Nd:YAG) laser technology in treating benign prostatic hyperplasia (BPH) was initially described in 1992 by Costello and colleagues,[1] representing the first published description of laser prostatectomy.

Shortly thereafter, Gilling and colleagues[2] described the use of holmium: YAG (Ho:YAG) in the ablation of prostate tissue, and although holmium laser technology had well-established applications in treating urinary calculi, this was its first application in treating the prostate. They developed a combination approach using holmium to create a channel in the prostate and the Nd:YAG to coagulate the prostate (holmium laser ablation of the prostate, or HoLAP). However, they discovered that holmium could be used alone and had fewer side effects, but the process was slow and tedious with the 60 W laser unit currently available.

This group then expanded on the technique by combining holmium laser resection of the prostate (HoLRP) with mechanical morcellation (holmium laser enucleation of the prostate, or HoLEP).[3] Since then, a plethora of studies have been published touting the procedure and it has slowly gained popularity, particularly outside the United States.[4] Outcomes have been as good as

traditional methods, with recently published 10-year data showing sustained results over time. HoLEP has distinct advantages over other surgical approaches, including efficacy despite prostate size, low morbidity, and shorter hospitalizations. The American Urological Association's guidelines on the treatment of BPH include HoLAP and HoLEP, and dedicated CPT codes exist for each procedure.[5] This article describes the holmium wavelength and its benefits in prostate surgery, discuss indications of surgery, describes the surgical technique of both the modern HoLAP and HoLEP and suggested postoperative care, and reviews published studies supporting both techniques as excellent treatments for men experiencing bladder outlet obstruction secondary to the prostate.

PHYSICS

Both Ho:YAG and Nd:YAG are crystals used as active laser media in solid-state lasers. Solid-state lasers use a solid rather than liquid or gas medium to derive optical gain within the laser. The benefits of Ho:YAG over Nd:YAG laser are partly related to their differences in wavelength. The holmium wavelength (2140 nm, nonvisible/infrared) is absorbed by water. The depth of penetration is 0.5 mm, and if the laser is more than that distance from the target (ie, prostate), it has no effect on tissue and the energy is dissipated in the water. Nd:YAG has a shorter wavelength (1064 nm),

Financial Disclosures: Dr Lerner has the following financial disclosures: Lumenis, Inc: Preceptor, Consultant; Boston Scientific, Inc: Preceptor. Dr Tyson has no financial disclosures.
a Section of Urology, VA Boston Healthcare System, Boston, MA, USA
b Boston University School of Medicine, 12 Water Street, Hingham, Boston, MA 02043, USA
c Dartmouth Medical School, Hanover, 5 Rope Ferry Road #6112, Hanover, NH 03755, USA
* Corresponding author. Boston University School of Medicine, 12 Water Street, Hingham, Boston, MA 02043.
E-mail address: lerner_lori@hotmail.com (L.B. Lerner).

resulting in deeper tissue penetration and more thermal injury.

Ho:YAg has the additional advantage of being a pulsed solid-state laser, which leads to a shorter absorption length.[2] Both holmium and YAG have excellent hemostatic properties and can be used in normal saline, negating issues related to hyponatremia and operative time, which are described later.

The drawbacks of the Nd:YAG are that the tissue effects can cause edema, heating of the irrigant fluid, and deeper tissue injury, leading to prolonged catheter time, delayed clinical improvement, and irritative symptoms that can be severe and persistent.[2] Therefore, YAG has fallen out of favor and lasers such as holmium and potassium titanyl phosphate (KTP) have become the preferred wavelengths.[3]

Holmium energy is delivered through small, flexible fibers and is controlled with precision by the operating surgeon. Energy is stored within the laser resonator and released in a pulsed fashion, controlled with a foot pedal. Energy travels along the laser fiber through internal reflection that bounces the energy down the fiber. Specialized clear lens protective eyewear is recommended for the operating physician and those working with the fiber. For the patient, having the eyes closed or blocked by a sheet is sufficient. The machine is key-controlled and easy to use. Regular maintenance is recommended to ensure proper functioning, and blast shield replacements should be kept in stock.

Hemostasis

The hemostatic effects of holmium are believed to be related to the physics of the laser energy. How the laser energy interacts with the tissue reflects primarily the wavelength, time of energy application, and the energy density (fluence). The wavelength and interaction with the target tissue determines the efficiency with which the energy is transferred to the tissue. The holmium wavelength has a high absorption in water.

For the prostate, which is a tissue type that has a high density of water, the wavelength has a very favorable absorption coefficient, implying good tissue conductance of thermal energy.[6] The energy is absorbed by water in the prostate cells and the tissue is heated to 100°C, effectively causing vaporization/ablation. Coagulation occurs if the tissue is heated to temperatures greater than 70°C but less than 100°C.

Holmium energy is delivered through a fiber that can be controlled to produce either ablation or coagulation. By lowering the fluence, either

through decreasing the energy pulse or pulling the fiber tip away from the tissue, the tissue temperature is lowered and ablation does not occur; rather, the heat is absorbed into the tissue, resulting in coagulation.[7] These properties come into effect when treating the prostate, regardless of whether the patient is on anticoagulant medication. The water content of the cells is no different, and therefore the hemostatic properties are the same. Given its hemostatic properties, no limitations exist to its use on patients taking blood thinners. Patients are sent home the same day of surgery or the following morning after an overnight observation.

Surgical Indications

Any patient who has voiding symptoms secondary to bladder outlet obstruction is a candidate for holmium surgery. Patients who have glands less than 60 g can be considered for HoLAP or HoLEP. However, gland sizes greater than 60 g are best suited for HoLEP, because ablation would be time-consuming. Basically, patients who urologists would consider good candidates for transurethral resection of the prostate (TURP) or open prostatectomy can undergo holmium surgery.

In addition, patients on anticoagulation medication are treated effectively with holmium, even when taking therapeutic levels of coumadin or platelet aggregation inhibitors, such as clopidogrel bisulfate or aspirin. Overall bleeding, regardless of coagulation status at surgery, is much reduced in all patients compared with that seen during transurethral resection (TUR) and open procedures. Because normal saline is used during resection, TUR syndrome risk is eliminated. Fluid absorption is minimal given coagulation of the blood vessels with tissue resection. These decreases in risk for operative effects may allow more fragile elderly patients to undergo definitive therapy for which they might otherwise not be deemed medically fit.

Instruments and Settings

HoLEP is an endoscopic approach that follows principles similar to those of open prostatectomy. In essence, the laser fiber becomes the finger that is used in open surgery. A standard setup includes a 26F resectoscope with laser bridge, 30° lens, 5F ureteral catheter, 80 or 100 W holmium laser unit, and a 550-μm end-fire laser fiber. Olympus and Storz have resectoscope adaptors that can be used, whereas other companies such as Wolf have dedicated laser resectoscopes.

The laser is set at 2 J and 40 or 50 Hz, depending on the total wattage of the laser unit. For tissue retrieval, necessary equipment includes a morcellator, morcellator tubing, tissue retrieval sock, retrieval loop, long nephroscope lens, and percutaneous nephrolithotomy grasping instruments.

Various practitioners have used slightly modified equipment choices, including a 28F resectoscope, 7F ureteral catheter, and an offset lens for use with morcellation that can be placed within the same resectoscope sheath. Use of the lens resectoscope adaptor (as is the authors' preference), negates the need to exchange the resectoscope for a nephroscope during morcellation.

For HoLAP, the equipment used is similar, except that no morcellation/tissue retrieval instruments are necessary. The 550-μm side-fire fiber is used. This fiber is surrounded by a casing that makes the outside diameter larger than the end-fire fiber, and therefore no ureteral catheter is necessary if a laser bridge is used. The most common settings are those used for HoLEP at 2 J and 40/50 Hz. Although other settings have been described, the most recent trend has been to use these.

Surgical Technique: Holmium Laser Enucleation of the Prostate

The urethra is dilated with sounds, if indicated, and a resectoscope is placed. The laser fiber is passed through the ureteral catheter, which is then advanced through the laser bridge. The ureteral catheter helps stabilize the fiber and prevent bouncing. The catheter should be extended no more than a millimeter or two from the end of the scope to prevent obstruction of view. The laser fiber should be out beyond the edge of the catheter, but kept in fairly close control. The hands are positioned on the scope as shown in **Fig. 1**, which allows for better movement and rotation of the scope during the procedure.

Incisions are made in the 5 and 7 o'clock positions to the level of the surgical capsule, which is easily identified by the presence of parallel fibers, a distinct difference from the "fluffy" appearance of the prostate. Incisions are extended from the bladder neck to the verumontanum. A sweeping motion is used to create a wide groove. Once the two grooves have been created, the fiber is used to enucleate the middle lobe along the surgical capsule in a retrograde fashion from the veru toward the bladder neck. The beak of the scope can be used to peel the adenoma along the capsule, toward the bladder neck, by placing the beak underneath the lobe and pushing upwards. Those on 5α-reductase inhibitors may not peel well, because the capsule in these men is much more adherent to the adenoma.

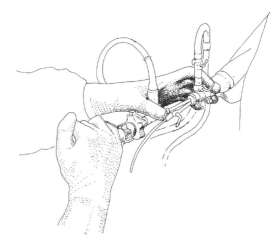

Fig. 1. Hand position during holmium laser enucleation of the prostate. (*Courtesy of* Charles F. Foltz, VA Boston Healthcare System, Boston, MA.)

Bleeding can be controlled by defocusing the fiber over the bleeding site and holding the fiber in place for several seconds. The settings can be changed to 2.5 to 3 J and 35 to 40 W for coagulation, if desired. If the bleeding is recalcitrant, treating the tissue around the site may be successful.

Once the middle lobe is resected, attention is directed to the lateral lobes. The urinary sphincter is identified and a groove is made along the capsule at the level of the veru beneath the apex of the prostate and continued laterally and anteriorly. The scope is used to negotiate the turn, rotating and pushing the scope along the capsule. The fiber is kept constant and fixed and is used to separate the adenoma from the capsule. Again, a peeling motion can be used, with the scope lifting and pushing the gland off the capsule toward the bladder neck. This technique will likely not be successful in patients on 5α-reductase inhibitors. With small prostates, this lateral motion can be continued up along the anterior surface and across the midline to the opposite side.

For larger prostates, the scope is turned to the 12 o'clock position and a midline incision made in the prostate from the bladder neck to the level of the veru, again down to the capsule. The incision is widened with the same sweeping back and forth motion, creating a trough. The incisions are then connected from the lateral edge to 12 o'clock and retrograde enucleation is performed.

Morcellation

Once all three lobes have been enucleated and passed into the bladder, the laser bridge is exchanged for the morcellator bridge. If no morcellator bridge is available, the resectoscope is exchanged for a rigid nephroscope. Normal saline irrigation is essential in this portion of the procedure, and the bladder must be kept full. The morcellator is passed through the working channel of the offset lens, and the prostate pieces engaged. Depression of the pedal halfway initiates the suction component of the morcellator. Once the lobe is engaged, the morcellator and scope are pulled back to the bladder neck and directed up off the bladder floor. Positioning the morcellator at the bladder neck, which is more fixed, helps avoid inadvertent engagement of the bladder wall, particularly with large, floppy bladders. The pedal is depressed fully and the reciprocating blades morcellate and suction the tissue through the device, which is collected in a retrieval sock and sent to pathology. Pieces that are small or cannot be morcellated can be collected through the retrieval loop or stone grasping instruments.

Surgical Technique: Holmium Laser Ablation of the Prostate

A laser bridge is recommended for ablation because it keeps the fiber in a predictable location and prevents bouncing. The 550-μm side-fire fiber is advanced through the bridge and out through the end of the scope until the solid line is visible. This line must been seen throughout ablation to avoid injury to the resectoscope and lens. The aiming beam must be identified (70° angle from the fiber) and tissue ablation begun, keeping the fiber close to, but not touching, the prostate. The fiber should be rotated slowly, with the surgeon avoiding going too fast, which is a common mistake. The surgeon must allow sufficient time for the energy to be absorbed; rapid rotations only heat the irrigant and do not ablate tissue.

Surgeons tend to develop an approach that works well for them, with the goal being to ablate all adenoma until prostatic capsule is visualized circumferentially from the bladder neck to the veru. The authors start with troughs at 5 and 7 o'clock, ablating the middle lobe to capsule, then proceeding to the lateral lobes. Starting at the bladder neck, adenoma is ablated to capsule, using the handpiece to rotate the fiber over the surface of the lateral lobe from the middle lobes troughs to 12 o'clock, gradually moving distally toward the veru. Once capsule is visible throughout, the contralateral lobe is addressed.

Postoperative Care

Whether HoLEP or HoLAP was performed, the authors leave a catheter in place overnight, generally a 20F standard two-way catheter. Overstretching of the bladder during the procedure may cause transient detrusor dysfunction, and an overnight catheter reduces the risk for a return visit to the emergency department. Other urologists remove the catheter the same day, but generally only after HoLAP. If a patient was performing self-catheterization or was in urinary retention preprocedure, experts recommend leaving the catheter in place for 3 to 5 days and having it removed at home by the patient or in clinic after a voiding trial. Most patients are discharged the same day as the procedure or the following morning after an overnight observation. Patients who are therapeutically anticoagulated may be kept overnight, but rarely is three-way irrigation required. Patients are seen at 4 weeks for measurement of uroflow and post-void residual. Further follow-up after that point is case-specific.

Bladder Recovery

Depending on the stage of bladder decompensation before surgery, some recovery process of the bladder is expected. Like those that would be encountered after a TURP or open prostatectomy, the symptoms include short-term exacerbation of irritative voiding symptoms, transient incontinence (stress and/or urge), retrograde ejaculation, urethral strictures, and urinary retention. Dysuria is uncommon with holmium laser treatments.

The stress symptoms are similar to those encountered after an open prostatectomy, given the volume of tissue removed with HoLEP, which is greater than that for TURP and ablative techniques. The prostatic fossa is often large postprocedure, and can lead to urine trapping and leakage with stress maneuvers in the short-term. In addition, the resectoscope is positioned across the urinary sphincter for a longer duration than in TURP and the authors believe transient sphincter dysfunction can occur. However, as with TURP and open procedures, most patients resolve their voiding issues with time and bladder recovery. Anticholinergic medication should be used in patients who have urge symptoms. The duration of recovery is individual and this should be stressed to patients before surgery.

HOLMIUM LASER ENUCLEATION OF THE PROSTATE: TRICKS, TIPS, AND TRIBULATIONS
Don't Start with Mt. Everest!

The most important tip is to start with prostates no larger than 60 g until the technique has been mastered. In fact, for the first 10 cases, glands smaller than 40 g are ideal. Once the technique is understood, then larger glands can be worked on and many potential problems can be avoided altogether, or easily addressed. An option to trilobar enucleation is to begin with 5 and 7 o'clock incisions and middle lobe enucleation with an end-fire fiber, followed by lateral lobe ablation with a side-fire fiber. Once the urologist is comfortable with the incisions and middle lobe, the surgeon can progress to the lateral lobes.

Undermining of the Bladder Neck

With standard TURP, because the loop works from the top down, surgeons have a clear view of the bladder neck during resection. With HoLEP, by staying on the capsule and working in a retrograde fashion, the bladder neck can be undermined. Most of the time, this is not dangerous or even problematic, but can lead to fluid extravasation around the bladder in the pelvis. This issue can be easily avoided by identifying the lobes at risk for undermining and thereby modifying the technique. Lobes at risk are those with a sharp upwards angle into the bladder (high bladder neck), requiring that the lobe be lifted extensively. It can be challenging to direct the fiber upwards under the lobe. In cases like this, the surgeon should either leave a rim of prostate tissue and make a more superficial incision plane during enucleation to reduce the angle, or remove the lobe working from lateral to medial in a V formation. Once the most distal portion of the lateral lobe is free, the lobe will flip upwards and the degree of the angle will be reduced, making it easy to resume the back and forth sweeping motion with the fiber.

Middle Lobe that Extends into the Bladder and Splays the Trigone

Provided that the surgeon stays on capsule, no injury should occur to the ureteral orifices. The resection may be close to the orifices, but injury is unlikely. Even if mucosa near or surrounding the orifices is ablated, penetration of the holmium energy is so superficial that injury, stricture, or obstruction is low risk. To the authors knowledge, no significant ureteral injuries have occurred with HoLEP.

Middle Lobe Just Proximal to Veru

When making incisions at the 5 and 7 o'clock positions, the portion of the gland just proximal to the veru can be large and posterior. The scope often must be towed down and a straight incision made to open up the gland. Once this cut has been made, the resectoscope can be used to retract the lobes and then the incision continued to the capsule.

Anterior 12 O'Clock Position

Most urologists early in the learning phase find this incision to be challenging. Often, the incision is not carried distal enough because of concern for injuring the sphincter. If the incision is too short, the lobe will not advance toward the bladder, making the retrograde enucleation difficult, or two parallel incisions will be made. Familiarity with the procedure makes this incision easier to perform.

Urethral Mucosa at Anterior Distal Edge

If the anterior incision is not made distal enough, or the lateral incision not extended enough anteriorly, urethral mucosa at the anterior position over the veru will prevent advancement. This occurrence is best identified by pulling the scope back to the veru and looking up to 12 o'clock; it is often easy to see the mucosa pulling and an incision can be made under direct visualization. Once the mucosa is incised, the planes become obvious and the remainder of the case is generally straightforward.

Creation of Two Incisions

Surgeons must make sure the lateral and anterior incisions match. Creating two parallel incisions can create confusion, disorientation, and inefficiency. If the surgeon stays on capsule throughout, this is avoided. If two incisions are made, the surgeon must get orientation, find the bridge between the two incisions, incise the bridge, and get back on track. Starting with small prostates will help with this portion of the learning curve.

Difficulty with Suction

Unlike TURP where the scope is off the prostate bed, with HoLEP the scope is towed down. Because the suction ports are located underneath the resectoscope, times may occur during the procedure when the undersurface of the scope is in contact with the prostate and suctioning of fluid does not occur. Removing the suction tubing and allowing for gravity drainage is the best course of action. Once the middle lobe is removed, this generally does not occur because the channel is then more open.

Morcellation: Poor Visualization from Bleeding

Poor visualization caused by bleeding is rare, but can be frustrating. Depressing the pedal of the morcellator part way to flush the bladder often helps, as does compression of the prostatic fossa with the scope. The bladder can also be filled to capacity, which may compress any bleeding vessels. Once the piece is engaged in the morcellator, visualization is generally good. If visualization remains poor, the pieces can be left and the patient brought back to the operating room in a few weeks. The lobes are large, will float around in the bladder, and are unlikely to obstruct, and therefore no Foley is required. Morcellation of these retained lobes is often easy and quick.

Engagement of Bladder Mucosa with the Morcellator

The mucosa of the prostate lobes is present on the resected lobes and, when morcellating, differentiating between bladder mucosa and prostatic urethral mucosa can sometimes be worrisome. These mucosa can be defined by engaging the lobe and then, before morcellation, turning and rotating the lobe, which clearly shows the resected edges. If the bladder mucosa is inadvertently engaged, the suction tubing should be removed from the morcellator and the device gently pulled free of the mucosa. Any bleeding is often minimal and can be left alone or treated with the laser. Bladder injury can be easily avoided if strict rules are followed. One should avoid "chasing pieces" and allow the lobe to come to the morcellator, ensure the bladder is full, and position the morcellator off the bladder floor back near the bladder neck.

Morcellator Does not Seem to be Morcellating

Depending on the composition of the prostatic tissue, some lobes morcellate more quickly than others. If the pieces are not morcellating, the tissue may need to be reengaged. With the pedal depressed, the morcellator can be pulled gently in and out of the scope, which frees the lobe and then reengages it in a different location. If the tissue is clearly not cutting, it may be time to change the blades. Each set of blades is good for approximately 8 to 10 cases.

Inability to Engage Pieces into the Morcellator

Small round pieces may not seed into the morcellator blades. If the piece has a rough edge, the lobe should be engaged at this location. If it is round in all directions, the piece should be retrieved with the retrieval loop or a stone grasper.

Inability to Remove Pieces Beyond the Sphincter

When using the retrieval loop or stone graspers, the piece must be kept close to the scope and the scope used to keep the sphincter open. The normal curve of the urethra must be followed rather than trying to pull the piece straight out. Once the piece is distal to the sphincter, a finger can be placed in the perineum to help advance the piece through the urethra. Very large pieces can be removed in this fashion.

COMPLICATIONS

In a retrospective analysis of 206 patients, the most common intraoperative complications identified were bladder mucosal injury (2%), incomplete tissue morcellation (2%), capsular perforation (1.5%), blood transfusions (1%), and creation of false passages in the bladder neck (0.5%).[8] Postoperative complications included recatheterization rates approaching 8%, bladder neck contractures (4%), urethral strictures (2%), and clot retention (2%). And although meaningful comparisons to other surgical modalities, such as TURP, are difficult given the intrinsic bias of retrospective study designs, the morbidity rates of these early published reports suggested some advantages over TURP, especially for larger prostates.

A subsequent prospective cohort study involving 268 patients, however, found a much high incidence of capsular perforation (10%), superficial mucosal injury (4%), and ureteral orifice injury (2%), with transfusion rates of less than 1%.[9] However, postoperatively, the commonest complication identified was transient urinary incontinence (10%). The high incidence of transient urinary incontinence is believed to be secondary to more complete tissue removal with partial weakening or stretching of the external sphincter,[10] with most cases resolving within 1 to 6 months.[11]

Other postoperative complications of HoLEP include urinary tract infection, epididymitis, bulbar strictures, bladder neck contractures, and bleeding with clot retention.

DISCUSSION

The long-held gold standard for endoscopic surgery for BPH is TURP. However, this procedure has significant limitations, with complication rates approaching 15%.[12] The penetration of the cautery loop is 6 mm, thereby increasing risks for erectile dysfunction, scarring, burns, and strictures.[13] Also, water (hypotonic fluid) is used as opposed to normal saline, limiting surgeons to a resection time of 60 minutes, which is the threshold at which most patients who absorb irrigant will avoid significant hyponatremia. However, hyponatremia can still occur, even when strict time limits are observed with TUR syndrome, occurring in approximately 1% to 2% of patients.

Bleeding after TURP is common and expected, with blood transfusion rates reported to be as high as 6.4%. Because of these issues, patients who are anticoagulated and are unable to stop their blood thinners are at risk with TURP and may not be considered candidates for surgical therapy. Lastly, patients who have large prostates (generally >100 g) are often not offered TURP, or may require a staged approach or open surgery. Patients are kept in-house on irrigation until the urine is clear, which generally occurs within 1 to 3 days. Rebleeding is common at 10 to 14 days when the layer of ischemic tissue sloughs, and can be particularly problematic in patients who have returned to therapeutic doses of their blood thinners. These issues, combined with the myriad other potential complications, have led urologists to look for alternative surgical approaches. Thus, laser therapies with their reduced morbidity have emerged to challenge conventional TURP.

OUTCOMES OF HOLMIUM LASER ENUCLEATION OF THE PROSTATE COMPARED WITH TRANSURETHRAL RESECTION OF THE PROSTATE
Urodynamics

In a randomized controlled trial of 61 patients, urodynamic relief of obstruction was better at 6 months in patients undergoing HoLEP compared with TURP. Detrusor pressures (Pdet) at maximum urinary flow (Q_{max}) at 6 months was 20.8 cm H_2O in the HoLEP group compared with 40.7 cm H_2O in the TURP arm ($P<.001$).[14] This effect, however, disappeared by 12 months, because Pdet was comparable between groups. This improved relief in urodynamic obstruction is mostly attributable to greater tissue retrieval with HoLEP compared with TURP. These data are the only ones published, suggesting an advantage of HoLEP over TURP at relieving urodynamically proven obstruction.

A recent systematic review found that although HoLEP had comparable results with TURP regarding International Prostate Symptom Score (IPSS), Quality of life scores, and Q_{max}, it was superior with regard to immediate postoperative parameters, such as duration of catheterization, length of hospitalization, and degree of blood loss.[15] Prostate-specific antigen decrease after HoLEP has been shown to correlate well with the weight of adenoma resected and is a good

surrogate for volume reduction in the absence of transrectal ultrasonography or histology.[16] However, volume assessment using transrectal ultrasound pre- and postoperatively has shown significant reductions in prostate volume after HoLEP.

Length of Operation

In contrast, pooled estimates of difference favored TURP over HoLEP regarding length of operation.[15] The most likely explanation for this observation is twofold. First, early in the evolution of HoLEP, additional time was required for the fragmenting of prostatic tissue into pieces small enough to allow evacuation through the resectoscope sheath,[17] a technical aspect that has drastically improved since the introduction of soft tissue mechanical morcellation.[18] Second, more tissue is resected during HoLEP,[14,19,20] and thus more time is needed. However, once the influence of tissue retrieval (morcellation or irrigation) was accounted for, tissue removal was more efficient in the HoLEP arms.[14]

Histology

The coagulation and vaporization effects of HoLEP are well documented, leading many to question the tissue quality for histopathologic examination and cancer detection. In a prospective study of 80 consecutive tissue specimens, Naspro and colleagues[21] found that tissue quality between techniques were comparable in all respects. In each cohort, rates of incidental prostatic adenocarcinoma and high-grade prostatic intraepithelial neoplasia were similar. The major histologic alterations secondary to resection and coagulation were limited to the external surfaces of enucleated tissues, and architectural and cytologic artifacts were observed without any significant differences between HoLEP and TURP.

Adverse Events

In a systematic review of all adverse events in four well-designed randomized controlled trials, rates of urethral strictures, stress incontinence, blood transfusions, and reinterventions were comparable between the techniques, but the composite complication rate favored HoLEP over TURP (8% vs 16%).[15] Rates of urethral strictures (2%–3%), recatheterization (0%–16%), blood transfusions (0%–1%), urinary retention (5%), reinterventions (0%–2%), and stress incontinence (1%–2%) all tended to be equal or lower in the HoLEP arms compared with TURP.[14,17,19,20] However, bladder mucosal injuries (0%–18%) are higher in HoLEP groups but are usually benign and may reflect differences in surgeon experience.

Transurethral Resection Syndrome

In addition to techniques such as bipolar TURP and other laser modalities, one of the most lauded advantages of HoLEP is its ability to be used with normal saline irrigation, removing the threat of TUR syndrome. In fact, no report of TUR syndrome after HoLEP has been found in the literature. Preoperative weight of prostate, total irrigation time, amount of irrigation fluid used, and weight of resected tissue all directly influence the amount of fluid absorbed during HoLEP.[22] This study showed a drop in hemoglobin, but no change in serum electrolytes. A study by Kuntz and colleagues,[17] however, showed a mild drop in serum sodium of approximately 1.1 mmol/L in the HoLEP arm. Others have found postoperative decreases in serum sodium to be closer to 3 mm/L, although none of these had clinical significance.

LEARNING CURVE/TEACHING

HoLEP and HoLAP provide attractive alternatives to TURP for all the reasons presented. However, although HoLAP is easy to learn and only requires a few cases to become proficient, this is not the case with HoLEP. The HoLEP learning curve is the main impediment to its widespread application, and several studies have looked to better define this issue. The best illustration of the HoLEP learning curve is the observation that enucleation efficiency as defined by grams of tissue enucleated per minute increases proportionally to surgeon experience. Seki and colleagues[23] found that the average enucleation efficiency for the first 10 cases was 0.29 g/min, compared with 0.75 g/min by the 70th case ($P<.01$), suggesting a learning curve of at least 50. El-Hakim and colleagues[24] determined that a senior resident who was supervised by an experienced urologist felt adept with the procedure after 27 cases. Shah and colleagues[25] determined that enucleation efficiency and percentage of tissue resected reached a plateau at 50 cases, suggesting that although most surgeons can perform the procedure earlier, their mastery of the technique takes a bit longer.

These studies and others identify increases in operative and morcellation efficiency/tissue removal, decreases in operative time, intraoperative complications, conversion rates, and improved patient outcomes and comfort with the procedure as end points of the learning curve.[3,23,24]

Shah and colleagues[25] also suggested that urologists can also learn in a largely independent manner. In a prospective cohort study of the first 162 patients treated by a residency-trained urologist who had previously assisted with only four prior HoLEP procedures, complication rates and micturition parameters were similar between early and late cases. The two most technically difficult steps identified were the initial apical enucleation and the incision of the remaining anteroapical mucosal attachment of the lateral lobes.[24,25] The investigators suggested that these initial difficulties were overcome faster with intense review of unedited video recordings and discussions with an expert who could provide guidance in navigating the most technically difficult aspects of the operation.

Although rates of intraoperative and early postoperative complications may have slightly improved with experience, comparisons between their first 50 cases (group 1) and last 62 cases (group 3) showed no significant differences in complications or efficacy parameters (Q_{max}, post-void residual, and American Urological Association scores). Taken together, these data argue that even in self-taught methods of learning, HoLEP has excellent patient safety profiles and acceptable rates of early complications.

Only one study has provided data on long-term outcomes from cases performed during the initial learning curve. In a retrospective analysis of 118 cases, 4 of the first 50 (8%) required reoperation during the 5 years of follow-up, whereas only 1 of the subsequent 68 required reoperation during the same period of follow-up.[26] Rates of urethral stricture, bladder neck contracture, and meatal stenosis were similar among both groups and approximated 1% to 2% at 5 years.

Training programs and proctoring are critical for most urologists. Industry-sponsored standardized training programs have been developed to provide the education, exposure, and teaching that the new HoLEP practitioner requires. In addition, new HoLEP practitioners should perform the procedure regularly to truly maximize learning and decrease complications. In the authors' experience, performing no fewer than two procedures per month is vital. In fact, this number is low, and new practitioners should attempt to perform at least one case a week, or two in one day, to reinforce learning and skills. Urologists who do not have the patient load to maintain regular operative frequency will have a longer learning curve and experience more complications.

HEMOSTASIS AND ANTICOAGULATION

Several studies have examined oral anticoagulation with HoLEP. Elzayat and colleagues[27] published a series on 14 patients who underwent HoLEP while fully therapeutic on oral anticoagulation (mean International Normalized Ratio, 2.0) and reported that two patients (14.2%) required blood transfusions in the postoperative period. In the same study, the authors reported that of 34 patients who underwent low molecular weight heparin substitution for oral anticoagulation before TURP, 5 (14.7%) required blood transfusion compared with only 1 of 33 patients (3%) who discontinued their oral anticoagulation altogether in the preoperative period. The transfusions rates reported by these authors were lower than rates reported in cohort studies performed with TURP, leading the HoLEP researchers to conclude that HoLEP is a safer alternative to TURP in patients at risk for bleeding.

A study performed by the authors of this article showed no transfusions in any of their 76 patients, 13 of whom were taking coumadin and 25 of whom were taking aspirin.[28]

SEXUAL FUNCTION

Only two randomized clinical trials involving HoLEP have specifically addressed sexual function in patients undergoing surgical treatment for BPH.[29,30] Both studies showed a slight postoperative improvement in erectile function as measured by the international index of erectile function (IIEF), a validated sexual function questionnaire. In both studies, however, this finding was statistically insignificant and also true for patients randomized to the TURP and open prostatectomy arms. Furthermore, whether these slight improvements in erectile function are related to the preoperative cessation of finasteride or α-blockers or to an improvement in lower urinary tract symptoms is uncertain.

Briganti and colleagues[30] did, however, uncover a significant deterioration in postoperative orgasmic function for both HoLEP and TURP, as measured with the IIEF. Although comparisons between HoLEP and TURP were statistically insignificant, orgasmic function was decreased at 12 and 24 months after both techniques. This decrease in orgasmic function is believed to be primarily related to the high prevalence of retrograde ejaculation (up to 76% at 6 months).[31,32] Despite the significant decrease in the orgasmic function domain, the other IIEF domains such as intercourse satisfaction, sexual desire, and overall satisfaction were unaffected, indicating that patients do not seem to be bothered by retrograde ejaculation with respect to their overall sexual experience.

SIZE COMPARISONS

Larger prostates take longer to enucleate and morcellate; however, procedure efficiency increases with prostate size, as described by Shah and colleagues[9] Perioperative complications do not vary with size, except for a higher incidence of superficial bladder mucosal injury and stenotic complications in larger prostates, likely related to a longer time of morcellation increasing the chances of bladder injury, and longer duration of urethral instrumentation. Reported outcomes are similar and independent of prostate size; Q_{max}, post-void residual, IPSS, and quality of life score all improved significantly after HoLEP. Postoperative management is similar irrespective of prostate size.

HOLMIUM LASER ENUCLEATION OF THE PROSTATE COMPARED WITH OPEN PROSTATECTOMY

Increasing evidence shows that compared with open prostatectomy, HoLEP is a safer and more economical surgical treatment of large adenomas, particularly in prostates larger than 100 g. In a well-designed, randomized trial of 120 patients, HoLEP was found to have lower perioperative morbidity than open prostatectomy; no differences were seen in micturition parameters, sexual function, or continence.[33]

Despite an increase in operating time (136 vs 91 min) and overall lower tissue retrieval (84 vs 96 g), HoLEP was associated with shorter hospitalizations (70 vs 251 h), and shorter durations of catheterization (31 vs 194 h). The mean decrease in hemoglobin was also lower in the HoLEP cohort (1.9 vs 2.8 g/dL; $P<.0001$), and no patient required blood transfusion (compared with 13% in the open prostatectomy arm). Regarding micturition parameters (post-void residual, Q_{max}, and IPSS), no differences were identified between groups up to 5 years follow-up.[34] A separate and slightly smaller randomized controlled trial (n = 81) found that bladder mucosal injuries and postoperative dysuria were higher in the HoLEP groups ($P<.001$), but all other perioperative data were comparable.[29] Taken together, these findings suggest some short- and long-term advantages of HoLEP over open prostatectomy, especially when treating large prostates.

In addition to lower perioperative morbidity and long-term efficacy that is similar to open prostatectomy, some data suggest that HoLEP is more economical than open prostatectomy.[35] A relatively recent hospitalization economic impact study found that average perioperative costs in U.S. dollars associated with HoLEP and open prostatectomy were $2356.50 and $2868.90, respectively (excluding the salaries of the urologist and anesthetist). The costs related to the use of the operating room were higher in the HoLEP group, constituting 25% of the total cost of HoLEP (compared with 16% for open prostatectomy). The average operating room set-up/disposables/fiber costs were significantly less in the open prostatectomy group. Despite this, HoLEP offered a overall perioperative net cost savings of 9.6%, which was mostly attributable to the shorter hospital stays.

SUMMARY

Holmium laser applications of the prostate are safe and efficacious. Although HoLAP is easy to learn, once HoLEP is mastered, the technique is straightforward. Patient outcomes are at least comparable with other transurethral approaches; the less-invasive nature of HoLEP provides potential advantages over open techniques. The steep learning curve for HoLEP should be viewed as what would be expected in mastering any new endoscopic or laparoscopic surgical technique. Preceptorships are essential to avoid some of the pitfalls, or at least to learn how to negotiate them once encountered. Experts who use HoLEP find the procedure enjoyable, surgically enhancing in regard to skills, and superior to other methods of prostate reduction. The authors believe HoLEP is a size-independent gold standard. When indicated, HoLAP is easy and likewise rewarding with excellent clinical outcomes.

REFERENCES

1. Costello AJ, Bowsher WG, Bolton DM, et al. Laser ablation of the prostate in patients with benign prostatic hypertrophy. Br J Urol 1992;69(6):603–8.
2. Gilling PJ, Cass CB, Malcolm AR, et al. Combination holmium and Nd:YAG laser ablation of the prostate: initial clinical experience. J Endourol 1995;9(2):151–3.
3. Gilling PJ, Kennett K, Das AK, et al. Holmium laser enucleation of the prostate (HoLEP) combined with transurethral tissue morcellation: an update on the early clinical experience. J Endourol 1998;12(5):457–9.
4. Tanagho EA, McAninch JW, editors. Smith's general urology. 17th edition. Lange Medical Books/McGraw Hill; 2008. p. 354–5.
5. AUA guidelines on the management of benign prostatic hyperplasia: diagnosis and treatment recommendations. American Urological Association Education and Research, Inc, 2003. Available at: www.auanet.org. Accessed July 30, 2009.
6. Te AE. The development of laser prostatectomy. BJU Int 2004;93:262–5.
7. Jansen ED, van Leeuwen TG, Motamedi M, et al. Temperature dependence of the absorption coefficient of water for midinfrared laser radiation. Lasers Surg Med 1994;14:258–68.
8. Kuo RL, Paterson RF, Siqueira TM Jr, et al. Holmium laser enucleation of the prostate: morbidity in a series of 206 patients. Urology 2003;62(1):59–63.
9. Shah HN, Mahajan AP, Hegde SS, et al. Peri-operative complications of holmium laser enucleation of the prostate: experience in the first 280 patients, and a review of literature. BJU Int 2007;100(1):94–101.
10. Elhilali MM. Editorial comment: day-case holmium laser enucleation of the prostate for gland volumes of <60 mL: early experience. BJU Int 2003;91:64.
11. Elzayat EA, Habib EI, Elhilali MM. Holmium laser enucleation of the prostate: a size-independent new 'gold standard'. Urology 2005;66(Suppl 5):108–13.
12. Mebust WK, Holtgrewe HL, Cockett AT, et al. Transurethral prostatectomy: immediate and postoperative complications. A cooperative study of 13 participating institutions evaluating 3,885 patients. J Urol 1989;141:243–7.
13. Barba M, Fastenmeier K, Hartung R. Electrocautery: principles and practice. J Endourol 2003;17(8): 541–55.
14. Tan AH, Gilling PJ, Kennett KM, et al. A randomized trial comparing holmium laser enucleation of the prostate with transurethral resection of the prostate for the treatment of bladder outlet obstruction secondary to benign prostatic hyperplasia in large glands (40 to 200 grams). J Urol 2003;170(4 Pt 1):1270–4.
15. Tan A, Liao C, Mo Z, et al. Meta-analysis of holmium laser enucleation versus transurethral resection of the prostate for symptomatic prostatic obstruction. Br J Surg 2007;94(10):1201–8.
16. Tinmouth WW, Habib E, Kim SC, et al. Change in serum prostate specific antigen concentration after holmium laser enucleation of the prostate: a marker for completeness of adenoma resection? J Endourol 2005;19(5):550–4.
17. Kuntz RM, Ahyai S, Lehrich K, et al. Transurethral holmium laser enucleation of the prostate versus transurethral electrocautery resection of the prostate: a randomized prospective trial in 200 patients. J Urol 2004;172(3):1012–6.
18. Tan AH, Gilling PJ. Holmium laser prostatectomy: current techniques. Urology 2002;60(1):152–6.
19. Montorsi F, Naspro R, Salonia A, et al. Holmium laser enucleation versus transurethral resection of the prostate: results from a 2-center, prospective, randomized trial in patients with obstructive benign prostatic hyperplasia. J Urol 2004;172(5 Pt 1):1926–9.
20. Gupta N, Sivaramakrishna, Kumar R, et al. Comparison of standard transurethral resection, transurethral vapour resection and holmium laser enucleation of the prostate for managing benign prostatic hyperplasia of >40 g. BJU Int 2006;97(1):85–9.

21. Naspro R, Freschi M, Salonia A, et al. Holmium laser enucleation versus transurethral resection of the prostate. Are histological findings comparable? J Urol 2004;171(3):1203–6.

22. Shah HN, Kausik V, Hegde S, et al. Evaluation of fluid absorption during holmium laser enucleation of prostate by breath ethanol technique. J Urol 2006;175(2):537–40.

23. Seki N, Mochida O, Kinukawa N, et al. Holmium laser enucleation for prostatic adenoma: analysis of learning curve over the course of 70 consecutive cases. J Urol 2003;170(5):1847–50.

24. El-Hakim A, Elhilali MM. Holmium laser enucleation of the prostate can be taught: the first learning experience. BJU Int 2002;90(9):863–9.

25. Shah HN, Mahajan AP, Sodha HS, et al. Prospective evaluation of the learning curve for holmium laser enucleation of the prostate. J Urol 2007;177(4):1468–74.

26. Elzayat EA, Elhilali MM. Holmium laser enucleation of the prostate (HoLEP): long-term results, reoperation rate, and possible impact of the learning curve. Eur Urol 2007;52(5):1465–71.

27. Elzayat E, Habib E, Elhilali M. Holmium laser enucleation of the prostate on anticoagulant therapy or with bleeding disorders. J Urol 2006;175:1428–32.

28. Tyson MD, Lerner LB. Safety of holmium laser enucleation of the prostate in anticoagulated patients. J Endourol 2009;23(8):1343–6.

29. Naspro R, Suardi N, Salonia A, et al. Holmium laser enucleation of the prostate versus open prostatectomy for prostates >70 g: 24-month follow-up. Eur Urol 2006;50(3):563–8.

30. Briganti A, Naspro R, Gallina A, et al. Impact on sexual function of holmium laser enucleation versus transurethral resection of the prostate: results of a prospective, 2-center, randomized trial. J Urol 2006;175(5):1817–21.

31. Gilling PJ, Aho TF, Frampton CM, et al. Holmium laser enucleation of the prostate: results at 6 years. Eur Urol 2008;53(4):744–9.

32. Meng F, Gao B, Fu Q, et al. Change of sexual function in patients before and after Ho:YAG laser enucleation of the prostate. J Androl 2007;28(2):259–61.

33. Kuntz RM, Lehrich K. Transurethral holmium laser enucleation versus transvesical open enucleation for prostate adenoma greater than 100 gm.: a randomized prospective trial of 120 patients. J Urol 2002;168(4 Pt 1):1465–9.

34. Kuntz RM, Lehrich K, Ahyai SA. Holmium laser enucleation of the prostate versus open prostatectomy for prostates greater than 100 grams: 5-year follow-up results of a randomized clinical trial. Eur Urol 2008;53:160–8.

35. Salonia A, Suardi N, Naspro R, et al. Holmium laser enucleation versus open prostatectomy for benign prostatic hyperplasia: an inpatient cost analysis. Urology 2006;68(2):302–6.

Minimally Invasive Therapy of Lower Urinary Tract Symptoms

Robert F. Donnell, MD

KEYWORDS

- Benign prostate hyperplasia
- Lower urinary tract symptoms • TUMT • TUNA • Botox

MINIMALLY INVASIVE THERAPIES

The establishment of guidelines, pharmacologic therapies, improved understanding of lower urinary tract symptoms (LUTS) versus benign prostate hyperplasia (BPH), respect for patient-centered goals, and improved discrimination of the patient with occult prostate cancer[1] have empowered change in the management of LUTS. These new tools have allowed urologists to act on the recognized limitations of transurethral prostatectomy (TURP) as a historical gold standard and search for "ideal therapies" that provide durable, noninvasive treatments with an improved relief of symptoms at a decreased complication rate and cost and that simultaneously correct BPH-associated morbidities. Requisite to the chronic, progressive nature of BPH, the ideal therapy would also prevent future BPH-associated morbidities.[2] These ideal therapies are not practical at this point in the evolution of therapy, thus the current goal of interventional therapy is to restore the comfort and well-being of patients.[3]

Symptom progression is the bane of any treatment modality and is the most common manifestation of the progressive nature of BPH. Once a patient demonstrates symptom progression beyond watchful waiting or pharmaceutical therapy he requires counseling to evaluate appropriate treatment options in light of age-related risks, comorbid medical conditions, and the complexities associated with multiple medications.[4] Potential risk factors have been identified for symptom progression, urinary retention, and prostate surgery such as prostate-specific antigen (PSA),[5–7] obstructive symptom score,[5,6] bother score,[6] prostate volume,[6,7] decreased flow rate,[6] and increased postvoid residual (PVR)[6] and transitional zone volume.[5] Prostate volume and PSA were the best predictors of acute urinary retention, and PSA was the best predictor of prostate surgery (for all indications).[7] Emerging literature suggests a relationship between the metabolic syndrome and the development of BPH, with a 56% increased total prostate annual growth rate and a 34% increased transition zone annual growth rate noted in men with metabolic syndrome compared with men without the metabolic syndrome.[8] Prognostic parameters and their ability to predict progression may be important in the future of LUTS management and selection of therapy.

Patient selection for therapy has been difficult to assess in light of different patient expectations, payer sources, health care resources, and the evolution of technology. There is evidence that in the United States, the majority of men in a commercially available insurance plan chose watchful waiting in the first year, 18.7% of men chose an α-blocker, and only 2% of men chose a surgical or minimally invasive therapy.[9] Race and social economic status may also play a role in patient treatment selection based on studies reporting that surgical intervention was more common in black men[10] and black beneficiaries were 17% less likely to receive minimally invasive surgical treatment (MIST) than whites in 2005.[11]

The author has no disclosures.

The Department of Urology, The Medical College of Wisconsin, 9200 W. Wisconsin Avenue, Milwaukee, WI 53226, USA

E-mail address: rdonnell@mcw.edu

Urol Clin N Am 36 (2009) 497–509
doi:10.1016/j.ucl.2009.08.003
0094-0143/09/$ – see front matter © 2009 Published by Elsevier Inc.

Octogenarians have a significantly increased rate of surgical complications compared with younger patients (39% vs 22%, P<.05) and would theoretically benefit from minimally invasive therapies. However, the most frequent indications for surgery in octogenarians are urinary retention (55% of octogenarians vs 38% of younger men) or gross hematuria (7% vs 1.2%) and these indications are not associated with minimally invasive therapies as often as LUTS (38% of octogenarians vs 59% of younger men).[12] There is evidence that the skill set of the urologist plays a significant role in the management options offered to patients as practitioners closer to completion of their residency training are more likely to include a minimally invasive technique. The most common minimally invasive therapies offered were transurethral microwave thermotherapy (TUMT) (55%) and transurethral needle ablation (TUNA) (33%).[13]

A review of Medicare data from 1999 to 2005 indicated that the net result of all these influences resulted in a 44% increase in the total BPH procedures driven by a 529% increase in the number of MISTs (from 11,582 to 72,887). These data correspond to a 439% increase in the rate of MIST procedures from 136 to 678 procedures per 100,000 males during this period. During this same period the TURP rate decreased approximately 5% per year and by 2005 TURP accounted for only 39% of the surgical treatment procedures and MIST procedures accounted for 57%.[11] Age, anesthetic risk, grade of obstruction, prostate volume, serum PSA value, treatment-related complication rate, presence of an indwelling catheter, and neurologic disorders should be taken into consideration when choosing an appropriate treatment.[14]

TUMT

Microwave as a therapy for the prostate has evolved since first introduced by Yerushalmi and colleagues in 1985.[15] Microwave frequencies fall within the range of 300 to 3000 MHz and are absorbed as they propagate through tissue, producing changes in the tissue that result in heat. Analogous to ultrasound, higher frequencies do not penetrate the tissue so deeply. Similar to ultrasound, increasing the energy output (capacity to perform work) of the microwave signal increases the amount of power (work/time) that irradiates the tissue. When the prostate tissue absorbs this energy, heat is produced, thus the more energy absorbed, the greater the heat created. In TUMT, an external power source creates microwaves between the frequencies of 900 and 1100 MHz. All approved units employ a microwave antenna incorporated into a urethral catheter. Continued improvement in antenna design has refined the focus of the energy within the prostate transition zone, and resultant treatment temperatures have progressed sequentially from less than 45°C (hyperthermia) to greater than 45°C (thermotherapy) (the minimum temperature to destroy prostate cells reliably), to temperatures greater than 70°C (thermoablation). Thermoablation produces cavities in the prostate and is reported to result in greater improvements in symptoms and objective parameters. The goal of microwave therapy is to provide efficacious treatment with less patient risk than that of TURP.

Patients who are potential candidates for TUMT should meet the criteria for treatment according to the American Urological Association (AUA) guidelines for BPH.[16] This would include men with moderate-to-severe LUTS of BPH who failed medical therapy, do not want medical therapy, or cannot or will not consider surgery. A patient's decision to undergo TUMT is typically determined by his perceived balance between a one-time method requiring minimal anesthetic, reduced risks compared with TURP, and an improved efficacy compared with medical therapy. However, urologists must recognize that there is an array of microwave devices and that these design differences affect appropriate patient selection. Urologists must be familiar with factors such as antenna length and design that determine the location of the preferential focus and the minimum and maximum size of the prostate that can be reliably treated.

The rapid evolution of technology and the inherent differences in device design preclude grouping outcomes of all devices into a single conclusion without careful understanding of the individual device characteristics. For example, the limited energy output of the Prostasoft 2.0 produced an initial symptomatic improvement, but the objective parameters failed to improve compared with baseline, and up to 66% of men required supplemental treatment.[17–19] In contrast, the higher energy output of the Prostasoft 3.5 was associated with a decrease in the international prostatic symptom score (IPSS) of 11 points (from 20 to 9.3) and an increase in the maximum urinary flow rate of 5 mL/s (9.4 mL/s to 14.6 mL/s) at 6 months after treatment.[20] The higher energy microwave was also associated with a longer indwelling urinary catheter time of 18 days but was not associated with serious complications. Additional investigators[21] have noted similar improvements with other higher energy devices (Targis, Prostate Solutions Inc.), reporting significant symptomatic improvement up to 24 months.

In these studies, the mean maximum flow rate increased from 7.3 mL/s to 14.5 mL/s at 6 months, the mean PVR decreased from 199 mL to 34.8 mL at 6 months, and both parameters remained stable at 12 months. The authors also noted that the prostate volume decreased from 57 cm^3 to 42 cm^3, cavitation was observed in 77% of patients and only 13% of patients required retreatment within 1 year. High-energy devices also allowed clinicians to expand the indications for the device. Originally, TUMT was thought to be insufficient therapy for patients presenting with urinary retention despite the general patient characteristics most attractive to the use of a minimally invasive therapy. Many of these patients were older, had a larger prostate volume, and had more surgical comorbidities. However, the high-energy TUMT devices have reported a catheter-free rate of 82% to 91% in selected patients, although most also must continue medical therapy.

Although it can be difficult to recruit patients to sham controlled and randomized clinical trials, a limited number of these studies involving TUMT are available. When compared with sham (the catheter was placed but the antenna was not powered), there was a reported average decrease in symptom scores of 11 points (compared with 5 points with sham) at 6 months in 220 patients.[22] When high-energy TUMT was compared with terazosin (52 participants), the literature indicates that α-blockers provide a more rapid improvement in IPSS, peak flow, and quality of life (QOL) at 2 weeks compared with TUMT, although by 4 months TUMT demonstrated superior outcomes (IPSS score 35%, Q_{max} 22%, QOL 43% better in TUMT compared with α-blockers), was associated with fewer adverse events (7 of 51) compared with α-blockers (17 of 52), and TUMT maintained its effectiveness compared with terazosin for at least 18 months.[23] Newer α-blockers are associated with fewer side effects and a randomized investigation of neoadjuvant and adjuvant α-blockade combined with TUMT demonstrated highly significant improvement in symptoms as early as 2 weeks after therapy compared with TUMT alone, and at 12 weeks the 2 groups exhibited comparable symptom reduction. Thus, earlier relief of symptoms may be possible and may improve patient satisfaction with TUMT.[24]

When compared with the historical gold standard, TURP, the magnitude and durability of the symptom score and the maximum flow rate improvements were greater after TURP.[25] However, TURP was associated with a 9.4% to 19.9% complication rate, and required an anesthetic, postoperative hospitalization, and a 2% yearly re-operation rate. In contrast, TUMT resulted in a lower incidence of retrograde ejaculation, erectile dysfunction, TURP syndrome, clot retention, transfusion requirement, was rarely was associated with strictures but had a 7% yearly re-operation rate, and the average catheter time with high-energy TUMT was 3 to 14 days.[26,27] Similarly, the ProstaLund Feedback Treatment (ProstaLund Operations AB, Uppsala, Sweden) has been compared with TURP and has not shown inferior outcomes, but selection and reporting bias and a limited number of patients inhibit meaningful use of these data.[28] Few trials have directly compared TUMT with other minimally invasive procedures,[29] although short-term studies of individual procedures suggest similar improvement in symptoms and flow rate.[30]

Limitations imposed by the lack of large-scale multi-institution trials were addressed in a pooled analysis of 6 multicenter studies of cooled thermotherapy, involving 541 men whose baseline measures were comparable across the studies.[32–35] At 3 months, the AUA symptom score had improved by a mean of 11.6 (55%), Q_{max} by a mean of 4.0 (51%), and QOL by a mean of 2.3 (53%). These improvements were maintained for 48 months with only slight attenuation (corresponding mean changes of 43%, 35%, and 50%) and were highly statistically significant ($P<.0001$–0.01). A satisfactory level of improvement (at least 25%) was observed at all points in more than 85% of patients for AUA symptom score and QOL and in more than 65% of patients for Q_{max}.[31] This large, long-term pooled analysis confirms the results observed for TUMT in smaller and shorter-term studies.

There is evidence that TUMT results in relatively small changes in PSA (mean decrease of 0.27 ng/mL at 1 year) and prostate volume (mean decrease of 3.80 cm^3 at 1 year), supporting the concept that prostate volume reduction is not a significant factor in symptom relief and that prostate function is unaltered after TUMT. In the absence of a well-defined mechanism of action and the observation that TUMT is associated with an increased retreatment rate compared with TURP it becomes clear that prognostic parameters indicating long-term response are critical to the success of this technology. Ideally, these parameters that would improve patient selection because they would predict men at risk for retreatment and thus reduce the risks and expense associated with exposure to serial treatments. When investigators examined the prognostic value of age, PSA, and prostate volume, they found that improvement occurred in all subgroups of patients, but a PSA level greater than 4 ng/mL was observed to predict an unsatisfactory symptom score and maximum urinary flow rate at 3 or more years in patients who initially demonstrated a satisfactory response to treatment. For the first time, the authors offered prognostic indicators for eventual failure in the patient after initial success, adding to the previous studies where PSA was an identified risk for deterioration in symptoms and flow rate,[36] episodes of acute urinary retention,[7,37] and prostate growth in all response groups.[38] Logically, patients with elevated baseline PSA levels may need more careful long-term follow-up to assess the need for retreatment.

During the procedure patients commonly experience mild perineal warmth, mild pain, and a sense of urinary urgency. However, only 5% of patients reported their pain as being severe during Targis therapy. It is the authors' experience that all patients required a prostate anesthetic block and pretreatment oral analgesics.

The main risks of TUMT include urinary retention,[39] infection (1%–13%), and postoperative pain. The increased risk for infection following TUMT may be related to the length of catheter dwell time and necrotic tissue sloughing. Erectile dysfunction following TUMT appears to be related to the energy protocol of the device used, with higher-energy TUMT protocols resulting in a greater incidence of erectile dysfunction (18.2%) compared with low-energy protocols (no reported incidence).[29,40] Retrograde ejaculation occurs less often in TUMT compared with the reported rate for TURP (0%–28% of patients after TUMT, 48%–90% of patients after TURP). Overall, patients' sexual satisfaction appears to be greater among those who have undergone TUMT rather than TURP, with 55% of patients undergoing microwave thermotherapy reported as being very satisfied, compared with a 21% rate among patients after TURP.[39] Clinicians are cautioned that the risk of acute myocardial infarction is not negligible using TUMT. TURP and TUMT are associated with a higher incidence of mortality caused by acute myocardial infarction, (especially more than 2 years after therapy) compared with the general population.[41] A recent report also indicates that the risk of hypertension and cerebrovascular accident is also increased with TUMT.[42] Other rare complications have been reported following TUMT; these include, but are not limited to, bladder perforation, bowel irradiation, chronic pain, urethral injury, prostatitis, urethral tear, anal irritation, and urethral stricture. Some patients have experienced serious injuries following TUMT, including damage to the penis and urethra, and have required colostomies or partial amputation of the penis. In December 2000, the US Food and Drug Administration issued a warning about these injuries[43,44] and identified the following risk factors that may contribute to these side effects;

- Incorrect placement or undetected migration of the treatment catheter or the rectal temperature sensors
- Failure of the physician to remain with the patient throughout the entire treatment duration
- Failure to pause treatment when the patient is communicating serious pain
- Oversedation of the patient, which compromises his ability to communicate pain
- Treatment of patients who have undergone prior radiation therapy to the pelvic area
- Treatment of patients whose prostate sizes are outside the ranges specified in the labeling
- Leakage from the balloons used to retain the urethral catheter or the rectal temperature sensor in the correct anatomic position

Of all nonablative thermal therapies, TUMT is the best documented.[45] The literature has reported that TUMT is safe when properly supervised by a physician and is an effective minimally invasive alternative treatment for symptomatic BPH. TUMT can be performed in a 1- to 2-hour office visit without intravenous sedation, but the urologist must be cognizant of the reports concerning myocardial infarction, hypertension, and stroke when using this therapy as an alternative for patients who are at high surgical and anesthetic risk. It is not effective for patients with a large median lobe or a very large prostate, and it results in less significant improvement in urinary flow patterns than TURP. Cost-effectiveness analysis has suggested that TUMT has lower costs,[46] but long-term analysis of the cost-benefit scheme in light of the risk for serial treatments is required.

TUNA OF THE PROSTATE

TUNA of the prostate radiates radiofrequency (RF) energy to create heat in the target tissue, resulting in coagulation necrosis. The RF energy is a 456-kHz signal compared with frequencies in the megahertz range for microwave, and this lower frequency is responsible for the differences in tissue interaction, including a greater depth of penetration of tissue. The radiated energy, the duration of treatment, the size of the electrodes, and the depth of the electrode are adjusted to create the desired prostate lesion, therefore clinicians are cautioned not simply to compare the power levels (5–10 W)[47] used in RF to microwave therapies. The delivery system uses a 22F rigid cystoscope system to deploy 2 needles at a 90° angle from the axis of the cystoscope and a 40° angle from each other. The needles are covered with insulated sheaths that protect the prostate urethra yet allow the physician to vary the depth of the penetration of the exposed portion of the needle. The RF energy creates temperatures of 70 to 110°C, and treatment times are 2.5 to 3 minutes per lesion. The prostate is treated every 1 to 1.5 cm along the length of the prostate gland. Because the prostate urethra is insulated from the RF energy, the pain-sensitive region is preserved, which is believed to be critical to minimize anesthesia requirements and reduce postoperative complications of irritative voiding and hematuria. Histologically, the Precision Plus TUNA unit (Boston Scientific, Natick, MA, USA) produced a coagulation defect with necrosis that ranged from 1.2 cm by 0.7 cm to 1.7 cm by 1 cm. The current product release (Prostiva, Medtronic, Minneapolis, MN, USA) is designed to create similar lesions in a shorter period of time when compared with the original TUNA device. Gadolinium-enhanced magnetic resonance imaging at 1 week following treatment demonstrated that the lesions produced by Prostiva are consistent with necrosis, the lesions were prominent in the bladder neck and lateral lobes but still confined to the prostate, and the mean lesion volume was 7.56 cm³ or 11.28% of the mean prostate volume from this series. Thus, continued product development appears to have shortened treatment time required to produce comparable ablative lesions,[48] which is beneficial given the need to tolerate the rigid cystoscope.

Similar to TUMT, TUNA of the prostate is most commonly used (1) when pharmaceutical therapy no longer provides sufficient relief and (2) as a primary therapy for the patient who is not interested in medical therapy and unwilling to undergo a TURP. Two articles[49,50] detail the outcomes for RF ablation for men with urinary retention; although the total number of men treated was only 58, 78% to 79% of men were treated successfully.

Approved devices for RF ablation of the prostate are available from a single manufacturer, and the manufacturer's published indications for use include men older than 50 years with prostate sizes between 20 and 50 cm.[51] The early outcome reports for TUNA of the prostate indicated symptom score improvement, increased peak urinary flow rate, and decreased post-void residuals at 2-year follow-up that exceeded outcomes expected from medical therapy,[52] but short-term follow-up identified that 4 to 25% of patients in several small series (range 30–45 patients, total

216 patients) required TURP as a rescue therapy.[49,50,53,54] Subsequent reports from Zlotta[49] reported the baseline characteristics with a mean follow-up of 63 months for a multicenter study involving 188 consecutive patients with symptomatic BPH treated with the TUNA II or TUNA III catheters under local anesthesia. The mean IPSS improved from 20.9 to 8.7 ($P<.001$) and 78% of men experienced at least 50% improvement; the mean urinary peak flow rate increased from 8.6 mL/s to 12.1 mL/s ($P<.01$, t-test), and 24% of men experienced at least a 50% improvement. The mean PVRs decreased from 179 mL to 122 mL (both $P<.001$). The term RF ablation implies the destruction of significant volumes of tissue, yet the mean prostate volume and PSA levels did not change significantly (53.9 vs 53.8 cm³ and 3.3 vs 3.6 ng/mL, respectively at 5 years, both P values >0.05, t-test). Rescue therapies included medical treatment in 12 patients (6.4%), a second TUNA in 7 patients (3.7%), and surgery in 22 of 186 patients (11.1%). Of these patients, 23.3% required additional treatment at 5-year follow-up following the original TUNA procedure.[55] The American counterpart to Zlotta's European study also detailed the outcomes and durability of TUNA 5 years after treatment.[56] Patients treated with TUNA had statistically significant improvement at all annual evaluations compared with baseline data in the 5-year follow-up. At 5 years, IPSS scores decreased from 24 to 10.7, QOL scores improved from 11.8 to 3.8, and peak flow rate improved from 8.8 mL/s to 11.4 mL/s.

Subsequent international studies concerning men who had failed medical therapy before TUNA echoed the higher need for retreatment with RF ablation of the prostate. Rosario and colleagues[57] reported the 10-year follow-up for 71 men in whom treatment failure was defined as an impaired QOL caused by LUTS or progression of LUTS requiring additional therapy. The authors reported a failure rate of 83% at a median of 20 months, although 20% of men realized adequate relief from α-blockers once again when the α-blocker therapy was resumed. According to this report only 17% of men remained symptom free up to 10 years after TUNA of the prostate. Of those men who required intervention after TUNA, 46% underwent TURP, 3% underwent incision of the bladder neck, and only one participant selected another minimally invasive therapy. In contrast to earlier reports of the potential 40% to 50% cost savings attributed to TUNA versus TURP,[58] and the similar costs of TUNA compared with a 5-year regimen of single drug therapy (with 5α-reductase inhibitor or tamsulosin therapy),[59] the authors concluded that in the long term, the serial treatments following TUNA increased the cost of health.[60] This report supported an earlier meta-analysis of 35 studies (9 comparative, 26 noncomparative) that concluded the long-term failure rate of TUNA is significantly greater than TURP (odds ratio (OR) 7.44 [2.47, 22.43]). The authors concluded that the body of evidence that supported the introduction of TUNA into clinical practice was of moderate- to low quality, thus the role of TUNA in the care of the BPH patient and its cost-effectiveness could not be well defined.[61] More recent reports have questioned the cost-effectiveness of all minimally invasive therapies, not only TUNA, although the models used were valid for the health system in the United Kingdom.[62] Of the TUNA cases in the United States, 86% seem to be performed in office-based clinics in contrast with practice patterns in Europe,[11,45] which needs to be considered when interpreting costs of care. In summary, more recent data suggest that the long-term outcomes for TUNA of the prostate may not be so durable as the outcomes achieved with TURP, and the cost of therapy may be controversial, but the decreased morbidity makes TUNA a useful treatment option in select patients.

TUNA often relieves BPH symptoms within 2 to 6 weeks and most patients are able to resume regular activity in 24 to 72 hours. Postoperative urinary retention is reported in 13% to 41% of patients and typically resolves in 48 to 72 hours. A second period of catheterization may be required in 12% of patients. Patients often do not notice improvement in their voiding symptoms for 2 to 6 weeks,[58] and may require 2 to 3 months to realize significant relief of symptoms.

Side Effects

- Irritative voiding symptoms occur in up to 40% of patients, are typically self-limiting, and often resolve in 7 days but may last as long as 4 weeks
- Dysuria
- Urinary retention
- Hematuria
- Urethral stricture rate less than 2%
- The incidence of erectile dysfunction is rare (<2%)
- Impotence is reported in approximately 3% of patients, and deterioration in function is reported slightly more often
- Urinary incontinence is not reported
- Little evidence suggests that retrograde ejaculation occurs; marginal decreases in ejaculatory fluid are reported

INJECTION THERAPY

Injection of therapeutic material into the prostate was first investigated more than 100 years ago. Injecting therapeutic agents into the prostate for the relief of LUTS caused by BPH is intriguing. The technology would theoretically allow physicians to select a therapeutic agent or combination of agents to target specific patient factors such as excessive growth (static component), increased smooth muscle tone (dynamic component), or altered innervation. In addition, dosing based on prostate volume may treat a wider range of patients, and the technology required is already commonly employed. Ethanol is the most extensively studied injectable to date.[63] Studies concerning ethanol are clinically based, and typically involve small numbers of patients. Goya and colleagues[64] reported outcomes of 34 patients with a mean prostate volume of 49.3 cm^3 who were followed for a median of 4.3 years. Dehydrated ethanol (mean dose 6.4 mL) was injected into the prostate with endoscopic guidance after combined sacral and urethral anesthesia. Patients required catheterization for a mean of 7.6 days. Patients demonstrated a statistically significant decrease in mean IPSS (21.8 points to 13.1 points) and the mean QOL index decreased from 5.0 points before injection to 2.8 points after 3 years ($P<.001$); however, this was not an "intent to treat" analysis and data for 17 patients were not included. The improvements in mean peak urine flow rate (8.3 mL/s before injection to 12.7 mL/s after therapy) and decreased mean residual urine volume (93 mL to 28 mL after injection) were significant, with results that exceeded those expected of medical therapies. The prostate volume did not vary significantly in the 3-year follow-up. There were no major complications and after 3 years of follow-up 59.0% of patients did not require additional therapy. Mutaguchi and colleagues[65] also reported successful outcomes in a smaller series of Japanese men, although approximately 25% of the men in this series had known prostate cancer and larger prostate glands, which may influence differences in their findings that the prostate volume decreased 28.1% at 6 months (statistically significant) unlike previous studies. The mean injected ethanol volume was 22.7% of the prostate volume, which was similar to Goya's study and did not account for the discrepancy. More recent studies concerning transurethral ethanol injection in men with high-risk comorbidities and persistent symptoms or retention support the outcomes noted in earlier studies and report statistically significant improvements in IPSS score and QOL scores, mean PFRs (6.0

pretreatment to 15.2 mL/min), and PVR (baseline value of 290.6 ± 14.14 mL to 4.2 ± 14.10 mL) at 1-year follow-up (P<.001).[66]

Following the initial success reported in smaller trials, Grise and colleagues[67] reported a multi-center, prospective, European study involving 115 men treated with a specialized injection system, the ProstaJect (AMS, Minnetonka, MN, USA). The treatment dosages were based on prostate volume, prostatic urethral length, and presence of a median lobe. At 12 months, follow-up data were available for 94 men, and similar to Goya's study, the average prostate volume was 45.9 cm[3], but the average volume of ethanol injected was 14 mL, which is approximately 30% of prostate volume. The improvements in IPSS and QOL at 1-year follow-up were significant and had decreased by more than 50%. The average peak urinary flow rate (which had improved by 35%) was sustained through 12-month follow-up and the average prostate volume reduction was 16%. Postoperatively, 98% of patients voided spontaneously 4 days following treatment. Adverse events included pain or irritative voiding symptoms in 26% of patients, hematuria in 16%, with retrograde ejaculation, and erectile dysfunction in less than 3% of patients. During the 1-year follow-up, 7% of patients required TURP. Two patients experienced serious adverse events (bladder necrosis) requiring urinary diversion and a ureteral implantation. As a result the injection procedure was modified, and the needle placement was moved more distally in the prostate urethra and away from the bladder neck. Similar to other therapies, the improvement in outcome parameters did not correlate with the reduction in prostate volume, suggesting that the mechanism of action is not limited to relief of the mechanical component of BPH. Similar reports describing specialized injection systems and randomly assigned doses of 15%, 25%, or 40% of prostate volume by transrectal ultrasound also found statistically significant improvements in symptom score, urine flow rate, and PVRs at 6 months following injection. The authors did not identify a dose-related response to injection therapy. Although the authors report that adverse events were generally mild or moderate, the prevalence of side effects was noteworthy, including hematuria (42.9%), irritative voiding symptoms (40.3%), pain/discomfort (25.6%), and urinary retention (22.1%), but no serious adverse events.[68]

Accurate control of the injected volume would theoretically improve the injection process. Investigators[69] combined a custom polymer whose viscosity improved the visibility of the injected material under ultrasound, inhibited runback along the needle, and prevented spread to extraprostatic tissue. The authors tested injecting gel (3% polymer and 97% ethanol) using a volume comparable to previous studies (21.5% of prostate volume) with the transrectal, transurethral, and transperineal approaches. The improvements in the IPSS, QOL scores, and maximum urinary flow rates were statistically significant for all approaches, but the transrectal and the transperineal routes were well tolerated under local anesthetic, which was a significant advantage compared with the spinal anesthesia required for the transurethral route. There were no extraprostatic injuries or adverse effects.

A case report has indicated that it is possible to develop bladder calculus as a result of calcification of sloughed tissue from the prostate after ethanol injection.[70]

BOTULINUM TOXIN

Most injectants produce prostate necrosis but prostate gland volume reduction is controversial and the degree of LUTS relief varies. Anhydrous ethanol was the most widely studied injectable, but large-scale trials identified significant side effects, leaving the field to continue to search for other effective agents.[71]

The potential for an intraprostatic injection of botulinum toxin-A (Botox-A) to provide relief of LUTS caused by BPH was first studied in the rat prostate and demonstrated selective denervation and prostate atrophy at all doses of Botox.[72,73] Later studies demonstrated increased apoptotic activity in the glandular and the stromal component of the prostatic tissue.[74] There are seven botulinum neurotoxins and all block acetylcholine release presynaptically in the neuromuscular junction, which results in a temporary denervation, but each toxin subtype produces different durations of paralysis determined by the different half-life of each subtype.[75] The onset of muscle weakness occurs within a few days, reaches maximal effect within 2 weeks, then decreases after several more weeks to a stable level of symptoms. Recovery from Botox requires resprouting of terminals from the axon, followed by slow recovery of the ability of the neuron to release acetylcholine.[76,77] The Botox dose affects the intensity of denervation and the duration of the initial and plateau periods.[76,78–81]

Maria and colleagues[82] reported the results of a randomized placebo-controlled study in 30 consecutive men with BPH comparing 4 mL of saline solution in 15 men versus 200 U of Botox-A in 15 men. Symptom scores decreased 65% from baseline (which was statistically significant) at 20 months after transperineal Botox injection with transrectal ultrasound guidance. The maximum urinary flow rate improved from 8.1 mL/s to 15.4 mL/s and the mean PVR decreased from 126 mL to 21 mL. The PSA decreased 51% from baseline, which mirrors a reported decrease in the average prostate volume from 51 to 17 mL.

Subsequent studies of Botox involved small numbers of participants, the route of injection varied, and the injection dose was not standardized. However, all studies uniformly reported successful outcomes, with rapid relief of symptoms often within 1 week, reaching maximal relief in less than 1 month, and the response was durable for a minimum of 6 months. These studies included men with LUTS refractory to α-blocker therapy[73,83] and men who were considered poor surgical risk treated with 200 U of Botox for their complaints of urinary retention or markedly increased PVRs.[84] At a mean follow-up of 10 months no patient developed recurrence of his symptoms or retention.[84] The mean prostate volume decreased 13.3% to 18.8%, the symptom scores improved 52.6% to 73.1%, and the QOL index improved 44.7% to 61.5%. The maximal flow rate increased significantly by 39.8% to 72%.[73] Botox also seemed to decrease voiding pressure.[84]

When the dose of Botox was controlled for the pretreatment prostate volume, the symptom scores and QOL indices improved by more than 30% in 76% of men. Although 29% of men did not experience a change in prostate volume, two-thirds of these men realized an improvement greater than 30% in maximum flow rate, LUTS, and QOL, and no adverse effects were noted.[73,85] Further, the time interval to improved voiding seems shorter than the interval associated with other MIST therapies.[82,86]

MIST II is a randomized, stage trial sponsored by the National Institutes of Health of Botox injection of 100 or 300 U transrectally. Although the study was not powered to show differences in dose levels, the study did show that Botox was safe and provided relief of LUTS. The AUA symptom scores decreased from 18.6 to 12.5 in the 100-U group and the AUA symptom score improved from 19.8 to 11.2 in the 300-U group at 12 weeks. These changes reflect 32.4% and 42.1% improvements in the AUA symptom score. The Q_{max} also improved from baseline values of 10.2 mL/s (in the 100-U group) and 9.6 mL/s (in the 300-U group) to 12.3 and 12.4 mL/s at 12 weeks, respectively. These improvements in maximum urine flow rate represent an improvement of 25.6% to 28.4%. The authors reported that 73% of men in the 100-U group and 81% of men in the 300-U group met efficacy criteria and no participant experienced severity grade 4 or 5 toxicity events. Events of severity grade 2 to 3 were reported by 17% of men in the 100-U arm and 18% in the 300-U arm.[87]

Botox-A seems to be the first therapeutic agent to target the static and dynamic components of obstruction. Its use inhibits the autonomic efferent effects on prostate growth and contraction and also inhibits the abnormal afferent effects on prostate sensation. Although the mechanism is not yet fully understood, the clinical outcomes for the concurrent administration of Botox and α-blockers has been interpreted to suggest that the adrenergic influence is reinforced by the anticholinergic effect of Botox-A. Nitric oxide would thus be involved in a Botox-A action mechanism in BPH.[88] Clinically, investigators[89] have noted that storage symptoms improved more than the voiding symptoms and have postulated that the inhibitory effect on the smooth muscle tone and aberrant sensory function might also be important. The use of Botox for the relief of LUTS requires a better understanding of the optimal dose, the duration of effect, and the mechanisms by which Botox-A affects the prostate. Botox-A use in prostate disease is currently off-label.[90]

URETHRAL STENT

Urethral stents for the relief of LUTS have interested urology investigators for decades. Stent technology in cardiac, vascular, and gastrointestinal areas stimulated desire for a BPH device with similar advantages. Prostate stents were attractive as an option for the patient with urinary obstruction whose comorbid condition precluded safe consideration of a TURP.[91] Stents can be broadly classified into permanent and temporary stents. The permanent stents were designed to serve as scaffolding for eventual urethral epithelization to reduce encrustation. The placement of a urethral stent can be accomplished under a local anesthetic, is intended to be immediately effective, and catheterization following treatment is not required in the properly selected patient.

The reported experience with the UroLume endourethral prosthesis (AMS, Minnetonka, MN, USA) demonstrated that stent technology could provide relief of moderate-to-severe LUTS. Although only 11 of the original 62 patients were available at the 12-year follow-up, the available results were informative. The symptom score improved from 20.4 before placement to 6.82 at 5 years and increased to 10.82 at 12 years. Urinary peak flow rates improved from 9 mL/s before placement to 11.7 mL/s at 5 years and 11.5 mL/s at 12 years. Most informative was the rate of stent removal. Twenty-nine percent of stents were removed in the first 2 years, 11% in years 3 to 5, and 6% by year 10; 34% of men died from unrelated causes with the stent in place. Early stent explantation was reported to be primarily a result of poor case selection, or stent malposition/migration, and stents explanted remote from placement were removed because of symptom progression.[92]

A comprehensive review of the literature (1989–2005) concerning the UroLume stent for men with BPH identified 20 case series involving 990 men, but only 10 studies assessed symptoms before stent placement. All studies reported decreases in symptom scores, Madsen-Iversen score (22.2 to 7.9) or IPSS (22.4 to 12.4), and peak urine flow rates improved from 8.9 mL/s to 13.1 mL/s. When the authors combined the outcomes for catheter-dependent men, 84% voided spontaneously after stent insertion. However, the stent failed within the first year in at least 16% of these men and stent migration was the most common cause of failure (37% of men who failed). Most patients initially experienced perineal pain or irritative voiding symptoms following stent placement. The authors concluded that the literature lacked sufficient follow-up to support conclusions on stent durability beyond 1 year, thus they stated that stents should be considered only in patients at high risk.[93] A competing product, the Memotherm stent (Bard Nordic, Helsingborg, Sweden), also demonstrated utility in high-risk patients who were in urinary retention. Similar to many UroLume studies the study population was small, the follow-up was limited, and 13% of patients required stent removal in the first year;[94] however; it has been suggested that when a stent needs to be removed, the Memokath (Pnn Medical, Kvistgaard, Denmark) design allows for easier removal.[95]

Temporary stents are being investigated as a means to treat the transient bladder outlet obstruction frequently observed after minimally invasive thermotherapy procedures aimed at treating benign prostatic obstruction, with biodegradable and retrievable stents shown as successful modalities for this indication.

By using a prostatic stent to simulate transurethral resection of the prostate, it has been possible to assess the risk of postresection incontinence in patients with combined severe bladder outlet obstruction and severe overactive bladder before the operation. However, larger controlled clinical studies are needed to corroborate the value of the test.

Prostatic obstruction can induce severe overactive bladder in some cases. The stent test indicates that patients who do not leak and experience reduced symptoms when they are relieved of their outlet obstruction can be advised to have a transurethral resection of the prostate.[96]

Stents have not achieved their theoretical benefits and their use remains limited. A typical man treated with a stent will have comorbid medical issues that require a single intervention without anesthesia. Most patients experience discomfort and irritative voiding symptoms following stent placement; not all men realize improvement in their symptoms; stents can migrate or obstruct; and they can be a complication in the face of urinary tract infections. If stent removal is necessary, the patient who cannot tolerate a complicated procedure is required to undergo a procedure rather than mechanical drainage of the bladder. Although the impact of stents on sexual activity is reported to be minimal, with 62% to 80% of patients reporting antegrade ejaculation, the comorbid medical conditions in the typical patient suggest that this population is less likely to realize benefit. Stents do not necessarily protect from the progressive nature of BPH, and there may be questions concerning the hyperplastic nature and carcinogenic properties of an indwelling stent . Therefore, stents should be used only in those who cannot tolerate other procedures or as a temporizing procedure until a more definitive procedure can be performed. The key to obtaining optimal outcomes in men with BPH is careful patient selection and proper stent deployment.[95]

SUMMARY

Minimally invasive therapy devices reflect the continued evolution of the technologies in the quest to realize a noninvasive efficacious product with long-term durability and a low side-effect profile. Minimally invasive therapies can improve symptoms in the properly selected patient, but the literature suggests that the degree and durability of improvement have not achieved the goals physicians expect. No single minimally invasive therapy is appropriate for all patients and the urologist is advised to select appropriately. Patient selection is critical and the urologist is obliged to share with the patient the quality of relief versus the durability of outcomes of the minimally invasive devices. Multicenter randomized research activity seems most active in injection therapy with agents such as Botox. The current state of health care demands lower-cost efficacious therapies; because of its low capital expenditure, injection therapy will likely be the focus of research in these therapies.

REFERENCES

1. Jones JS, Follis HW, Johnson JR. Probability of finding T1a and T1b (incidental) prostate cancer during TURP has decreased in the PSA era. Prostate Cancer Prostatic Dis 2009;12(1):57–60.
2. Gonzalez RR, Kaplan SA. First-line treatment for symptomatic benign prostatic hyperplasia: is there a particular patient profile for a particular treatment? World J Urol 2006;24(4):360–6.
3. Hoznek A, Abbou CC. Impact of interventional therapy for benign prostatic hyperplasia on quality of life and sexual function. Curr Urol Rep 2001; 2(4):311–7.
4. Benign prostatic hyperplasia in elderly men. What are the special issues in treatment? Postgrad Med 1997;101(5):141–3 [148, 151–4 passim].
5. Djavan B, Fong YK, Harik M, et al. Longitudinal study of men with mild symptoms of bladder outlet obstruction treated with watchful waiting for four years. Urology 2004;64(6):1144–8.
6. Wiygul J, Babayan RK. Watchful waiting in benign prostatic hyperplasia. Curr Opin Urol 2009;19(1): 3–6.
7. Roehrborn CG, McConnell JD, Saltzman B, et al. PLESS Study Group. Proscar long-term efficacy and safety study. Storage (irritative) and voiding (obstructive) symptoms as predictors of benign prostatic hyperplasia progression and related outcomes. Eur Urol 2002;42(1):1–6.
8. Ozden C, Ozdal OL, Urgancioglu G, et al. The correlation between metabolic syndrome and prostatic growth in patients with benign prostatic hyperplasia. Eur Urol 2007;51(1):199–203 [discussion: 204–6].
9. Black L, Naslund MJ, Gilbert TD Jr, et al. An examination of treatment patterns and costs of care among patients with benign prostatic hyperplasia. Am J Manag Care 2006;12(4 Suppl):S99–110.
10. Fowke JH, Murff HJ, Signorello LB, et al. Race and socioeconomic status are independently associated with benign prostatic hyperplasia. J Urol 2008; 180(5):2091–6 [discussion: 2096].
11. Yu X, Elliott SP, Wilt TJ, et al. Practice patterns in benign prostatic hyperplasia surgical therapy: the dramatic increase in minimally invasive technologies. J Urol 2008;180(1):241–5.
12. Nadu A, Mabjeesh NJ, Ben-Chaim J, et al. Are indications for prostatectomy in octogenarians the same as for younger men? Int Urol Nephrol 2004;36(1): 47–50.
13. Ercole B, Lee C, Best S, et al. Minimally invasive therapy for benign prostatic hyperplasia: practice patterns in Minnesota. J Endourol 2005;19(2): 159–62.
14. Miano R, De Nunzio C, Asimakopoulos AD, et al. Treatment options for benign prostatic hyperplasia in older men. Med Sci Monit 2008;14(7):RA94–102.
15. Yerushalmi A, Fishelovitz Y, Singer D, et al. Localized deep microwave hyperthermia in the treatment of poor operative risk patients with benign prostatic hyperplasia. J Urol 1985;133(5):873–6.
16. Available at: www.auanet.org/content/guidelines-and-quality-care/clinical-guidelines.cfm?sub=bph.
17. de la Rosette JJ, D'Ancona FC, Debruyne FM. Current status of thermotherapy of the prostate. J Urol 1997;157(2):430–8.
18. Wasson JH, Reda DJ, Bruskewitz RC, et al. A comparison of transurethral surgery with watchful waiting for moderate symptoms of benign prostatic hyperplasia. The Veterans Affairs Cooperative Study Group on Transurethral Resection of the Prostate. N Engl J Med 1995;332:75–9.
19. Nawrocki JD, Bell TJ, Lawrence WT, et al. A randomized controlled trial of transurethral microwave thermotherapy. Br J Urol 1997;79:389–93.
20. de la Rosette JJ, Francisca EA, Kortmann BB. Clinical efficacy of a new 30-min algorithm for transurethral microwave thermotherapy: initial results. BJU Int 2000;86(1):47–51.
21. Hoffman RM, Monga M, Elliot SP, et al. Microwave thermotherapy for benign prostatic hyperplasia. Cochrane Database Syst Rev 2007;(4):CD004135.
22. Tan AH, Nott L, Hardie WR, et al. Long-term results of microwave thermotherapy for symptomatic benign prostatic hyperplasia. J Endourol 2005;19(10): 1191–5.
23. Djavan B, Roehrborn CG, Shariat S. Prospective randomized comparison of high energy transurethral microwave thermotherapy versus alpha-blocker treatment of patients with benign prostatic hyperplasia. J Urol 1999;161(1):139–43.
24. Djavan B, Shariat S, Fakhari M. Neoadjuvant and adjuvant alpha-blockade improves early results of high-energy transurethral microwave thermotherapy for lower urinary tract symptoms of benign prostatic hyperplasia: a randomized, prospective clinical trial. Urology 1999;53(2):251–9.
25. Larson TR. Rationale and assessment of minimally invasive approaches to benign prostatic hyperplasia therapy. Urology 2002;59(Suppl 2A):12–6.
26. Vesely, Stepan, Knutson, Tomas, Dicuio, Mauro, et al. Transurethral microwave thermotherapy: clinical results after 11 years of use. J Endourol 2005; 19(6):730–3.
27. Puppo P. Long-term effects on BPH of medical and instrumental therapies. Eur Urol 2001;39(Suppl 6):2–6.
28. Walmsley K, Kaplan SA. Transurethral microwave thermotherapy for benign prostate hyperplasia: separating truth from marketing hype. J Urol 2004; 172(4 Pt 1):1249–55.
29. Arai Y, Aoki Y, Okubo K, et al. Impact of interventional therapy for benign prostatic hyperplasia on quality of life and sexual function: a prospective study. J Urol 2000;164:1206–11.

30. Madersbacher S, Marberger M. Is transurethral resection of the prostate still justified? BJU Int 1999;83:227–37.

31. Trock BJ, Brotzman M, Utz WJ, et al. Long-term pooled analysis of multicenter studies of cooled thermotherapy for benign prostatic hyperplasia: results at three months through four years. Urology 2004;63:716–21.

32. Djavan B, Seitz C, Roehrborn CG, et al. Targeted transurethral microwave thermotherapy versus alpha-blockade in benign prostatic hyperplasia: outcomes at 18 months. Urology 2001;57:66–70.

33. Thalmann GN, Mattei A, Treuthardt C, et al. Transurethral microwave therapy in 200 patients with a minimum followup of 2 years: urodynamic and clinical results. J Urol 2002;167:2496–501.

34. Larson TR, Blute ML, Bruskewitz RC, et al. A high efficiency microwave thermoablation system for the treatment of benign prostatic hyperplasia: results of a randomized, sham-controlled, prospective, double-blind, multicenter clinical trial. Urology 1998;51:731–42.

35. Blute ML, Larson T. Minimally invasive therapies for benign prostatic hyperplasia. Urology 2001; 58(Suppl 6A):33–41.

36. Roehrborn CG, Boyle P, Bergner D, et al. Serum prostate-specific antigen and prostate volume predict long-term changes in symptoms and flow rate: results of a four-year, randomized trial comparing finasteride versus placebo. PLESS Study Group. Urology 1999;54:662–9.

37. Roehrborn CG, Malice M, Cook TJ, et al. Clinical predictors of spontaneous acute urinary retention in men with LUTS and clinical BPH: a comprehensive analysis of the pooled placebo groups of several large clinical trials. Urology 2001;58:210–6.

38. Roehrborn CG, McConnell J, Bonilla J, et al. Serum prostate specific antigen is a strong predictor of future prostate growth in men with benign prostatic hyperplasia: PROSCAR long-term efficacy and safety study. J Urol 2000;163:13–20.

39. Fitzpatrick JM. Minimally invasive and endoscopic management of benign prostatic hyperplasia. In: Wein AJ. editor, 9th edition. Campbell-Walsh urology. vol. 3. Philadelphia: Saunders Elsevier: 2007. p. 2803–44.

40. Francisca EA, d'Ancona FC, Hendriks JC, et al. Quality of life assessment in patients treated with lower energy thermotherapy (Prostasoft 2.0): results of a randomized transurethral microwave thermotherapy versus sham study. J Urol 1997;158(5):1839–44.

41. Hahn RG, Farahmand BY, Hallin A, et al. Incidence of acute myocardial infarction and cause-specific mortality after transurethral treatments of prostatic hypertrophy. Urology 2000;55(2):236–40.

42. Larson BT, Mynderse LA, Somers VK. Blood pressure surges during office-based transurethral microwave therapy for the prostate. Mayo Clin Proc 2008;83(3):309–12.

43. U.S. Food and Drug Administration. Microwave therapy warning. JAMA 2002;284(21):2711.

44. FDA Public Health Notification: Serious injuries from microwave thermotherapy for benign prostatic hyperplasia October 11, 2000.

45. d'Ancona FC. Nonablative minimally invasive thermal therapies in the treatment of symptomatic benign prostatic hyperplasia. Curr Opin Urol 2008; 18(1):21–7.

46. Blute M, Ackerman SJ, Rein AL, et al. Cost effectiveness of microwave thermotherapy in patients with benign prostatic hyperplasia: part II—results. Urology 2000;56:981–7.

47. Schulman CC, Zlotta AR, Rasor JS, et al. Transurethral needle ablation (TUNA). Safety, feasibility, and tolerance of a new office procedure for treatment of benign prostatic hyperplasia. Eur Urol 1993;24: 415–23.

48. Huidobro C, Larson B, Mynderse S, et al. Characterizing Prostiva RF treatments of the prostate for BPH with gadolinium-enhanced MRI. ScientificWorldJournal 2009;9:10–6.

49. Zlotta AR, Peny MO, Matos C, et al. Transurethral needle ablation of the prostate: clinical experience in patients in urinary acute retention. Br J Urol 1996;77(3):391–7.

50. Millard RJ, Harewood LM, Tamaddon K. A study of the efficacy and safety of transurethral needle ablation (TUNA) treatment for benign prostatic hyperplasia. Neurourol Urodyn 1996;15(6):619–28.

51. Available at: http://professional.medtronic.com/interventions/rf-ablation/overview/index.htm.

52. Schulman CC, Zlotta AR. Transurethral needle ablation of the prostate for treatment of benign prostatic hyperplasia: early clinical experience. Urology 1995;45(1):28–33.

53. Kahn SA, Alphonse P, Tewari A, et al. An open study on the efficacy and safety of transurethral needle ablation of the prostate in treating symptomatic benign prostatic hyperplasia: the University of Florida experience. J Urol 1998;160(5):1695–700.

54. Rodrígo Aliaga M, López Alcina E, Monserrat Monfort JJ, et al. [Treatment of benign hyperplasia of the prostate using thermal transurethral needle ablation (TUNA)]. Actas Urol Esp 1997;21(7): 649–54 [in Spanish].

55. Zlotta AR, Giannakopoulos X, Maehlum O, et al. Long-term evaluation of transurethral needle ablation of the prostate (TUNA) for treatment of symptomatic benign prostatic hyperplasia: clinical outcome up to five years from three centers

56. Hill B, Belville W, Bruskewitz R, et al. Transurethral needle ablation versus transurethral resection of the prostate for the treatment of symptomatic benign prostatic hyperplasia: 5-year results of a prospective,

randomized, multicenter clinical trial. J Urol 2004; 171(6 Pt 1):2336–40.

57. Rosario DJ, Woo H, Potts KL, et al. Safety and efficacy of transurethral needle ablation of the prostate for symptomatic outlet obstruction. Br J Urol 1997; 80(4):579–86.

58. Naslund MJ, Stitcher MF. A cost comparison of TUNA vs TURP [abstract]. J Urol 1997;157(Suppl): 155.

59. Naslund MJ, Carlson AM, Williams MJ. A cost comparison of medical management and transurethral needle ablation for treatment of benign prostatic hyperplasia during a 5-year period. J Urol 2005;173(6):2090–3 [discussion: 2093].

60. Rosario DJ, Phillips JT, Chapple CR. Durability and cost-effectiveness of transurethral needle ablation of the prostate as an alternative to transurethral resection of the prostate when alpha-adrenergic antagonist therapy fails. J Urol 2007;177(3): 1047–51.

61. Bouza C, López T, Magro A, et al. Systematic review and meta-analysis of transurethral needle ablation in symptomatic benign prostatic hyperplasia. BMC Urol 2006;6:14 1186.

62. Lourenco T, Armstrong N, N'Dow J, et al. Systematic review and economic modelling of effectiveness and cost utility of surgical treatments for men with benign prostatic enlargement. (Winchester, England). Health Technol Assess 2008;12(35):169–515, iii, ix–x, 1–146.

63. Saemi AM, Plante MK. Injectables in the prostate. Curr Opin Urol 2008;18(1):28–33.

64. Goya N, Ishikawa N, Ito F, et al. Transurethral ethanol injection therapy for prostatic hyperplasia: 3-year results. J Urol 2004;172(3):1017–20.

65. Mutaguchi K, Matsubara A, Kajiwara M, et al. Transurethral ethanol injection for prostatic obstruction: an excellent treatment strategy for persistent urinary retention. Urology 2006;68(2):307–11.

66. Magno C, Mucciardi G, Gali A, et al. Transurethral ethanol ablation of the prostate (TEAP): an effective minimally invasive treatment alternative to traditional surgery for symptomatic benign prostatic hyperplasia (BPH) in high-risk comorbidity patients. Int Urol Nephrol 2008;40(4):941–6.

67. Grise P, Plante M, Palmer J, et al. Evaluation of the transurethral ethanol ablation of the prostate (TEAP) for symptomatic benign prostatic hyperplasia (BPH): a European multi-center evaluation. Eur Urol 2004;46(4):496–501.

68. Plante MK, Marks LS, Anderson R, et al. Phase I/II examination of transurethral ethanol ablation of the prostate for the treatment of symptomatic benign prostatic hyperplasia. J Urol 2007;177(3):1030–5 [discussion: 1035].

69. Larson BT, Netto N, Huidobro C, et al. Intraprostatic injection of alcohol gel for the treatment of benign prostatic hyperplasia: preliminary clinical results. ScientificWorldJournal 2006;6:2474–80.

70. Ikari O, Leitao VA, D'ancona CA, et al. Intravesical calculus secondary to ethanol gel injection into the prostate. Urology 2005;65(5):1002.

71. Plante MK, Folsom JB, Zvara P. Prostatic tissue ablation by injection: a literature review. J Urol 2004; 172(1):20–6.

72. Doggweiler R, Zermann DH, Ishigooka M, et al. Botox-induced prostatic involution. Prostate 1998; 37(1):44–50.

73. Chuang YC, Tu CH, Huang CC, et al. Intraprostatic injection of botulinum toxin type-A relieves bladder outlet obstruction in human and induces prostate apoptosis in dogs. BMC Urol 2006;6:12.

74. Chuang YC, Chiang PH, Huang CC, et al. Botulinum toxin type A improves benign prostatic hyperplasia symptoms in patients with small prostates. Urology 2005;66(4):775–9.

75. Davletov B, Bajohrs M, Binz T. Beyond Botox: advantages and limitations of individual botulinum neurotoxins. Trends Neurosci 2005;28(8):446–52.

76. Blitzer A, Sulica L. Botulinum toxin: basic science and clinical uses in otolaryngology. Laryngoscope 2001;111:218–26.

77. O'Day J. Use of botulinum toxin in neuro-ophthalmology. Curr Opin Ophthalmol 2001;12:419–22.

78. Bell MS, Vermeulen LC, Sperling KB. Pharmacotherapy with botulinum toxin: harnessing nature's most potent neurotoxin. Pharmacotherapy 2000;20: 1079–91.

79. Brashear A. The botulinum toxins in the treatment of cervical dystonia. Semin Neurol 2001;21:86–90.

80. Mahant N, Clouston PD, Lorentz IT. The current use of botulinum toxin. J Clin Neurosci 2000;7:389–94.

81. Tsui JKC. Botulinum toxin as a therapeutic agent. Pharmacol Ther 1996;72:13–24.

82. Maria G, Brisinda G, Civello IM, et al. Relief by botulinum toxin of voiding dysfunction due to benign prostatic hyperplasia: results of a randomized, placebo-controlled study. Urology 2003;62(2): 259–64.

83. Chuang YC, Chancellor MB. The application of botulinum toxin in the prostate. J Urol 2006;176(6 Pt 1): 2375–82.

84. Kuo HC. Prostate botulinum A toxin injection – an alternative treatment for benign prostatic obstruction in poor surgical candidates. Urology 2005;65(4):670–4.

85. Chuang YC, Chiang PH, Huang CC, et al. Botulinum toxin A improves refractory benign prostatic hyperplasia symptoms [abstract]. J Urol 2004; 171(Suppl):1524.

86. Wein AJ. Prostate botulinum A toxin injection—an alternative treatment for benign prostatic obstruction in poor surgical candidates. J Urol 2005;174(5):1903.

87. ED Crawford, R Donnell, K Hirst, et al. 12-week results of a phase II trial of 100 and 300 units

botulinum neurotoxin type A (BoNT-A) for the management of benign prostatic hyperplasia. The AUA Annual Meeting, Chicago (IL). April 2009.

88. Park DS, Cho TW, Lee YK, et al. Evaluation of short term clinical effects and presumptive mechanism of botulinum toxin type A as a treatment modality of benign prostatic hyperplasia. Yonsei Med J 2006;47(5):706–14.

89. Chuang YC, Chiang PH, Yoshimura N, et al. Sustained beneficial effects of intraprostatic botulinum toxin type A on lower urinary tract symptoms and quality of life in men with benign prostatic hyperplasia. BJU Int 2006;98(5):1033–7.

90. Ilie CP, Chancellor MB. Perspective of Botox for treatment of male lower urinary tract symptoms. Curr Opin Urol 2009;19(1):20–5.

91. Klein LT, Kaplan SA. Prostatic stents for benign prostatic hyperplasia. J Long Term Eff Med Implants 1997;7(1):101–14.

92. Masood S, Djaladat H, Kouriefs C, et al. The 12-year outcome analysis of an endourethral wallstent for treating benign prostatic hyperplasia. BJU Int 2004;94(9):1271–4.

93. Armitage JN, Cathcart PJ, Rashidian A, et al. Epithelializing stent for benign prostatic hyperplasia: a systematic review of the literature. J Urol 2007; 177(5):1619–24.

94. Uchikoba T, Horiuchi K, Satoh M, et al. Urethral stent (Angiomed-Memotherm) implantation in high-risk patients with urinary retention. Hinyokika Kiyo 2005;51(4):235–9.

95. Vanderbrink BA, Rastinehad AR, Badlani GH. Prostatic stents for the treatment of benign prostatic hyperplasia. Curr Opin Urol 2007;17(1):1–6.

96. Knutson T. Can prostate stents be used to predict the outcome of transurethral resection of the prostate in the difficult cases? Curr Opin Urol 2004; 14(1):35–9.

Treatment of Bladder Diverticula, Impaired Detrusor Contractility, and Low Bladder Compliance

Charles R. Powell, MD[a],*, Karl J. Kreder, MD[b]

KEYWORDS

- Urinary bladder • Diverticulum
- Benign prostatic hyperplasia • Bladder neoplasms
- Urinary bladder neck obstruction

Ever since Rokitansky noted that bladder diverticula resulted from urethral obstruction in 1849, urologists have associated the treatment of the bladder outlet with the treatment of diverticula,[1] but until 1906 there were only 5 cases of bladder diverticula described in the American literature.[2] Large series on bladder diverticula are not reported in the literature as commonly as they were in the first part of the twentieth century. The largest contemporary series from the last 10 years reports on 25 patients,[3] and studies from 1940 to 1967 describe as many as 285 patients.[2,4,5] This may lead one to speculate that the problem is not as prevalent, or that interest for this clinical entity in the scientific community has waned. The authors believe diverticula of the bladder have become less prevalent in North America, perhaps because of more treatment options for benign prostatic hyperplasia (BPH) and a tendency to recognize and treat BPH earlier. Therefore, a review of the available data is important for the modern practicing clinician, who may not see the condition frequently. The authors' experience, lessons from contemporary literature, and experience from earlier literature are examined to provide a background for the modern clinician to make informed treatment decisions. Many exciting new approaches to diverticula have been described recently, such as improved imaging technology and urodynamic studies to guide the decision to perform bladder outlet-reducing surgery and better plan the surgical approach. New surgical approaches involving laparoscopy and robotic surgery have also become available. However, the principles guiding the decision to operate remain the same.

ETIOLOGY AND INCIDENCE

There are 2 categories of bladder diverticula: congenital diverticula, which present primarily in childhood; and acquired diverticula, which are typically seen in adulthood.

Congenital diverticula usually present in boys less than 10 years of age, and the incidence is estimated to be 1.7%.[6] These are believed to be caused by insufficient muscle backing of the ureterovesical junction, and usually present in the same location near the ureterovesical junction (so-called Hutch diverticula). The bladder is

Disclosures: No external funding was received for the preparation of this manuscript. Charles Powell – none, Karl Kreder – Pfizer (meeting participant, no financial), Astellas (meeting participant, no financial), Medtronic (safety monitor, no financial).
[a] Department of Urology, Indiana University School of Medicine, 535 Barnhill Drive, Suite 420, Indianapolis, IN 46202-5289, USA
[b] Department of Urology, University of Iowa, 200 Hawkins Drive, 3 RCP, Iowa City, IA 52242-1089, USA
* Corresponding author.
E-mail address: crpowell@iupui.edu (C.R. Powell).

Urol Clin N Am 36 (2009) 511–525
doi:10.1016/j.ucl.2009.08.002
0094-0143/09/$ – see front matter

seldom trabeculated, and bladder outlet obstruction is not believed to play a significant role.

Acquired diverticula, on the other hand, present in men during the sixth to seventh decade and are often asymptomatic. Various estimates on the incidence in men range from 1% to 8%.[7,8] Diverticula are typically discovered in men during a workup for lower urinary tract symptoms. Bladder diverticula occur uncommonly in women.[9] When discovered in female patients, they are most commonly attributed to urethral obstruction as a result of bladder neck hypertrophy. This review focuses primarily on diverticula in men; however, the principles and techniques for treating women are the same.

In men, diverticula are believed to be caused primarily by bladder outlet obstruction. This high pressure voiding over time results in a herniation of the bladder mucosa through the smooth muscle layer (muscularis propria). Because of this, diverticula are often thin walled and lack the ability to contract; thus causing stasis of urine, also serving as a nidus for stone formation and infection. Urine stasis has been proposed as a risk factor for tumor formation, and several investigators have reported tumors arising from these diverticula.[10–18] Diverticula may be single or multiple, and classically appear posteriorly on the bladder near the ureteral orifices, making dissection and excision treacherous. Acquired bladder diverticula have been reported less frequently in modern urologic practice, possibly as a result of advances in the management of bladder outlet obstruction caused by BPH.

BPH AND DIVERTICULA

Because diverticula are often attributed to bladder outlet obstruction, the role of benign prostatic enlargement (BPE) consequent to BPH must be considered. The natural history of BPH/BPE is progressive, such that trabeculation of the detrusor muscle progresses to the development of cellules, and finally bladder diverticula with deposition of connective tissue throughout the detrusor muscle, ultimately leading to its decompensation if left untreated.[6,19]

Although causality is commonly implied, there is only circumstantial evidence linking BPH to formation of diverticula. BPH has been noted to be present in 70% of patients with diverticula, compared with bladder neck contracture, which was seen in 12%, and urethral stricture in 12%.[20] Two other important considerations are bladder neck hypertrophy as a primary cause of obstruction and bladder neck contracture following transurethral resection of the prostate (TURP) or radical prostatectomy. Iatrogenic diverticulum

formation should also be considered following ureteral reimplantation, and cystotomy and bladder closure. Early work in fetuses has led to the theory that diverticula are located posteriorly at the transition between the thick muscle fibers of the trigone and the thinner fibers of the lateral bladder wall.[21] Other investigators make anecdotal reference to the increased incidence of inguinal and diaphragmatic hernias in adult patients with bladder diverticula, but no data are given to support these observations.[2]

CONCERN FOR MALIGNANCY IN THE DIVERTICULUM

Bladder diverticula are known to promote stasis and urinary retention. Some investigations have suggested this increases the risk for malignancy, and the incidence of tumor in a bladder diverticulum has been as high as 10% to 13%.[14,22] The study by Melekos and colleagues[22] was retrospective, and reviewed a population of men with a mean age of 69 years, all with bladder diverticula, from 1987. This incidence varies widely by author, however, and others have reported incidence of malignancy in individuals with bladder diverticula ranging from 2%[23] to 5.5%.[18] These series seem to include similar patients, all of whom had been diagnosed with bladder diverticula in the fifth or sixth decade, and most are men. Most seem to be from referral hospitals. Because all available studies are retrospective, the possibility of bias must be considered. By comparison, transitional cell carcinoma of the bladder in the general population ranges in incidence from 1% to 2%.[24] Lifetime incidence in North America from Surveillance, Epidemiology and End Results (SEER) data (and referenced by the Urologic Diseases in America project) is 3.5% for men and 1.13% for women.[25] Early reports of tumor arising from diverticula demonstrated poor survival, with 2-year survival ranging from 16% to 58%.[11,26] One possible explanation for the aggressive behavior of cancer in diverticula is the lack of muscle therein, such that cancer cell penetration into the lamina propria constitutes invasive disease. More recent reports, however, have shown 5-year survival rates of 72%,[10,13] possibly as a result of earlier detection. Because of the low numbers of patients having both tumors and bladder diverticula, well-powered, prospective, randomized trials do not exist, leading to considerable debate as to how asymptomatic diverticula should be managed when encountered.

Earlier investigators reached a very different conclusion than contemporary investigators. In the largest series to date, Kelalis and colleagues[5] at the Mayo Clinic reviewed their experience from 1955 to 1964 with 285 patients having bladder diverticula. Nineteen of 285 (7%) were noted to harbor malignancy. A subset of 8 patients had been diagnosed with diverticula 1.5 to 16 years before malignancy was diagnosed and were initially treated with outlet-reducing surgery alone. All of those patients subsequently died, and overall, 13 of 19 died within the first year after tumor diagnosis. These patients were treated with partial or radical cystectomy, leading the investigators to "unhesitatingly recommend prophylactic excision" when diverticula are encountered. More recently, Montague and Boltuch[15] described a 90% 2-year survival rate; 62% of these patients were found to have noninvasive, Ta lesions.

Some investigators have now concluded that the presence of a bladder diverticulum poses no greater risk of de novo malignancy and prophylactic bladder diverticulectomy is not warranted.[27] The authors believe that because of the improved prognosis in more contemporary series, prophylactic diverticulectomy is not warranted, but rather periodic surveillance on these patients with voided cytology and cystoscopy is advised. The risk of intervention has to be weighed against the potentially increased risk of missing a malignancy. When high-grade or invasive tumor is found, however, aggressive treatment should be undertaken, including diverticulectomy combined with intravesical chemotherapy or radical cystectomy.[10] Moreover, because there is no muscle or serosa backing the diverticulum harboring a tumor, there is some debate as to whether T1 tumors should be treated differently from conventional transitional cell carcinoma of the bladder.[22] It is clear that great care must be taken during biopsy and transurethral resection (TUR) if cystoscopic management is undertaken, because the thin wall of the diverticulum makes bladder perforation more likely.

Transitional cell carcinoma is the most common histologic type of tumor found in diverticula, with incidence from 80% to 100% of all diverticular tumors, followed by squamous cell carcinoma (7%–15%) and adenocarcinoma (0%–15%).[6,10,11,14–16,18] Patients with tumor in the diverticulum most commonly present with hematuria followed by urinary tract infection.[15]

In an effort to further understand the conditions under which malignancy arises from within diverticula, some investigators have examined histologic changes seen in the epithelium of benign diverticula. When Gerridzen and colleagues reviewed their series of 48 cases, they found that only 19% of the diverticula removed demonstrated normal mucosa, whereas 69% demonstrated chronic inflammation, and 13% revealed squamous metaplasia.[20] Kelalis and colleagues[5] noted that 26 of 31 benign diverticulum specimens demonstrated chronic inflammation, cellular infiltration, squamous metaplasia, or leukoplakia. It seems that the mucosa found within diverticula is not normal.

CLINICAL EVALUATION

The workup for patients with suspected diverticula shares components with the workup for lower urinary tract symptoms (LUTS), with some important differences. Medical history, American Urological Association (AUA) symptom index score, physical examination including digital rectal examination, urinalysis, and prostate-specific antigen (PSA) (if the patient has a 10-year or more life expectancy) should be undertaken on initial evaluation.[28] Urinary cytology is useful given the possibility of tumor arising from the diverticulum. In addition, serum creatinine is advised for the workup of bladder diverticula, given the chronic nature of the disorder and possibility of concomitant hydronephrosis, which was noted to be present in 6.9% of 115 patients with diverticula from 1 series.[4] Some investigators believe upper tract imaging to assess for hydronephrosis is important, although the AUA BPH guidelines do not recommend this for the workup of BPH.[6,28] McConnell and colleagues[28] noted in the 1994 Agency for Health Care Policy and Research (AHCPR) meta-analysis that 7.6% of BPH patients had evidence of hydronephrosis, and of those, 33.6% were noted to have renal insufficiency. This was a compilation of 25 investigations including more than 6000 BPH patients evaluated with intravenous pyelogram (IVP) and served as the template for the most recent 2003 AUA Guideline on BPH.[29] The authors perform upper tract imaging on all diverticula because some have been known to cause hydronephrosis. Our study of choice is a computed tomography (CT) scan with contrast, because this gives excellent detail of the bladder and diverticula, and information on the proximity of the distal ureter for posterior diverticula.

Appropriate imaging classically has included cystogram and IVP. In some instances, this can detect diverticula and filling defects suggestive of a tumor or blood clot (Fig. 1). A filling defect in the area of the bladder neck can denote a large median lobe of the prostate, as shown in Fig. 2. J-hooking of the ureter is 1 finding suggestive of significant BPH (see Fig. 2). CT urogram with three-dimensional reconstruction of the ureters and bladder has replaced cystography and IVP where available (Fig. 3), and conventional CT can

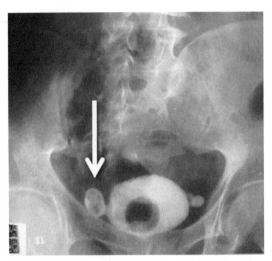

Fig. 1. A cystogram is not only useful for detecting diverticula, which often will remain opacified after bladder emptying but also filling defects that represent tumor as demonstrated by the *arrow* in this film. (*Courtesy of* P.S. Talwar, MD, Department of Radiology, University of Illinois at Chicago Medical Center.)

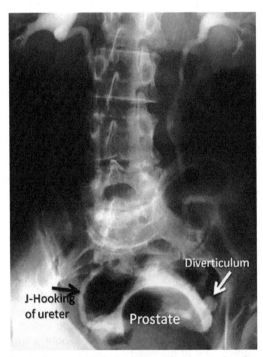

Fig. 2. A filling defect at the bladder neck often denotes a large median lobe of the prostate. Lateral deviation of the ureters, known as J-hooking, is demonstrated in this IVP. (*Courtesy of* P.S. Talwar, MD, Department of Radiology, University of Illinois at Chicago Medical Center.)

be used where three-dimensional reconstruction is not available. CT is more sensitive for detection of bladder and ureteral stones (**Fig. 4**) than plain radiography.[30] In many cases, CT can be used to measure the size of the ostium leading to the diverticulum (**Fig. 5**A), or determine the size of a median lobe of the prostate (**Fig. 5**B). CT with delayed excretory phase cuts can help the clinician localize the ureters relative to the diverticulum and thereby aid in the decision on whether to place preoperative stents (**Fig. 6**). It is important to recognize that diverticula can be multiple. The CT in **Fig. 7** demonstrates hydronephrosis bilaterally. This patient presented with renal failure, which improved significantly with intravenous fluid hydration and Foley catheterization before surgery. If CT is unavailable, if there is a contraindication to intravenous contrast, or if ionizing radiation is undesirable to the patient, ultrasound can be considered. It is useful to determine if hydronephrosis is present, but its limitations should be recognized. Ultrasound gives less anatomic detail about the location of the diverticulum relative to the ureters. It is not as sensitive as CT when used to detect ureteral stones although newer techniques have enhanced ultrasonographic imaging of calculi.[31–33] Magnetic resonance imaging is a useful imaging modality to detect hydronephrosis, but is not as sensitive at detecting stones as CT.[34] Retrograde pyelography is also useful, and can be done at the time of cystoscopy.

Cystoscopy is indicated in all patients with suspected bladder diverticula. It is the most sensitive modality for detecting tumors within the diverticulum. Cytology should also be done.[6,18] Cystoscopy combines the ability to locate the diverticulum, determine if stone exists in the diverticulum, and gauge the size of the ostium connecting the diverticulum to the bladder. When tumor is suspected within a bladder diverticulum whose lumen cannot be envisioned because of a narrow os, contrast imaging using CT scanning can be helpful as can the use of the flexible ureteroscope.

Voiding cystourethrography (VCUG) is useful for determining if the diverticulum empties when voiding, an important factor in patients suffering from recurrent urinary tract infections. VCUG also detects vesicoureteral reflux. **Fig. 8** demonstrates the importance of obtaining lateral views during VCUG, because the diverticulum is not always evident on anterioposterior (AP) views.

Urodynamic studies are helpful in imaging diverticula and determining their association with causative conditions such as bladder outlet obstruction, detrusor overactivitiy, and impaired detrusor contractility. It would be fair to say that videourodynamics is the method of choice when

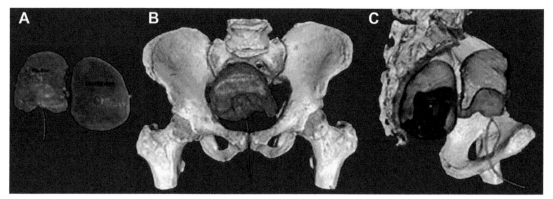

Fig. 3. CT urogram with three-dimensional reconstruction of the ureters and bladder can demonstrate the size and location of the diverticulum (*A, B*). A lateral view is helpful in judging its position relative to the rectum and other structures (*C*). (*Courtesy of* F.N. Joudi, MD, Department of Urology, University of Iowa.)

evaluating bladder diverticula.[35] Investigators from Spain have used urodynamic data to compare men with bladder diverticula with similar men with BPH.[36] Men with BPH alone exhibited significant differences when compared with 24 men with bladder diverticula. Postvoid residual was greatly increased (45 mL vs 221 mL, $P<.008$), and the incidence of urinary retention was also increased in the diverticula cohort (6.1% vs 25%, $P<.01$), as was the incidence of urinary tract infection (3.1% vs 21.7%, $P<.004$). Urethral resistance was noted to be much higher in the diverticula group (36.5 cm H_2O vs 48.5 cm H_2O, $P = .04$), and evidence of abdominal straining was also noted more frequently in men with diverticula (23.9% vs 50%, $P = .02$). Some of these patients received surgical treatment: 11 underwent a bladder outlet procedure alone, whereas 8 received both a bladder outlet procedure and diverticulectomy. The only significant difference between the groups was a decrease in postvoid dribbling in those undergoing diverticulectomy and the bladder outlet procedure (75%) compared with only 10% of the patients undergoing bladder outlet procedure alone. **Fig. 9** provides an example of a urodynamic tracing from a man with a diverticulum, elevated voiding pressure, and postvoid residual. High voiding pressures may be more noticeable with a narrow-neck diverticulum than with a wide-mouth diverticulum. The diagnostic steps described earlier are summarized in the algorithm in **Fig. 10** for rapid reference.

TREATMENT OF THE DIVERTICULUM

Three questions that need to be addressed when developing a treatment plan for patients diagnosed with bladder diverticula are:

- is surgery on the prostate necessary?

- is surgery on the diverticulum necessary?
- if both are indicated, should the procedures be staged or simultaneous?

Observation

The least invasive option for the management of diverticula is observation. If the patient chooses observation, periodic cystoscopy and cytology to detect any malignant transformation are recommended.[6,18] The authors also perform periodic upper tract imaging with ultrasound if no surgical intervention is planned, and we prefer CT with contrast if surgery is a possibility to determine the relationship of the ureters to the diverticulum. The clinician should be aware of the data from earlier large series in which tumor has been noted to develop in the diverticulum years later and that those investigators concluded that the poor prognosis of these patients warrants prophylactic diverticulectomy.[5,10] There is an equally compelling view from more contemporary investigators, however, supporting the observation approach.[27] Although the possibility of malignant transformation is

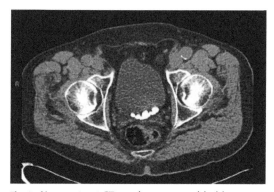

Fig. 4. Noncontrast CT can demonstrate bladder stones with a high degree of sensitivity.

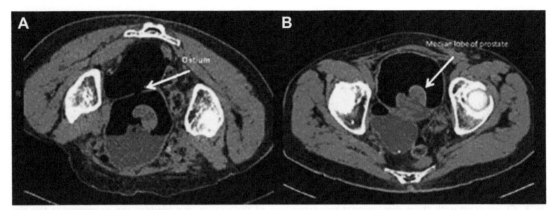

Fig. 5. CT is useful to measure the ostium of the diverticulum (*A*) and the size of the median lobe of the prostate (*B*), helping the clinician counsel the patient about the need for TURP or open prostatectomy.

a critical issue, the issue of progressive bladder decompensation should also be considered, and has been demonstrated to occur in animal and human models.[19] This is monitored in our clinic with periodic uroflowmetry and postvoid residual measurements.

Surgical Treatment of the Bladder Outlet

Bladder outlet obstruction is implicated in most cases of bladder diverticula. Over time, this can lead to histologic changes to the detrusor muscle and ultimately to detrusor decompensation.[19] Early surgical reduction of bladder outlet obstruction may slow and possibly reverse this disabling phenomenon, as was suggested in a 5-year cooperative prospective study of 556 men undergoing TURP for LUTS.[37] The men randomized to early TURP reported 85% better improvement in peak flow rate than those who underwent TURP later in the study. Moreover, there is some evidence that a poorly emptying bladder can be rehabilitated with a period of continuous, prolonged catheter drainage.[38] Patients with small diverticula that drain well may be well suited for treatment with TURP alone.

Medication for BPH is effective and can be considered. The patient should be aware of the potential need for ablative prostate surgery in the future and, because of this, should be followed periodically in a similar fashion to the patient who is being observed for diverticula (periodic cystoscopy and voided cytology, and postvoid residuals). Randomized prospective data do not exist comparing recurrence of diverticula when patients are treated medically versus surgically, but 1 series of 5 patients provides some anecdotal insight into this question.[39] The series included 2 patients treated medically for bladder outlet obstruction caused by BPH, and 1 later required

TURP. Other investigators have elected to stage the procedures, performing the TURP 1 week after the diverticulectomy to allow the bladder to heal, with good short-term results.[40]

One reasonable strategy to manage the bladder outlet is to consider whether there is urodynamic evidence for bladder outlet obstruction. Patients who have tried medical management with persistent evidence for obstruction should be considered surgical candidates. There is no randomized prospective evidence favoring a staged procedure. When bladder outlet surgery is indicated, techniques that have been described include TURP,[39–41] open prostatectomy,[42] potassium titanyl phosphate laser or holmium ablation, and holmium laser enucleation of the prostate.[43]

Table 1 summarizes some important series describing techniques and success rates, when

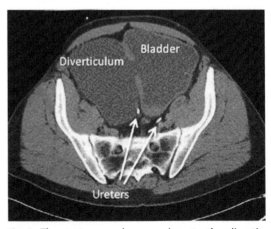

Fig. 6. The ureters can be very close to the diverticulum and a CT urogram with axial sections can be helpful in deciding if a patient will require stents preoperatively to help identify the ureters intraoperatively.

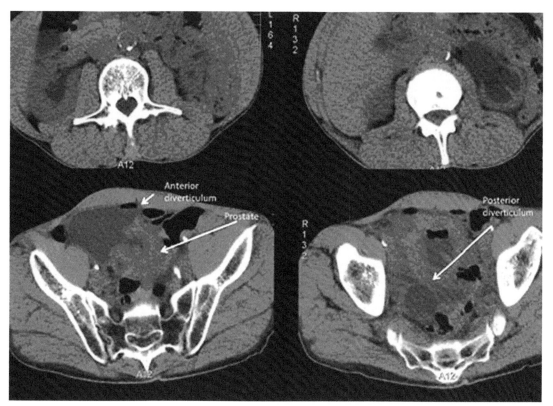

Fig. 7. Hydronephrosis was found bilaterally in this patient (*top left, top right*) who was noted to have a large anterior diverticulum (*bottom left*) and 1 located posteriorly adjacent to the rectum (*bottom right*). (*Courtesy of* D.C. Arnold, MD, Department of Urology, University of Illinois at Chicago Medical Center.)

available from early and contemporary literature. Only 1 study directly compared 2 techniques head-to-head.[44] This study by Porpiglia and colleagues[44] compared a series of 10 TURP procedures combined with laparoscopic bladder diverticulectomy with 13 simultaneous transvesical prostatectomy and open diverticulectomy procedures. Similar outcomes were obtained for postoperative urinary flow rates. Less blood loss, shorter hospital stay, and longer operative times characterized the laparoscopic approach. The authors have anecdotally seen patients who appeared to have the "pop-off" phenomenon showing no obstruction on urodynamic studies (as the increase in detrusor pressure during contraction is mitigated by the low resistance internal reservoir formed by the diverticulum), underwent diverticulectomy, and then returned within 6 months with clear-cut obstruction requiring TURP.

Surgical Treatment of the Diverticulum

After a plan has been made to treat the bladder outlet, a strategy must be devised to deal with

the diverticulum. Some investigators have concluded that excision of the diverticulum is not always necessary once bladder outlet surgery is done.[2,36] After 1 experience with 96 patients treated from 1932 to 1937, the investigators developed the following criteria for diverticulectomy: (1) large size with a tight orifice that causes it to drain poorly, (2) young men with poorly draining diverticula even if minimal symptoms exist, (3) stone present in the diverticulum, and (4) the presence of ureteral obstruction.[2] In their experience 6 of 29 (21%) were noted to have urinary retention postoperatively with postvoid residuals ranging from 100 to 200 mL in volume. Fifteen additional patients had a measureable residual less than 100 mL. In addition to these criteria, persistent infection, presence of tumor, ureteral reflux as seen in a Hutch diverticulum, and urinary retention have also been recognized as useful criteria that influence the decision to excise a diverticulum.[6,18] These indications for diverticulectomy are

- Presence of tumor
- Persistent infection
- Bladder stone

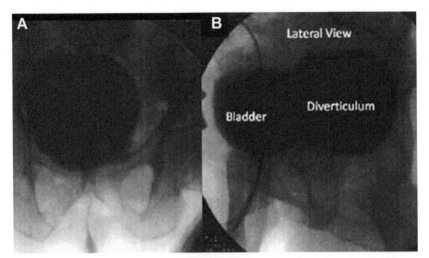

Fig. 8. The VCUG in AP view (*A*) does not demonstrate the diverticulum, but the lateral view shows a posterior diverticulum (*B*).

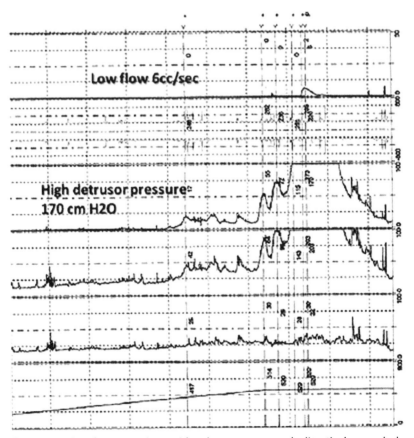

Fig. 9. This urodynamic tracing from a patient with a large narrow-neck diverticulum and elevated postvoid residual demonstrated obstruction with low flow (6 mL/s) and elevated voiding pressures (170 cm H_2O).

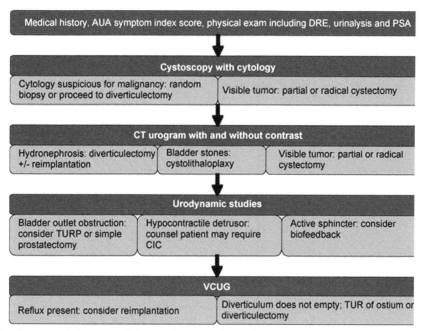

Fig. 10. An algorithm can help to recall the workup and determine which patients should have staged bladder outlet and diverticulectomy procedures or simultaneous procedures.

- Hydronephrosis on the side of the diverticulum
- Reflux on the side of the diverticulum
- Urinary retention including poorly draining diverticulum
- Troublesome LUTS including overflow incontinence

Techniques for Surgical Treatment of the Diverticulum

Methods for surgical bladder diverticulectomy include

- Transurethral incision of the diverticulum neck
- Open intravesical diverticulectomy and excision of mucosa
- Open extravesical diverticulectomy
- Laparoscopic diverticulectomy
- Robotically assisted laparoscopic diverticulectomy

TUR of the mouth of the diverticulum is the least invasive method described to aid in emptying, and fulguration of the mucosa of the diverticulum has been performed to cause scarring and shrinkage of the diverticulum.[45–47] One report in the Russian literature describes the diverticula as either decreased in size (55%) or no longer detectable at the postoperative visit (45%).[45] The technique

of removing only the mucosa was first performed in open fashion and described by Barnes in 1939, who indicated that even large diverticula can contract significantly.[48] Clayman and colleagues[49] concluded that the cystoscopic technique was "equally effective while being safer, faster, and less expensive" when compared with open techniques, and reported 5/6 patients had no residual diverticulum on repeat cystography. Although diverticula have been reported to decrease in size after this approach, the muscle backing will still be deficient, and a large diverticulum may still provide a low pressure outlet for voided urine, preventing complete emptying in some cases.[50] Moreover, it is unclear if this reduces the risk of malignancy. It has been noted by other investigators that this technique works poorly for large diverticula.[46,47]

The Technique of Transurethral Fulguration of a Bladder Diverticulum

Transurethral fulguration can be done with the rollerball using circular motions, spiraling laterally beginning at the middle of the diverticulum. When the mucosa can no longer be reached with the rollerball, the neck of the diverticulum can be incised with the rollerball or Collins knife on cutting current to expose more new mucosa.

Table 1
Series describing bladder diverticula

Author	Year	n	Technique	Number of Successful Outcomes	Complications
Abdel-hakim[40]	2007	13	Laparoscopic transperitoneal approach with 30 mL Foley balloon to aid in identifying diverticulum; 7 cases with BPH underwent TURP some time later, 3 cases with stricture underwent direct vision internal urethrotomy	13	1
Adot Zurbano[36]	2005	24	11 underwent TURP alone, 8 underwent TURP and excision of diverticulum (technique not specified)	Both methods comparable	Not given
Badawy[52]	2008	3	Pediatric series using extraperitoneal, transvesical approach with insufflation of the bladder	Not given	0
Thompson[2]	1940	96	14 underwent open prostatectomy alone; 96 others underwent diverticulectomy by an unspecified method	Not given	0
Kimbrough[8]	1941	30	Open diverticulectomy followed by bladder outlet procedure in most patients	Not given	2
Faramarzi-Roques[54]	2004	5	TURP followed by laparoscopic transperitoneal extravesical diverticulectomy	5	0
Gerridzen[20]	1982	48	Open diverticulum excision in 21, TCC in 5 of these	Not given	Not given
Fox[4]	1962	115	Combination of techniques for bladder outlet and diverticulum, all open, some staged	70	21

				Not given	Not given
Kelalis[5]	1967	286	31/286 received diverticulectomy for benign disease, an unknown number were treated with TURP alone, but 8 that did not get diverticulectomy initially developed tumors later	Not given	Not given
Macejko[41]	2008	2	TURP in 1, alpha blocker in 1, followed later by robot-assisted laparoscopic diverticulectomy	2	0
Myer[39]	2007	5	2 preoperative TURP, 2 postoperative TURP, 1 alpha blocker then transperitoneal robotic diverticulectomy assisted with cystoscopy	5	1
Porpiglia[3,a]	2004	25	12 underwent TURP followed immediately by transperitoneal laparoscopic diverticulectomy assisted with cystoscopy compared with 13 who underwent simultaneous open simple prostatectomy and bladder diverticulectomy	25	0
Shah[55]	2006	3	Simultaneous Holmium laser enucleation of the prostate followed immediately by extraperitoneal laparoscopic bladder diverticulectomy	3	0

[a] There is a similar series by the same author 2 years earlier with fewer patients that was not included in this table.

The classic approach involves an open extravesical approach or intravesical approach.[2,5,8,20] The advantage to the intravesical approach is less dissection and easier identification of all diverticula. It is limited by the presence of inflammation around the diverticulum, which sometimes can prohibit safe intravesical dissection. There is also a risk of incorporating ureter or peritoneal contents into the excised tissue or closure.[51]

The Technique of Extravesical Excision of a Bladder Diverticulum

The open extravesical approach is performed by first cleaning the peritoneum and bowel off the bladder. This involves a fair amount of perivesical dissection but minimizes the cystotomy incision that is necessary. Locating the diverticulum can be difficult at times, especially if inflammation is present and there are multiple diverticula. To aid in this, the authors place a Foley catheter in the bladder to fill it and make the diverticulum more prominent. The balloon of the Foley catheter can often be milked into the diverticulum from outside the bladder, further aiding the dissection. It is important to mark the edges of the diverticulum neck with stay sutures before incising it, because it is easy to excise some healthy bladder and mucosa without realizing it, reducing bladder capacity unintentionally.

The Technique of Intravesical Excision of a Bladder Diverticulum

The open intravesical approach is useful to minimize perivesical dissection and can be done by exposing only the dome of the bladder, marking the edges of the planned incision with stay sutures, and incising it. The diverticulum is often easier to identify from inside the bladder, and once the diverticulum is identified its furthest mucosal edge can be grasped and inverted into the bladder with an allis or Babcock clamp. The plane of dissection is between the mucosa and adventitial backing. Care must be taken to avoid incorporating ureter into the clamp or closing sutures if the diverticulum is noted to be near the ureter on preoperative imaging.

All of these approaches carry some risk of injury to the ureter if the diverticulum is located posteriorly, as it often is. The authors recommend preoperative stents if the preoperative CT urogram or pyelogram reveals that the ureters are close.

Use of Laparoscopy

The intravesical technique has been adapted by laparoscopic surgeons by insufflating the bladder with CO_2 and placing ports directly into the bladder.[52,53] This makes identification of all diverticula simpler. Multiple investigators have also reported on laparoscopic extravesical techniques.[3,40,54,55] There are some common elements to this technique, including identification of the diverticulum using a Foley catheter in the diverticulum and another catheter in the bladder to selectively fill and decompress it.[56] Some investigators have described an extraperitoneal approach to extravesical diverticulectomy, using dissection balloons to expose the space of Retzius before placing the camera.[55] Robotic assistance has also been described to aid in laparoscopic extravesical diverticulectomy in adults[39,41] and children.[57]

The open approach remains a reliable and proven method to improve bladder drainage, however, various laparoscopic approaches promise faster recovery and less postoperative pain with similar safety and intermediate-term results.[3,44]

THE FUTURE OF SURGICAL TECHNIQUES

Two novel surgical approaches to the pelvis and retroperitoneum have recently generated a good deal of excitement in the literature. Natural orifice translumenal endoscopic surgery (NOTES) and laparoendoscopic single-site surgery (LESS) promise minimally invasive access with fewer visible incisions or scars, but the techniques remain to be proven and are considered experimental at present.[58–60] To date, bladder diverticulectomy has not been reported using these techniques.

IMPAIRED DETRUSOR CONTRACTILITY AFTER DIVERTICULECTOMY

In certain cases, even with adequate management of bladder outlet obstruction and removal of the diverticulum, the patient is still unable to empty his bladder. This is typically caused by impaired detrusor contractility and is often accompanied by a poorly compliant bladder. This remains a difficult problem for the urologist to treat, and is commonly managed with clean intermittent catheterization or indwelling Foley catheter. In some cases where complications secondary to the indwelling catheter arise, urinary diversion is an option. Reduction cystoplasty can also be considered. Recently, however, investigators have noted success with other options. One report in the German literature has described improvement in urodynamic parameters after a 13-week period of continuous bladder drainage with suprapubic catheterization.[38] These investigators noted a significant reduction in urodynamic bladder capacity (691.8–496.8 mL) and mean postvoid residual reduction of 227 mL. It is not clear if this effect is durable. Others have noted significant improvement in nonobstructive urinary retention with sacral neuromodulation. No trial of sacral neuromodulation deals specifically with patients having diverticula, so the results need to be regarded with caution. Some factors that have been predictive of success with neuromodulation include the preoperative ability to void greater than 50 mL spontaneously and the presence of abnormal sphincter activity on electromyogram.[61,62] Patients suffering from impaired detrusor contractility after long periods of obstruction may respond to neuromodulation differently because presumably the cause of the urinary retention is different. Specific data are lacking on response rates for myogenic detrusor hypoactivity treated with sacral neuromodulation.

DECREASED BLADDER COMPLIANCE AFTER DIVERTICULECTOMY

A diverticulum acts as a pressure relief mechanism in some patients, particularly if the ostium is wide, because it has no muscle backing and can expand into the retroperitoneum with less resistance than a healthy bladder. It is commonly believed that the diverticulum forms in adults after a long period of obstructed voiding. Obstructed voiding has been demonstrated in human and animal models to lead to a noncompliant bladder.[19] When the diverticulum is removed, only the thick-walled bladder remains, potentially leaving a poorly compliant bladder. One group has performed detailed urodynamic studies on patients with diverticula and compared them with patients without diverticula, finding no difference in contractility between the 2 groups.[36] Compliance was not specifically mentioned. Differences included urethral resistance (which was noted to be much higher in the diverticula group) and evidence of abdominal straining (which was also noted more frequently in men demonstrating diverticula). The concern is valid, however, that after diverticulectomy, compliance may worsen. In addition to causing LUTS, poor compliance may jeopardize the kidneys over time.[28] For this reason it should not be ignored. A reasonable approach is to reassess voiding function following any procedure on a diverticulum, 1 urodynamic study, measurement of creatinine, urinary flow rate and post-void residual. Poor compliance can be managed with anticholinergic agents and clean intermittent catheterization when severe. Periodic botulinum toxin injections and surgical

enterocystoplasty are 2 other options if less invasive measures prove ineffective, but patients should be warned that these carry a risk for retention and mandatory clean intermittent catheterization. These measures are seldom necessary.

SUMMARY

Bladder diverticula are classically associated with bladder outlet obstruction, but the latter does not always cause the former. Careful investigation including cystoscopy, radiographic imaging of the upper tracts and bladder, and videourodynamic studies are important in planning surgical intervention. The decision to treat the bladder outlet, remove the diverticulum, or observe with regular surveillance has to be made with as much information as possible. Careful consideration should be given to the timing of bladder outlet surgery. Newer radiographic techniques and recently evolving minimally invasive approaches have reduced morbidity for these patients with similar outcomes.

REFERENCES

1. C.Rokitanskye Manual of pathological anatomy 1849;2:220. London: Sydenham Society; 1849.
2. Thompson GJ. The management of diverticulum of the bladder. Ninety-six patients treated by transurethral prostatic resection. Surg Gynecol Obstet 1940; 70:115–9.
3. Porpiglia F, Tarabuzzi R, Cossu M, et al. Is laparoscopic bladder diverticulectomy after transurethral resection of the prostate safe and effective? Comparison with open surgery. J Endourol 2004;18(1):73–6.
4. Fox M, Power RF, Bruce AW. Diverticulum of the bladder – presentation and evaluation of treatment of 115 cases. Br J Urol 1962;34:286–98.
5. Kelalis PP, McLean P. The treatment of diverticulum of the bladder. J Urol 1967;98(3):349–52.
6. Rovner ES. Bladder and urethral diverticula. In: Wein AJ, Kavoussi LR, Novick AC, et al, editors. Campbell-Walsh urology. Philadelphia: Saunders; 2007. p. 2361–90.
7. Burns E. Diverticula of the urinary bladder. Ann Surg 1944;119(5):656–64.
8. Kimbrough JC. The treatment of bladder diverticulum: report of 30 cases. J Urol 1941;45: 368–81.
9. Findlay HV, Riparetti PP. Diverticulum of the urinary bladder in a woman. Calif Med 1955;83(1):39–41.
10. Baniel J, Vishna T. Primary transitional cell carcinoma in vesical diverticula. Urology 1997;50(5): 697–9.
11. Faysal MH, Freiha FS. Primary neoplasm in vesical diverticula. A report of 12 cases. Br J Urol 1981; 53(2):141–3.

12. Garzotto MG, Tewari A, Wajsman Z. Multimodal therapy for neoplasms arising from a vesical diverticulum. J Surg Oncol 1996;62(1):46–8.

13. Golijanin D, Yossepowitch O, Beck SD, et al. Carcinoma in a bladder diverticulum: presentation and treatment outcome. J Urol 2003;170(5):1761–4.

14. Micic S, Ilic V. Incidence of neoplasm in vesical diverticula. J Urol 1983;129(4):734–5.

15. Montague DK, Boltuch RL. Primary neoplasms in vesical diverticula: report of 10 cases. J Urol 1976; 116(1):41–2.

16. Redman JF, McGinnis TB, Bissada NK. Management of neoplasms in vesical diverticula. Urology 1976;7(5):492–4.

17. Sousa Escandon A, Garcia R, Arguelles M, et al. Carcinosarcoma in a bladder diverticulum. A case report and literature review. Urol Int 2000;65(3): 169–72.

18. Yu CC, Huang JK, Lee YH, et al. Intradiverticular tumors of the bladder: surgical implications – an eleven-year review. Eur Urol 1993;24(2):190–6.

19. Levin RM, Haugaard N, O'Connor L, et al. Obstructive response of human bladder to BPH vs. rabbit bladder response to partial outlet obstruction: a direct comparison. Neurourol Urodyn 2000;19(5):609–29.

20. Gerridzen RG, Futter NG. Ten-year review of vesical diverticula. Urology 1982;20(1):33–5.

21. Watson E. Developmental basis for certain vesical diverticula. JAMA 1920;75(22):1473–4.

22. Melekos MD, Asbach HW, Barbalias GA. Vesical diverticula: etiology, diagnosis, tumorigenesis, and treatment. Analysis of 74 cases. Urology 1987; 30(5):453–7.

23. Das S, Amar AD. Vesical diverticulum associated with bladder carcinoma: therapeutic implications. J Urol 1986;136(5):1013–4.

24. Messing EM. Urothelial tumors of the bladder. In: Wein AJ, Kavoussi LR, Novick AC, et al, editors. Campbell-Walsh urology, vol. 3. 9th edition. Philadelphia: Saunders Elsevier; 2007. p. 2407–46.

25. Ries LAG, Eisner MP, Kosary CL, et al. editors. SEER cancer statistics review, 1975–2001. Bethesda (MD): National Cancer Institute; 2004. Available at: http://seer.cancer.gov/sr/1975_2001. Accessed April 5, 2009.

26. Lowe FC, Goldman SM, Oesterling JE. Computerized tomography in evaluation of transitional cell carcinoma in bladder diverticula. Urology 1989; 34(6):390–5.

27. Fellows FJ. The association between vesical carcinoma and diverticulum of the bladder. Eur Urol 1978;4(3):185–6.

28. McConnell JD, Barry MJ, Bruskewitz RC. Benign prostatic hyperplasia: diagnosis and treatment. Agency for Health Care Policy and Research. Clin Pract Guidel Quick Ref Guide Clin 1994;(8):1–17.

29. Roehrborn CG. Guideline on the management of benign prostatic hyperplasia (BPH). AUA guidelines volume 1, 2003. p. 2.

30. Linsenmeyer MA, Linsenmeyer TA. Accuracy of bladder stone detection using abdominal x-ray after spinal cord injury. J Spinal Cord Med 2004;27(5): 438–42.

31. Ulusan S, Koc Z, Tokmak N. Accuracy of sonography for detecting renal stone: comparison with CT. J Clin Ultrasound 2007;35(5):256–61.

32. Park SJ, Yi BH, Lee HK, et al. Evaluation of patients with suspected ureteral calculi using sonography as an initial diagnostic tool: how can we improve diagnostic accuracy? J Ultrasound Med 2008;27(10):1441–50.

33. Mendelson RM, Arnold-Reed DE, Kuan M, et al. Renal colic: a prospective evaluation of non-enhanced spiral CT versus intravenous pyelography. Australas Radiol 2003;47(1):22–8.

34. Silverman SG, Leyendecker JR, Amis ES Jr. What is the current role of CT urography and MR urography in the evaluation of the urinary tract? Radiology 2009;250(2):309–23.

35. Schafer W, Abrams P, Liao L, et al. Good urodynamic practices: uroflowmetry, filling cystometry, and pressure-flow studies. Neurourol Urodyn 2002; 21(3):261–74.

36. Adot Zurbano JM, Salinas Casado J, Dambros M, et al. [Urodynamics of the bladder diverticulum in the adult male]. Arch Esp Urol 2005;58(7):641–9 [in Spanish].

37. Flanigan RC, Reda DJ, Wasson JH, et al. 5-year outcome of surgical resection and watchful waiting for men with moderately symptomatic benign prostatic hyperplasia: a Department of Veterans Affairs cooperative study. J Urol 1998;160(1): 12–6 [discussion: 16–7].

38. Hamann MF, van der Horst C, Naumann CM, et al. [Functional results after temporary continuous drainage of the hypocontractile bladder. The potential rehabilitation of the detrusor]. Urologe A 2008; 47(8):988–93 [in German].

39. Myer EG, Wagner JR. Robotic assisted laparoscopic bladder diverticulectomy. J Urol 2007;178(6): 2406–10 [discussion: 2410].

40. Abdel-Hakim AM, El-Feel A, Abouel-Fettouh H, et al. Laparoscopic vesical diverticulectomy. J Endourol 2007;21(1):85–9.

41. Macejko AM, Viprakasit DP, Nadler RB. Cystoscope- and robot-assisted bladder diverticulectomy. J Endourol 2008;22(10):2389–91 [discussion: 2391–2].

42. Luttwak Z, Lask D, Abarbanel J, et al. Transvesical prostatectomy in elderly patients. J Urol 1997; 157(6):2210–1.

43. Kuntz RM, Ahyai S, Lehrich K, et al. Transurethral holmium laser enucleation of the prostate versus

transurethral electrocautery resection of the prostate: a randomized prospective trial in 200 patients. J Urol 2004;172(3):1012–6.

44. Porpiglia F, Tarabuzzi R, Cossu M, et al. Sequential transurethral resection of the prostate and laparoscopic bladder diverticulectomy: comparison with open surgery. Urology 2002;60(6):1045–9.

45. Martov AG, Moskalev A, Gushchin BL, et al. [Endoscopic treatment of bladder diverticula]. Urologiia 2001;6:40–4 [in Russian].

46. Orandi A. Transurethral fulguration of bladder diverticulum: new procedure. Urology 1977;10(1): 30–2.

47. Vitale PJ, Woodside JR. Management of bladder diverticula by transurethral resection: re-evaluation of an old technique. J Urol 1979;122(6):744–5.

48. Barnes RW. Surgical treatment of large vesical diverticulum: presentation of a new technique. J Urol 1939;42:794–801.

49. Clayman RV, Shahin S, Reddy P, et al. Transurethral treatment of bladder diverticula. Alternative to open diverticulectomy. Urology 1984;23(6):573–7.

50. Schulze S, Hald T. Voiding inability after transurethral resection of a bladder diverticulum. Scand J Urol Nephrol 1983;17(3):377–8.

51. Kaneti J. Transvesical diverticulectomy – pursestring and Foley catheter technique. Int Urol Nephrol 1990;22(6):525–9.

52. Badawy H, Eid A, Hassouna M, et al. Pneumovesicoscopic diverticulectomy in children and adolescents: is open surgery still indicated? J Pediatr Urol 2008;4(2):146–9.

53. Pansadoro V, Pansadoro A, Emiliozzi P. Laparoscopic transvesical diverticulectomy. BJU Int 2009; 103(3):412–24.

54. Faramarzi-Roques R, Calvet C, Gateau T, et al. Surgical treatment of bladder diverticula: laparoscopic approach. J Endourol 2004;18(1):69–72.

55. Shah HN, Shah RH, Hedge SS, et al. Sequential holmium laser enucleation of the prostate and laparoscopic extraperitoneal bladder diverticulectomy: initial experience and review of literature. J Endourol 2006;20(5):346–50.

56. Iselin CE, Winfield HN, Rohner S, et al. Sequential laparoscopic bladder diverticulectomy and transurethral resection of the prostate. J Endourol 1996;10(6):545–9.

57. Meeks JJ, Hagerty JA, Lindgren BW. Pediatric robotic-assisted laparoscopic diverticulectomy. Urology 2008;73(2):299–301 [discussion: 301].

58. Box G, Averch T, Cadeddu J, et al. Nomenclature of natural orifice translumenal endoscopic surgery (NOTES) and laparoendoscopic single-site surgery (LESS) procedures in urology. J Endourol 2008; 22(11):2575–81.

59. Gettman MT, Blute ML. Transvesical peritoneoscopy: initial clinical evaluation of the bladder as a portal for natural orifice translumenal endoscopic surgery. Mayo Clin Proc 2007;82(7):843–5.

60. Gettman MT, Box G, Averch T, et al. Consensus statement on natural orifice transluminal endoscopic surgery and single-incision laparoscopic surgery: heralding a new era in urology? Eur Urol 2008;53(6):1117–20.

61. Datta SN, Chaliha C, Singh A, et al. Sacral neurostimulation for urinary retention: 10-year experience from one UK centre. BJU Int 2008;101(2):192–6.

62. Goh M, Diokno AC. Sacral neuromodulation for non-obstructive urinary retention – is success predictable? J Urol 2007;178(1):197–9 [discussion: 199].

Genitourinary Pain Syndromes, Prostatitis, and Lower Urinary Tract Symptoms

Brian V. Le, MD, MA, Anthony J. Schaeffer, MD*

KEYWORDS

• Prostatitis • LUTS • Genitourinary pain • Interstitial cystitis

Benign prostatic hyperplasia (BPH) with associated lower urinary tract symptoms (LUTS), the focus of this issue of the *Urologic Clinics of North America*, is one of the most common conditions encountered by the practicing urologist. Indeed, as men age, the prevalence of BPH increases proportionally from 0% of men in their 30s to 88% of men in their 80s.[1] A certain subset of men with BPH have LUTS that are bothersome enough to seek evaluation. However, LUTS by themselves are not specific for BPH and other lower urinary tract processes may be associated with similar symptoms. Some men with LUTS also have pelvic pain. Urinary tract infection may coexist and compound these symptoms. As shown in **Fig. 1**, there is a cohort of men who have pain and infection, as well as LUTS, and any combination thereof.

The confluence of pain, infection, and voiding symptoms are commonly encountered in practice. Prostatitis, either acute or chronic bacterial, or chronic prostatitis (what is now called *chronic pelvic pain syndrome* [CPPS]) accounts for approximately 2 million outpatient visits per year in the United States.[2] Despite the prevalence of these symptoms, diagnosis, evaluation, and treatment of many of these genitourinary conditions remain difficult. Indeed, while research is underway to gain a clearer understanding of the pathophysiology, there are as yet no clear therapies for many of these disorders.

As with many other areas of medicine, the "treatment of pain" is particularly challenging because often the pain stems from multiple factors. Chronic pain disorders, such as fibromyalgia, inflammatory bowel syndrome, and interstitial cystitis, lead to reorganization of neurons involved in the processing of pain. Functional magnetic resonance studies done in our laboratory evaluating patients with CPPS and interstitial cystitis show distinct patterns in bilateral anterior insula and anterior cingulate cortex in patients experiencing chronic pelvic pain.[3] This article assesses the approach to evaluation and treatment of the patient population with LUTS and chronic pelvic pain, with or without infection.

The general principles in the approach to genitourinary pain syndromes are fairly similar: Clinicians should be attentive and responsive to the needs of the patient, validated questionnaires should be used to quantify symptoms and assess progress, treatable etiologies should be identified and

Research supported by National Institutes of Health–National Institute of Diabetes and Digestive and Kidney Diseases (NIH/NIDDK) grant U01 DK07003: Multi-Disciplinary Approach to the Study of Chronic Pelvic Pain (MAPP) Research Network.

Disclosures: Brian V. Le—no financial disclosures or conflicts of interest. Anthony J. Schaeffer—paid consultant for Alita Pharmaceuticals, Inc, NovaBay Pharmaceuticals, Inc, Exoxemis, Inc, CombinatoRx Inc, and Monitor Company Group, L.P.; meeting honoraria/travel reimbursement from The National Institutes of Health, Multidisciplinary Alliance Against Device-Related Infections (MADRI), The Scientific Consulting Group, Inc, and The American Austrian Foundation; editor and faculty honoraria and travel reimbursements from American Urological Association; author honorarium from Haymarket Media, Inc.

Department of Urology, Northwestern University, Feinberg School of Medicine, Chicago, IL, USA

* Corresponding author.

E-mail address: ajschaeffer@northwestern.edu (A.J. Schaeffer).

Urol Clin N Am 36 (2009) 527–536

doi:10.1016/j.ucl.2009.08.005

urologic.theclinics.com

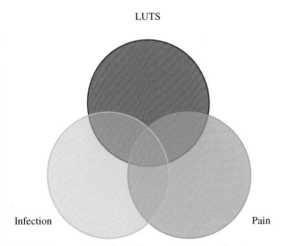

LUTS

Infection   Pain

Fig. 1. The overlap of voiding symptoms and pain are very common. Most genitourinary pain syndromes have a component of urinary symptoms (LUTS). Infection must be ruled out when evaluating the patient for treatment, as this subset may benefit from a course of antimicrobials.

treated, and multimodal approaches should be used for long-term management.

PROSTATITIS AND CHRONIC PELVIC PAIN SYNDROME
Epidemiology and Presentation

In 1995, the National Institutes of Health (NIH) developed a standard definition and classification of prostatitis syndromes, including a new category for asymptomatic patients with prostatic inflammation.[4] Prostatitis has been categorized into four clinical entities, with category III incorporating

CPPS. This serves as a framework for diagnosing, treating, and performing research in prostatitis syndromes (**Table 1**). The NIH categories are as follows:[5]

Category I: acute bacterial prostatitis (rare, 2%–5% of cases). Acute infection of the prostate gland marked by a combination of local symptoms (eg, dysuria, urinary frequency, and suprapubic/pelvic/perineal pain) and systemic symptoms (eg, fevers, chills, malaise); uropathogen typically identified as causal organism; responsive to antimicrobial therapy. Positive urine culture alone of 1000 or more colony forming units (cfu) per milliliter of urine is sufficient for confirming the diagnosis of acute bacterial prostatitis. Expressed prostatic secretions should not be obtained because of the theoretical concern for worsening sepsis.

Category II: chronic bacterial prostatitis (rare, 2%–5% of cases). Chronic infection of the prostate gland, characterized by intermittent local symptoms (eg, dysuria, urinary frequency, prostatic and suprapubic/pelvic/perineal pain); intermittent urinary tract infection ($\geq$1000 cfu/mL of urine); or postmassage urine bacteria counts at 10-fold increase over concentration in the urethral urine. Uropathogen is typically identified in expressed prostatic secretions; normally responsive to antimicrobial therapy.

Category III: chronic nonbacterial prostatitis/ CPPS (CP/CPPS) (common, 90%–95% of

---

Table 1
Interpretation of Meares-Stamey culture and microscopic data. NIH classification is based on the results of the four-glass localization cultures. Expressed prostatic secretions are considered positive if there is a 10-fold increase in uropathogen count (ie, colony forming units per milliliter) compared with VB1 and VB2

	NIH Classification of Prostatitis Syndrome				
Traditional Class	Bladder Urine Midstream (VB2) Specimen		Expressed Prostatic Secretions		NIH Classification (1995)
	Culture	WBC	Culture	WBC	
ABP	+	+	Not recommended		NIH category I
CBP	0	0	+[a]	+[b]	NIH category II
NBP	0	0	0	+[c]	NIH category IIIa
Prostadynia	0	0	0	0	NIH category IIIb
Not described			±	±	NIH category IV (asymptomatic)

Abbreviations: ABP, acute bacterial prostatitis; CBP, chronic bacterial prostatitis; NBP, nonbacterial prostatitis; WBC, white blood cell count.
 [a] Required.
 [b] Not required.
 [c] About 50% of patients have white blood cells in expressed prostatic secretions.

cases). Syndrome involving local symptoms (pelvic pain, urinary voiding symptoms, and ejaculatory symptoms); no identifiable uropathogen or infectious cause; treatment often fails to alleviate symptoms. The NIH Chronic Prostatitis Symptom Index (NIH-CPSI) questionnaire (**Fig. 3**) is the primary validated tool used to quantify the severity of category III prostatitis. Category III is subdivided into inflammatory (IIIA) and noninflammatory (IIIB) prostatitis based on the presence or absence of leukocytes in the expressed prostatic fluid or ejaculate.

Category IV: asymptomatic inflammatory prostatitis (prevalence unknown). Incidental observation of leukocytes in prostate secretions or prostate tissue obtained during evaluation for other disorders, (eg, for elevated prostate-specific antigen [PSA]). No infectious pathogens present; no treatment necessary.

Evaluation and Diagnosis

Acute and chronic bacterial prostatitis
Acute and chronic bacterial prostatitis are most commonly caused by *Escherichia coli*, identified in 65% to 80% of infections,[6] with *Pseudomonas aeruginosa*, *Serratia* spp, *Klebsiella* spp, and *Enterobacter aerogenes* making up another 10% to 15%.[7] Acute bacterial prostatitis is usually dramatic in its presentation, often presenting with both lower urinary tract infection and generalized sepsis.[1] Chronic bacterial prostatitis is usually associated with recurrent urinary tract infections bracketed by asymptomatic periods. Positive bacterial cultures from prostatic secretions (Meares, Stamey test, **Fig. 2**) confirm the diagnosis. Because of the possibility of urinary tract abnormalities in men with urinary tract infection, patients require CT and cystoscopy.

Chronic pelvic pain syndrome
The evaluation of CPPS involves administration of the NIH-CPSI questionnaire (**Fig. 3**), a history and physical examination (with a focus on genitourinary examination), digital rectal examination, urinalysis, and four-glass Meares-Stamey localization cultures. The four-glass localization test involves the sequential collection of urine and prostatic fluid specimens, before, during, and after prostatic massage, and provides fluid and culture data to enable correct categorization of CPPS (see **Fig. 2** and **Table 1**). Men with bacteria exclusively in the expressed prostatic secretions have CPPS and should be treated with appropriate antimicrobial therapy for a minimum of 4 weeks. Colony count in expressed prostatic secretions that exceed counts of midstream urine culture (VB2) by 10-fold or more are significant. Contamination from urethra is common. Therefore, it is essential that the number of colony forming units in the first 10 mL of urine (VB1) is known and that the expressed prostatic secretions or first 10 mL of urine after prostatic massage (VB3) exceeds the number of colony forming units in the VB1 by 10-fold or more.

In 1999, the NIH Chronic Prostatitis Collaborative Research Network (CPCRN) developed an instrument to measure the symptoms and quality of life of CPPS for use in research protocols as well as clinical practice. The result of this effort is the NIH-CPSI, which is administered as a questionnaire and has subsequently been validated in several studies.[8] Our recommendation is that this validated tool be incorporated into the evaluation to quantify initial symptoms and monitor response to therapy.

Treatment

Category I prostatitis
Treatment of acute bacterial prostatitis involves hospitalization if there is evidence of generalized sepsis necessitating blood and urine cultures plus parenteral antimicrobial therapy. Urinary drainage is necessary when patients present with urinary retention related to acute prostatic inflammation. It is reasonable to attempt gentle passage of a small Foley catheter. If catheter placement fails, a urologic consultation for suprapubic drainage should be initiated. Should patients fail to

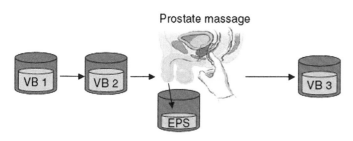

Prostate massage

VB 1 → VB 2 → EPS → VB 3

Fig. 2. Meares-Stamey four-glass test. The first 10 mL of urine (VB1) representing the urethral flora is collected. Then a midstream urine culture (VB2) representing the bladder flora is collected. At this point the physician performs a prostatic massage and collects the expressed prostatic secretions (EPS). The first 10 mL of urine after prostatic massage (VB3) is then collected. All are sent for culture and microscopic analysis.

NIH Chronic Prostatitis Symptom Index (NIH-CPSI)

Pain or Discomfort

1. In the last week, have you experienced any pain or discomfort in the following areas?   Yes   No

a. Area between rectum and testicles (perineum)   □ 1   □ 0

b. Testicles   □ 1   □ 0

c. Tip of the penis (not related to urination)   □ 1   □ 0

d. Below your waist, in your pubic or bladder area   □ 1   □ 0

2. In the last week, have you experienced: Yes   No

a. Pain or burning during urination?   □ 1   □ 0

b. Pain or discomfort during or after sexual climax (ejaculation)?   □ 1   □ 0

3. How often have you had pain or discomfort in any of these areas over the last week?

□ 0 Never
□ 1 Rarely
□ 2 Sometimes
□ 3 Often
□ 4 Usually
□ 5 Always

4. Which number best describes your AVERAGE pain or discomfort on the days that you had it, over the last week?

□ 1 □ 2 □ 3 □ 4 □ 5 □ 6 □ 7 □ 8 □ 9 □ 10

NO PAIN   PAIN   AS BAD AS YOU CAN IMAGINE

Urination

5. How often have you had a sensation of not emptying your bladder completely after you finished urinating, over the last week?

□ 0 Not at all
□ 1 Less than 1 time in 5
□ 2 Less than half the time
□ 3 About half the time
□ 4 More than half the time
□ 5 Almost always

6. How often have you had to urinate again less than 2 hours after you finished urinating, over the last week?

□ 0 Not at all
□ 1 Less than 1 time in 5
□ 2 Less than half the time
□ 3 About half the time
□ 4 More than half the time
□ 5 Almost always

Impact of Symptoms

7. How much have your symptoms kept you from doing the kinds of things you would usually do, over the last week?

□ 0 None
□ 1 Only a little
□ 2 Some
□ 3 A lot

8. How much did you think about your symptoms, over the last week?

□ 0 None
□ 1 Only a little
□ 2 Some
□ 3 A lot

Quality of Life

9. If you were to spend the rest of your life with your symptoms just the way they have been during the last week, how would you feel about that?

□ 0 Delighted
□ 1 Pleased
□ 2 Mostly satisfied
□ 3 Mixed (about equally satisfied and dissatisfied)
□ 4 Mostly dissatisfied
□ 5 Unhappy
□ 6 Terrible

Scoring the NIH Chronic Prostatitis Symptom Index Domains

Pain: Total of items 1a, 1b, 1c, 1d, 2a, 2b, 3 and 4 =
Urinary Symptoms: Total of items 5 and 6 =
Quality-of-Life Impact: Total of items 7, 8, and 9 =

Fig. 3. NIH-CPSI questionnaire. A requirement for diagnosis of CPPS is pain. The questionnaire also evaluates urinary symptoms, impact of symptoms, and quality of life.

improve clinically after 1 to 2 days, CT or MRI should be performed to rule out prostatic abscess, which requires surgical drainage. Prostatic abscess occurs primarily in immunocompromised patients, particularly men with HIV.[9] From 5% to 10% of men with acute bacterial prostatitis progress to chronic bacterial prostatitis.[10] Following resolution of symptoms and return of urine culture data, a 3- to 4-week course of outpatient antimicrobials is indicated.[5]

Category II prostatitis

Chronic bacterial prostatitis often responds to treatment with a 4- to 8-week course of prostate penetrating antimicrobials, such as fluoroquinolones or trimethoprim-sulfamethoxazole (TMP-SMX).[11,12] Fluoroquinolones demonstrate a 60% to 80% cure rate for category II prostatitis.[11,13] For those who fail treatment, usually with recurrence, investigational treatments, such as transurethral resection of the prostate,[14] or long-term suppressive antimicrobials may offer benefit.

Category III prostatitis

There are no formal guidelines for the management of CPPS and no proven therapies.[15] Though category III prostatitis has been broken down into inflammatory (IIIa) and noninflammatory (IIIb) prostatitis based on the presence or absence of leukocytes in expressed prostatic fluid, this has not proven to be of much clinical utility.[16,17] Numerous trials have failed to demonstrate efficacy of antimicrobials,[18–20] alpha-blockers,[18,21] anti-inflammatories, phytotherapy, biofeedback, thermal therapies,[22] and pelvic floor training.[5] A recently completed multicenter, randomized, double-blinded, placebo-controlled trial looking at alfuzosin for the treatment of chronic prostatitis–pelvic pain syndrome showed no benefit over placebo.[23]

If a patient has significant LUTS, goal-directed therapy should be considered and alpha-blockers may offer some benefit. Pelvic floor physical therapy may also be beneficial. Newer classes of medications, such as pregabalin used in the treatment of fibromyalgia and postherpetic neuralgia, show some promising preliminary data in this population as well.

Category IV: asymptomatic inflammatory prostatitis

No treatment is indicated for this category in the absence of symptoms, this diagnosis being primarily of research interest.

INTERSTITIAL CYSTITIS/PAINFUL BLADDER SYNDROME
Epidemiology and Presentation

Interstitial cystitis, also known as painful bladder syndrome, is a chronic bladder condition characterized by suprapubic pain and urinary symptoms of frequency, urgency, and nocturia, in the absence of infection and malignancy. It is predominantly found in women with a 10:1 female/male ratio and a prevalence of 0.01% to 0.50% in the female population.[24,25] In 1987, the National Institute of Diabetes and Digestive and Kidney Diseases (NIDDK) developed for research purposes consensus criteria for the diagnosis of interstitial cystitis.[26] These relatively conservative criteria facilitated identification of a homogenous population. However, in clinical practice, the diagnosis and subsequent treatment are often more individualized with less stringent criteria, most notably not requiring cystoscopy and hydrodistension under general anesthesia for the diagnosis of interstitial cystitis. Some advocate that the NIDDK criteria used alone are far too restrictive to be used in clinical practice and would underdiagnose as many as 40% of patients.[27] Despite these limitations, the NIDDK criteria have formed the basis for the diagnosis of interstitial cystitis, and have led to expanded research for this condition. The following are the NIDDK criteria for interstitial cystitis:[24,25]

Inclusion criteria

1. Cystoscopy: glomerulations and/or classic Hunner ulcer (examination for glomerulations must be done after hydrodistension under general anesthesia to 80–100 cm water for 1 to 2 minutes)
2. Symptoms: bladder pain and/or urinary urgency

Exclusion criteria

1. Bladder capacity greater than 350 mL on awake cystometry
2. Absence of an intense urge to void with the bladder filled to 100 mL during cystometry using a fill rate of 30 to 100 mL/min
3. Demonstration of phasic involuntary bladder contractions on cystometry using the fill rate described in number 2
4. Duration of symptoms less than 9 months
5. Absence of nocturia
6. Symptoms relieved by antimicrobials, urinary antiseptics, anticholinergics, or antispasmodics
7. Frequency of urination of less than eight times a day while awake
8. Diagnosis of bacterial cystitis or prostatitis within a 3-month period
9. Bladder or ureteral calculi
10. Active genital herpes
11. Uterine, cervical, vaginal, or urethral cancer
12. Urethral diverticulum
13. Cyclophosphamide or any type of chemical cystitis
14. Tuberculous cystitis
15. Radiation cystitis
16. Benign or malignant bladder tumors
17. Vaginitis
18. Age less than 18 years

The International Continence Society definition of painful bladder syndrome is "the complaint of suprapubic pain related to filling, accompanied by other symptoms such as increased daytime and night-time frequency, in the absence of proven urinary infection or other obvious pathology."[28]

Evaluation and Diagnosis

The patient with suspected interstitial cystitis should have a history and focused physical examination. The history should include review of fluid intake and output; diet (caffeine); pain and voiding symptoms; history of urinary tract infections, stones, or chemical cystitis; and sexual history (dyspareunia or abuse).[25] There are validated symptoms questionnaires, such as the O'Leary-Sant Questionnaire and Problem Index,[29] the University of Wisconsin Interstitial Cystitis Scale,[30] and the Pelvic Pain and Urgency/Frequency Patient Symptom Scale,[31] which may be useful in following patients with interstitial cystitis. Physical examination should focus on the genitourinary examination and include a pelvic examination in women and a digital rectal examination in men. Mandatory laboratory analysis involves a urinalysis and midstream urine culture to rule out infection and other etiologies of pain. In addition, we recommend cytology to rule out tumors, a symptom questionnaire, and a voiding diary, plus or minus cystoscopy with hydrodistension and biopsies. Optional evaluations include the potassium sensitivity test, which is used to detect abnormal permeability of the urothelium, as well as urodynamics and pelvic ultrasound.[25] The diagnosis of interstitial cystitis is established based on exclusion of other etiologies and significant findings based on history and cystoscopy.

Treatments

Conservative therapy, including dietary modification, stress reduction, keeping a voiding log and adjusting fluid intake as necessary, consciously trying to expand the interval of voids, and pelvic floor muscle training, may help some patients with mainly urinary symptoms.[32,33] Dietary modification involves identifying exacerbating foods and avoiding them. Some notable offenders include caffeine, alcohol, spicy foods, and urine acidifiers, such as cranberry juice.[1] Case control studies suggest that high levels of stress may exacerbate interstitial cystitis symptoms.[34] Thus, some advocate stress reduction. Though no microorganisms have been directly linked to interstitial cystitis, there are some who believe that they may play a role in the initiation and propagation of symptoms, and thus an empiric trial of antimicrobials is reasonable.[35]

Tricyclic antidepressants, amitriptyline being the most widely studied, have showed fairly good response rates, with 42% of patients noting a greater than 30% improvement in symptoms (a clinically relevant change) on validated questionnaires in a randomized control trial of amitriptyline compared with placebo.[36] Other noncontrolled studies have reported success rates from 64% to 90%, though response is less clearly defined.[37] The basis for amitriptyline's action is believed to be its central and peripheral anticholinergic

properties, its blockage of serotonin and norepinephrine reuptake, its sedative properties, and its antihistamine effects. The recommended dosage is 10 to 150 mg daily at bedtime titrated to response and side effects.

Other oral medications that have shown benefit in the treatment of interstitial cystitis include antihistamines, H1 and H2 antagonists, and long-term analgesics. Hydroxyzine (a first-generation H1 antagonist) in initial studies showed a dramatic response with improvements in almost all parameters by 30% or more[38]; subsequent controlled studies, including an NIDDK placebo-controlled trial, failed to confirm these findings.[39] Cimetidine, an H2 antagonist, showed significant improvement in symptom scores from 19 of 35 to 11 of 35 ($P<.001$) though no histologic changes on biopsy in a prospective, randomized, placebo-controlled trial. However, the etiology of this improvement remains unclear.[40] Most patients benefit from judicious pain management using nonsteroidal anti-inflammatory drugs, acetaminophen, antidepressants, anticonvulsants, and opioids.[41]

Use of pentosan polysulfate for the treatment of interstitial cystitis is based on the concept that interstitial cystitis results from defects in the epithelial permeability barriers, particularly the glycosylaminoglycan layer, allowing urinary constituents to enter the bladder wall and contribute to the inflammation and sensory stimulation of interstitial cystitis.[42] Pentosan polysulfate adheres to the luminal side of the bladder mucosa, thus enhancing or maintaining the permeability barrier of the bladder mucosa.[43] Two placebo-controlled multicenter trials in the United States[44] have demonstrated marginal evidence to support its use, with an improvement of 32% in the treatment group versus 16% with placebo. A subsequent randomized study, published by Nickels et al in 2005,[45] suggested a significant benefit with a 30% overall reduction in symptom scores, and a reduction in severity of symptoms. This response was not dose dependent; thus Nickels recommends the 300-mg dose, as higher doses are associated with increased side effects.

Intravesical therapy for interstitial cystitis has demonstrated limited success in randomized controlled trials. A recent Cochrane meta-analysis of intravesical treatments for interstitial cystitis reviewed dimethyl sulfoxide (DMSO), heparinoids, pentosan polysulfate, capsaicin and resiniferatoxin (RTX), BCG, and others. The primary outcome measures were pain and bladder capacity, with urinary symptoms as a secondary outcome measure. Two trials demonstrated no advantage of RTX over placebo.[46,47] One crossover trial showed benefit of intravesical DMSO over placebo and noted a 93% objective improvement versus 35% with saline, and 53% to 18% subjective improvement. However, all patients had fairly mild disease, and "improvement" was determined without a validated questionnaire.[48] Despite this, DMSO continues to be used in practice because of its overall safety and lack of side effects. BCG did seem to suggest a benefit in two trials, but the benefit was not statistically significant in either.[49,50] Pentosan polysulfate instillation did not result in significantly different pain symptoms, but did result in a minimal 33-mL increased bladder capacity, of unknown clinical significance.[51] Thus, of all the intravesical therapies, DMSO seems to be the most efficacious, though randomized controlled trials need to be conducted.

Surgical therapies may offer some benefit to the refractory patient. Neuromodulation with placement of sacral nerve stimulators have been mildly successful in some small uncontrolled trials.[52] These neuromodulation therapies appear promising, but require further investigation. As a last resort, urinary diversion and cystectomy are an option for the most severely afflicted patients, and the surgeon should be confident that the source of the pain is indeed from the bladder. The patient should be heavily counseled about quality-of-life issues involved in making such a decision, which should be made only after all other options have been exhausted. Additionally, pelvic pain can persist despite cystectomy in some patients.[53]

PELVIC FLOOR PAIN SYNDROME

Pelvic floor pain syndrome (PFPS) goes by many different names including *levator ani syndrome* and *pelvic floor dysfunction*, though it should not be confused with laxity of the pelvic floor in women. It is a condition characterized by pelvic/anorectal pain arising from spasm of the pelvic floor muscles. There is significant overlap between this condition, CPPS (category III prostatitis), and interstitial cystitis. As many as 50% of patients with CPPS report myofascial pain with palpation.[54] Up to 87% of women with a diagnosis of interstitial cystitis may demonstrate symptoms consistent with PFPS.[55] Though PFPS has been recognized to contribute to many of the above conditions and can exacerbate LUTS, treatment and research into this condition as a separate clinical entity have been limited. Evaluation consists of a history, genitourinary physical, urinalysis, and urine culture. The most notable findings on examination are myofascial trigger points, which are defined by

Simons and colleagues[56] as tender spots created by injury at the motor end plate as a result of acute, repetitive, or sustained muscle overloading.[57] Muscles of the pelvis must be examined carefully, with each muscle palpated separately, to gain some idea about their tenderness or spasm. Diagnosis is made based on positive examination findings with or without urinary symptoms.

Treatment of PFPS consists of combination of biofeedback exercises, physical therapy, and pain medications. No randomized controlled trials on PFPS have been conducted, but response rates with the combinations described above have noted response rates of 32% noting marked improvement and another 30% having modest improvement in symptoms.[57]

PROPOSAL FOR APPROACH TO THE PATIENT WITH LOWER URINARY TRACT SYMPTOMS AND PELVIC PAIN

We have briefly reviewed the main genitourinary pain syndromes: prostatitis including CPPS, interstitial cystitis, and PFPS. Though the genitourinary pain syndromes discussed have been broken down primarily along anatomic lines—interstitial cystitis being primarily a bladder problem, prostatitis a prostate problem, and PFPS attributed to the muscles of the pelvic floor—we continue to recognize the significant overlap among the various pain disorders. Other etiologies of pelvic pain, such as endometriosis, vaginismus, constipation, and irritable bowel syndrome, should be excluded from the differential before a genitourinary pain syndrome is diagnosed. In the evaluation of these pain syndromes, a broad symptomatic evaluation should be performed first, followed by confirmatory testing, to determine a particular patient's diagnosis. Though LUTS of urgency, frequency, and nocturia are often attributed to BPH, LUTS can manifest in a broad range of urologic conditions, including those associated with pain.

Here we propose a basic evaluation and a more comprehensive optional evaluation for patients with significant overlap among urinary and pelvic pain symptoms.

History
    History of urinary tract infections
    Sexual history including abuse
Physical examination
    Focus on muscles of the pelvic floor
    Complete genitourinary examination and digital rectal examination
Urinalysis with microscopic evaluation
Urine culture

Based on the findings of this basic evaluation, we advocate use of the appropriate validated symptom questionnaire and more specific studies based on the suspected diagnosis:

Appropriate symptom questionnaire

If prostatitis is suspected, we recommend the Meares-Stamey four-glass localization test

If interstitial cystitis is suspected, based on symptoms and other diagnoses excluded, cystoscopy under anesthesia with hydro-distension with or without biopsies should be strongly considered in patients with bothersome symptoms a minimum of 9 months. Additionally, a voiding diary should be used.

No further evaluation other than physical examination is required for PFPS

For specific populations, the following optional evaluations should be considered:

For patients with significant obstructive symptoms, or neurologic comorbidities, bladder scan, to assess postvoid resid-uals, and urodynamic studies may uncover a neurologic basis for the urinary symptoms

For patients with strong smoking history or hematuria, flexible cystoscopy should be performed to rule out malignancy

Once a working diagnosis is established, treat-ment should be instituted in a timely manner, not only to address the impact of symptoms on quality of life, but also to prevent central nervous system imprinting that can occur with chronic pain. Though large randomized controlled trials continue to be the standard of evidence, the heter-ogenous nature of the pelvic pain population means that treatments that do not statistically differ from placebo may still offer some benefit to an individual patient. Thus, therapy must be specifically tailored to the patient's symptoms and/or findings and outcomes must be closely monitored by appropriate means (eg, validated questionnaires or expressed prostatic secretion cultures). Additionally, pelvic floor rehabilitation and biofeedback, which have demonstrated limited benefit in randomized studies, continue to be used because of their low risk profile and potential benefits.

FUTURE DIRECTIONS

The role of the central nervous system in chronic pain is now appreciated. It is believed patients with chronic pain undergo measurable change in the brain anatomy function due to repetitive painful stimuli over time. This can lead to sensitization known as temporal summation of pain.[58] Dual-function medications that affect the central nervous system as well as inflammatory and pain pathways need further study. Preliminary data in our laboratory suggest that CPPS patients perform worse on gaming tests used to assess cognitive function. In the absence of a better understanding of its pathophysiology, at the very least we can phenotype patients to determine which organs are involved and whether the central nervous system has undergone imprinting such that they may benefit from dual therapy.

SUMMARY

Genitourinary pain syndromes present at the confluence of pain, infection, and urinary symp-toms. An important first step in the management of these chronic pain syndromes is to exclude more easily treated conditions, such as urinary tract infections or bladder outlet obstruction secondary to BPH, as well as other non-urologic conditions. The physical examination plays an important role in both palpation of the prostate and evaluation of the pelvic floor for muscular etiol-ogies that may benefit from physical therapy and biofeedback. Once these other diagnoses are excluded, the more difficult task of treating chronic pelvic pain can be addressed. Early institution of a symptom questionnaire will serve as a baseline while allowing for monitoring of progress through treatment. Educating the patient about the nature of the condition and setting realistic expectations for symptom improvement are essential. Instituting the appropriate therapy, providing enough time to determine a success or failure, and moving on to second- or third-line treatments based on thera-pies that have the strongest evidence to support their use is a prudent approach.

REFERENCES

1. Wein AJK, Louis R, Nowick AC, et al. Campbell Walsh urology. 9th edition. Philadelphia: Saunders Elsevier; 2007.
2. Collins MM, Stafford RS, O'Leary MP, et al. How common is prostatitis? A national survey of physician visits. J Urol 1998;159:1224–8.
3. Schaeffer AJ, Parks EL, Apkarian AV. Brain activity for spontaneous fluctuations of pain in urologic pelvic pain syndrome. Chicago (IL): AUA; 2009.
4. Krieger JN, Nyberg L Jr, Nickel JC. NIH consensus definition and classification of prostatitis. JAMA 1999;282:236–7.

5. Habermacher GM, Chason JT, Schaeffer AJ. Prostatitis/chronic pelvic pain syndrome. Annu Rev Med 2006;57:195–206.

6. Weidner W, Brunner H, Krause W. Quantitative culture of ureaplasma urealyticum in patients with chronic prostatitis or prostatosis. J Urol 1980;124:622–5.

7. Weidner W, Schiefer HG, Krauss H, et al. Chronic prostatitis: a thorough search for etiologically involved microorganisms in 1,461 patients. Infection 1991;19(Suppl 3):S119–25.

8. Litwin MS, McNaughton-Collins M, Fowler FJ Jr, et al. The national institutes of health chronic prostatitis symptom index: development and validation of a new outcome measure. Chronic Prostatitis Collaborative Research Network. J Urol 1999;162:369–75.

9. Leport C, Rousseau F, Perronne C, et al. Bacterial prostatitis in patients infected with the human immunodeficiency virus. J Urol 1989;141:334–6.

10. Lee YS, Han CH, Kang SH, et al. Synergistic effect between catechin and ciprofloxacin on chronic bacterial prostatitis rat model. Int J Urol 2005;12:383–9.

11. Schaeffer AJ, Darras FS. The efficacy of norfloxacin in the treatment of chronic bacterial prostatitis refractory to trimethoprim-sulfamethoxazole and/or carbenicillin. J Urol 1990;144:690–3.

12. Weidner W, Schiefer HG, Dalhoff A. Treatment of chronic bacterial prostatitis with ciprofloxacin. Results of a one-year follow-up study. Am J Med 1987;82:280–3.

13. Weidner W, Schiefer HG, Brahler E. Refractory chronic bacterial prostatitis: a re-evaluation of ciprofloxacin treatment after a median followup of 30 months. J Urol 1991;146:350–2.

14. Meares EM. Prostatitis syndromes: new perspectives about old woes. J Urol 1980;123:141–7.

15. Schaeffer AJ. Clinical practice. Chronic prostatitis and the chronic pelvic pain syndrome. N Engl J Med 2006;355:1690–8.

16. Schaeffer AJ, Datta NS, Fowler JE Jr, et al. Overview summary statement. Diagnosis and management of chronic prostatitis/chronic pelvic pain syndrome (CP/CPPS). Urology 2002;60:1–4.

17. Krieger JN, Jacobs RR, Ross SO. Does the chronic prostatitis/pelvic pain syndrome differ from nonbacterial prostatitis and prostatodynia? J Urol 2000;164:1554–8.

18. Datta NS. Role of alpha-blockers in the treatment of chronic prostatitis. Urology 2002;60(Suppl 6):27–8.

19. Nickel JC, Downey J, Clark J, et al. Levofloxacin for chronic prostatitis/chronic pelvic pain syndrome in men: a randomized placebo-controlled multicenter trial. Urology 2003;62:614–7.

20. Simmons PD, Thin RN. Minocycline in chronic abacterial prostatitis: a double-blind prospective trial. Br J Urol 1985;57:43–5.

21. Mehik A, Alas P, Nickel JC, et al. Alfuzosin treatment for chronic prostatitis/chronic pelvic pain syndrome: a prospective, randomized, double-blind, placebo-controlled, pilot study. Urology 2003;62:425–9.

22. Nickel JC, Siemens DR, Johnston B. Transurethral radiofrequency hot balloon thermal therapy in chronic nonbacterial prostatitis. Tech Urol 1998;4:128–30.

23. Nickel JC, Krieger JN, McNaughton-Collins M, et al. Alfuzosin and symptoms of chronic prostatitis-chronic pelvic pain syndrome. N Engl J Med 2008;359:2663–73.

24. Dawson TE, Jamison J. Intravesical treatments for painful bladder syndrome/interstitial cystitis. Cochrane Database Syst Rev 2007;(4):CD006113.

25. Nickel JC. Interstitial cystitis: characterization and management of an enigmatic urologic syndrome. Rev Urol 2002;4:112–21.

26. Gillenwater JY, Wein AJ. Summary of the national institute of arthritis, diabetes, digestive and kidney diseases workshop on interstitial cystitis, national institutes of health, Bethesda, Maryland, August 28–29, 1987. J Urol 1988;140:203–6.

27. Hanno PM, Landis JR, Matthews-Cook Y, et al. The diagnosis of interstitial cystitis revisited: lessons learned from the National Institutes of Health Interstitial Cystitis Database Study. J Urol 1999;161:553–7.

28. Abrams P, Hanno P, Wein A. Overactive bladder and painful bladder syndrome: There need not be confusion. Neurourol Urodyn 2005;24:149–50.

29. O'Leary MP, Sant GR, Fowler FJ Jr, et al. The interstitial cystitis symptom index and problem index. Urology 1997;49:58–63.

30. Goin JE, Olaleye D, Peters KM, et al. Psychometric analysis of the University of Wisconsin interstitial cystitis scale: implications for use in randomized clinical trials. J Urol 1998;159:1085–90.

31. Parsons CL, Dell J, Stanford EJ, et al. Increased prevalence of interstitial cystitis: previously unrecognized urologic and gynecologic cases identified using a new symptom questionnaire and intravesical potassium sensitivity. Urology 2002;60:573–8.

32. Chaiken DC, Blaivas JG, Blaivas ST. Behavioral therapy for the treatment of refractory interstitial cystitis. J Urol 1993;149:1445–8.

33. Parsons CL, Koprowski PF. Interstitial cystitis: successful management by increasing urinary voiding intervals. Urology 1991;37:207–12.

34. Rothrock NE, Lutgendorf SK, Kreder KJ, et al. Daily stress and symptom exacerbation in interstitial cystitis patients. Urology 2001;57(6 Suppl 1):122.

35. Warren JW, Horne LM, Hebel JR, et al. Pilot study of sequential oral antibiotics for the treatment of interstitial cystitis. J Urol 2000;163:1685–8.

36. van Ophoven A, Pokupic S, Heinecke A, et al. A prospective, randomized, placebo controlled, double-blind study of amitriptyline for the treatment of interstitial cystitis. J Urol 2004;172:533–6.

37. Hanno PM. Amitriptyline in the treatment of interstitial cystitis. Urol Clin North Am 1994;21:89–91.

38. Theoharides TC. Hydroxyzine in the treatment of interstitial cystitis. Urol Clin North Am 1994;21: 113–9.

39. Sant GR, Propert KJ, Hanno PM, et al. A pilot clinical trial of oral pentosan polysulfate and oral hydroxyzine in patients with interstitial cystitis. J Urol 2003; 170:810–5.

40. Thilagarajah R, Witherow RO, Walker MM. Oral cimetidine gives effective symptom relief in painful bladder disease: a prospective, randomized, double-blind placebo-controlled trial. BJU Int 2001;87:207–12.

41. Wesselmann U, Burnett AL, Heinberg LJ. The urogenital and rectal pain syndromes. Pain 1997; 73:269–74.

42. Parsons CL, Hurst RE. Decreased urinary uronic acid levels in individuals with interstitial cystitis. J Urol 1990;143:690–3.

43. Barrington JW, Stephenson TP. Pentosanpolysulphate for interstitial cystitis. Int Urogynecol J Pelvic Floor Dysfunct 1997;8:293–5.

44. Mulholland SG, Hanno P, Parsons CL, et al. Pentosan polysulfate sodium for therapy of interstitial cystitis. A double-blind placebo-controlled clinical study. Urology 1990;35:552–8.

45. Nickel JC, Barkin J, Forrest J, et al. Randomized, double-blind, dose-ranging study of pentosan polysulfate sodium for interstitial cystitis. Urology 2005; 65:654–8.

46. Chen TY, Corcos J, Camel M, et al. Prospective, randomized, double-blind study of safety and tolerability of intravesical resiniferatoxin (RTX) in interstitial cystitis (IC). Int Urogynecol J Pelvic Floor Dysfunct 2005;16:293–7.

47. Payne CK, Mosbaugh PG, Forrest JB, et al. Intravesical resiniferatoxin for the treatment of interstitial cystitis: a randomized, double-blind, placebo controlled trial. J Urol 2005;173:1590–4.

48. Perez-Marrero R, Emerson LE, Feltis JT. A controlled study of dimethyl sulfoxide in interstitial cystitis. J Urol 1988;140:36–9.

49. Mayer R, Propert KJ, Peters KM, et al. A randomized controlled trial of intravesical bacillus Calmette-Guérin for treatment refractory interstitial cystitis. J Urol 2005;173:1186–91.

50. Peters K, Diokno A, Steinert B, et al. The efficacy of intravesical Tice strain bacillus Calmette-Guérin in the treatment of interstitial cystitis: a double-blind, prospective, placebo controlled trial. J Urol 1997; 157:2090–4.

51. Bade JJ, Laseur M, Nieuwenburg A, et al. A placebo-controlled study of intravesical pentosanpolysulphate for the treatment of interstitial cystitis. Br J Urol 1997;79:168–71.

52. Peters KM, Carey JM, Konstandt DB. Sacral neuromodulation for the treatment of refractory interstitial cystitis: outcomes based on technique. Int Urogynecol J Pelvic Floor Dysfunct 2003;14:223–8.

53. Baskin LS, Tanagho EA. Pelvic pain without pelvic organs. J Urol 1992;147:683–6.

54. Shoskes DA, Berger R, Elmi A, et al. Muscle tenderness in men with chronic prostatitis/chronic pelvic pain syndrome: the chronic prostatitis cohort study. J Urol 2008;179:556–60.

55. Peters KM, Carrico DJ, Kalinowski SE, et al. Prevalence of pelvic floor dysfunction in patients with interstitial cystitis. Urology 2007;70:16–8.

56. Simons DG, Travell JG, Simons LS. Myofascial pain and dysfunction: the trigger point manual. 2nd edition. Baltimore (MD): Williams &Wilkins. 1999. vol. 1

57. Weiss JM. Pelvic floor myofascial trigger points: manual therapy for interstitial cystitis and the urgency-frequency syndrome. J Urol 2001;166:2226–31.

58. Klumpp DJ, Rudick CN. Summation model of pelvic pain in interstitial cystitis. Nat Clin Pract Urol 2008;5:494–500.

A Round Table Discussion: Case Studies of Patients with Lower Urinary Tract Symptoms

Jerry G. Blaivas, MD[a,b,*]

KEYWORDS

• Case studies • Male • LUTS • Videourodynamics

Box
Useful acronyms in discussing LUTS

AUASS: American Urologic Association BPH Symptom Score (also known as IPSS)

FBC: Functional bladder capacity, also called MVV – the largest voided volume recorded on a 24 hour bladder diary

MVV: The largest voided volume recorded on a 24 hour bladder diary

NBC index: Nocturnal blader capacity index a measure of nocturnal bladder capacity. The higher the number, the lower the bladder capacity at night compared to daytime bladder capacity

NP index: Nocturnal poluria index = NUV/24 hour urine volume

NUV: Nocturnal urine volume as recorded on a bladder diary

Neurourologic exam: Comprised of anal sphincter tone & control; bulbocavernosus reflex; and perianal sensation

pabd: Abdominal pressure

pdet: Detrusor pressure

pdet@Qmax: Detrusor pressure at maximum uroflow

pves: Vesical pressure

PVR: Post-void residual urine volume

Q: Uroflow

Qmax: Maximum uroflow

SIC: Intermittent self catheterization

UDS: Urodynamic study

USG: Ultrasound

UVJ: Ureterovesical junction

VOID: Shorthand method of depicting Qmax/voided volume/PVR; eg: VOID: 21/355/12 where Qmax = 21; voided volume; 355 and PVR = 12

VUDS: Videourodynamic study

---

[a] Weill Cornell Medical College, Department of Urology, 525 East 68th Street, New York, NY 10065, USA
[b] SUNY Downstate Medical School, Department of Urology, 450 Clarkson Avenue, Brooklyn, NY 11203, USA
* Corresponding author. Weill Cornell Medical College, 445 East 77th Street, New York, NY 10021.
E-mail address: jgblvs@gmail.com

Urol Clin N Am 36 (2009) 537–569
doi:10.1016/j.ucl.2009.08.006
0094-0143/09/$ – see front matter © 2009 Published by Elsevier Inc.

urologic.theclinics.com

The purpose of this article is to examine real-life case histories of men with routine and not so routine conditions underlying lower urinary tract symptoms (LUTS), and to demonstrate the utility of what has become our standard evaluation: repeated bladder diaries, urinary flow rate (Q), postvoid residual urine flow (PVR), cystoscopy, and videourodynamic studies (VUDS). A LUTS questionnaire (see article by Weiss elsewhere in this issue) is also routinely used, but in the interest of brevity, has not been included the questionnaires in the case reports. Each case history was sent to each of the other authors of this monograph who, on a case by case basis, answered queries and made relevant comments.

For years, videourodynamcs and cystoscopy routinely were conducted on all men who required treatment. Those invasive studies are now recommended only under the following circumstances: (1) men who elect invasive therapies, including minimally invasive surgical therapy (MIST); (2) men with hydronephrosis that could be due to outlet obstruction or low bladder compliance; (3) men with repeated very low flow rates and/or high PVR; (4) to confirm or diagnose a neurologic condition; and (5) men who have failed conservative therapies and desire further treatment.

From a physiologic viewpoint, the cause of LUTS is multifactorial, comprising at least 5 conditions: (1) urethral obstruction, (2) impaired detrusor contractility, (3) detrusor overactivity, (4) sensory urgency, and (5) polyuria; it is the purpose of the diagnostic evaluation to define these. Although LUTS have been subdivided into irritative and obstructive bladder symptoms, there is no correlation between these descriptive terms and the underlying physiology (as discussed in more detail in the article by Bushman). Storage symptoms include urinary frequency, urgency, urge incontinence, nocturia, and some kinds of pain. Voiding symptoms include hesitancy, straining, decreased stream, dysuria, and postvoid dribbling. **Table 1** lists LUTS and the possible underlying conditions causing each.

In this article, the patient evaluations and case histories are discussed among top experts who have authored articles in this issue: Dr Wade Bushman, Dr Stephen Petrou, Dr Lori Lerner,

Table 1
Causes of lower urinary tract symptoms

Symptom	Causes
Hesitancy weak/interrupted stream	Urethral obstruction Detrusor overactivity Impaired detrusor contractility Acquired voiding dysfunction
Urinary frequency	Polyuria Detrusor overactivity Small capacity bladder Acquired voiding dysfunction Low bladder compliance
Urgency urge incontinence	Detrusor overactivity Bladder inflammation/UTI
Stress incontinence	Sphincteric incontinence Stress hyperreflexia Low bladder compliance
Unaware incontinence	Detrusor overactivity Sphincteric incontinence Fistula
Nocturia	Nocturnal polyuria Detrusor overactivity Small capacity bladder Low nocturnal bladder capacity Global polyuria (24 h volume >40 mL/kg)
Nocturnal enuresis	Sphincter abnormality Detrusor overactivity Urinary retention
Postvoid dribble	Postsphincteric collection of urine

Dr Karl Kreder, Dr Charles Powell, Dr Matthew Rutman, Dr Kevin McVary, Dr Robert Donnell, Dr Gary Leach, and Dr Jeffrey Weiss.

CASE 1 (KM). OVERACTIVE BLADDER DOMINATED LUTS; TREATED WITH MEDICATION

Patient: KM is a 49-year-old executive with mixed storage and emptying symptoms.

History: He complains of urinary frequency, urgency, and nocturia and, when queried, admitted that he also has some hesitancy and weak stream, but the overactive bladder (OAB) symptoms dominated the clinical picture. These symptoms began about 6 to 12 months ago and have gradually worsened.

American Urological Association (AUA) symptom score: 27.

Physical examination: Prostate 25 g, smooth; right lobe slightly firmer than left.

Urinalysis: normal.

Questions for the panel: Do you require any more information before initiating treatment?

Answer:

All respondents wanted to see prostate-specific antigen (PSA) level, uroflow, and PVR. Only 40% thought a urine culture and/or urinary cytology was necessary, and 40% wanted to see a bladder diary. Dr McVary wanted to know whether there was a family history of prostate cancer and whether there were any risk factors for urethral stricture. Based on the digital rectal examination (DRE) he said "it sounds like a transrectal ultrasound (TRUS) prostate biopsy should be done." No one recommended upper tract imaging unless there was an elevated PVR.

Drs Kreder and Powell: "With the urinalysis being negative for leucine esterase and nitrite, we wouldn't pursue urinary tract infection as the cause but it could still be prostatitis. We would want a PSA so we don't miss the easy things—prostate cancer and prostatitis. If the PSA is elevated, we would recommend expressed prostatic secretions and culture and a prostate biopsy, especially of the firm area."

Back to the patient:

Neuro-urologic examination: normal (anal sphincter tone and control, perianal sensation, bulbocavernosus reflex)

Laboratory: PSA .7

VOID: 4/85/55 (The Q curve is seen in **Fig. 1**)

Voiding diary:

24-hour voided volume	1560 mL
Usual voided volume	90–120 mL
Maximum voided volume (MVV)	210 mL
Awake hours: # voids	8
Sleep hours: # voids	2
Nocturnal urine volume (NUV)	330 mL
Nocturia index (NUV/MVV)	1.6
Nocturnal polyuria index (NPi)-NUV/Total 24 hour volume	15%
Nocturnal bladder capacity (NBC) index	1.4

Comment: I consider the neuro-urologic examination—anal sphincter tone and control, perianal sensation, and the bulbocavernosus reflex—to be an essential part of the physical examination. It is almost always normal, but when it is not, it may be the only underlying clue to a neurologic lesion like cauda equina or Shy-Drager syndrome. It takes about 30 to 60 seconds to complete (and your finger is already in the rectum for the DRE)!

And the bladder diary! I don't know how anyone can treat these patients without one. Look at his. His MVV, which is his functional bladder capacity, is only 210 mL and most of his voids are between 90 and 120 mL. So his volume of 85 mL for the Q is only a bit lower than usual. If his usual voided volumes were 400 mL, for example, we'd more or less ignore this Q and repeat it.

Question for the panel: How would you treat him?

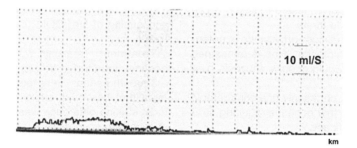

Fig. 1. KM. Uroflow.

Answer:

Dr Kreder: Start with tamsulosin 0.4 mg every bedtime and have a discussion about finasteride. If he is willing to take another pill and understands the uncertainty some feel about the higher incidence of high-grade cancers coming from the prostate cancer prevention trial, I would start that as well.

Dr Leach: Since his PSA is within normal limits AND Qmax is low and PVR low, I would consider a trial of α-blocker.

Dr Donnell: If he wanted treatment (and the PSA, and voiding diary supported), I would use α-blocker as the first line therapy.

Dr Lerner and Dr Bushman: α-Blocker.

Dr McVary: Offer α-blockers, with strict requests for follow-up in office in 6 to 8 weeks.

Dr Powell: I would empirically try α-blockers if PSA is normal. If still not better after 2 months on tamsulosin, would get urodynamic studies (UDS) and consider cystoscopy with repeat urinalysis (UA). He may be a candidate for daily tadalafil if he fails tamsulosin. I would continue tamsulosin.

Dr Rutman: Behavioral modification (fluid and caffeine reduction, bladder retraining), likely selective α-blocker (tamsulosin or uroxatral), possible antimuscarinic if still symptomatic (storage symptoms) despite α-blocker.

Dr Weiss: No treatment until additional information becomes available.

Question for panel: When initiating treatment do you consider any differences between commercially available α-adrenergic medications, that is, is one medication better for this patient than another?

Answer:

Dr Lerner and Dr Bushman: Only that tamsulosin and alfuzosin are easier to use because no need to titrate.

Dr Weiss: Terazosin is cheap, effective, and generally well titrated when begun with a dose pack card. If the patient develops or is at high risk for orthostatic hypotension, tamsulosin is my next line of therapy.

Dr Leach: I think all α-blocker medications are essentially equally efficacious, but generally I prescribe tamsulosin given less orthostatic hypotension and no need to titrate.

Dr Rutman: Yes, I discuss orthostatic hypotension, ejaculatory disturbance. If he is concerned about ejaculation, I would choose alfuzosin over tamsulosin.

Dr McVary: I most commonly use nontitratable α blockers but agree that generics requiring titrations are similar in efficacy.

Dr Kreder: Yes. I feel that tamsulosin is better for older men and those at risk for dizziness and

falls; otherwise, all are equally efficacious. If this man had no risk factors, terazosin is my drug of choice because a 100-day supply can be gotten for $19.00 while tamsulosin is $25.03 per 30-day supply, at the least expensive pharmacy Web site. Another difference is that alfuzosin is a good option for a young man with retrograde ejaculation on tamsulosin.

Dr Donnell: I believe that α-blockers are equal, and I prescribe based on patient's choice.

Back to the patient:

We did not treat him yet. We obtained cystoscopy and videourodynamic study (**Fig. 2**).

Cystoscopy: minimal bilobar prostatic encroachment, 1+ trabeculation, and small paraureteral bladder diverticulum.

The Schaefer and Abrams-Griffiths nomograms both show significant bladder outlet obstruction (**Fig. 3**A, B).

Question for panel: Does any of this information change your treatment plan?

Dr Weiss: This man has prostatic obstruction, small bladder capacity, and normal bladder contractility. I would begin an α-blocker, terazosin, titrated initially to 5 mg every bedtime.

Dr Leach: No.

Dr Kreder: Yes. The diverticulum should be carefully examined for tumor, and cytology sent yearly. Fulguration of the diverticulum should be offered, as it offers a minimally invasive way to ablate this small diverticulum. If he begins to develop urinary tract infections (UTIs) then discussion about diverticulectomy should take place. The patient is obstructed and can be started on α-blockers if not already taking them. If he is already on them or has tried them already, then I would offer him transurethral incision of the bladder neck, given the relatively small size of the prostate.

Question: How soon would you see him in follow-up after initiating treatment?

Answer: All respondents said 1 to 3 months.

Question: What efficacy outcomes measures would you use to assess outcomes?

Answer: There was no consensus at all except that 75% of the respondents said they would use the AUA symptom score as part of their assessment. All uses various combinations of symptom and quality of life (QOL) questionnaires, Q, and PVR.

Treatment: Terazosin was begun at 1 mg at bedtime and titrated to 4 mg every bedtime over a 3-month period. He noted a dramatic improvement that has been sustained for 5 years. The most striking difference was, "I only get up once at night (compared with) just about hourly." He also noted a dramatic decrease in the number and intensity of episodes of urgency and voids

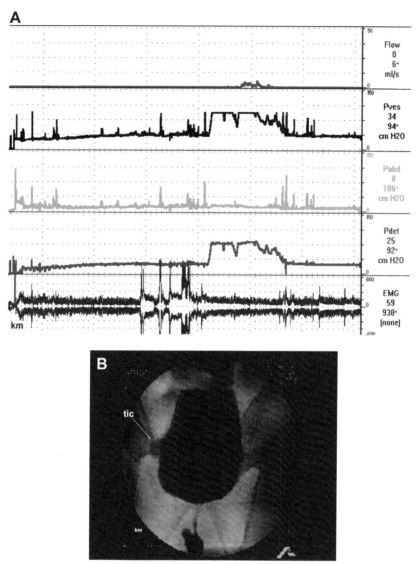

Fig. 2. (*A*) KM Urodynamic study. The pves tracing was subject to a software glitch that resulted in "graph clipping," which cut off the height of the curve. Nevertheless, it is apparent that he had a sustained detrusor contraction and pdet @ Qmax was 75 cm H_2O and Q max = 5 mL/s, indicating urethral obstruction. (*B*) KM. Voiding cystourethrogram exposed at Qmax, showing a narrowed prostatic urethra and a small right bladder diverticulum (tic).

with a much better stream. After about a year of treatment, he said "I'm back to normal…I can go to a meeting and I don't have to get up to urinate."

Comment: From a clinical perspective, KM was very much improved and very pleased with his treatment. The most striking improvement in symptoms is the marked improvement in urgency, bladder capacity, and nocturia. Although according to his diaries nocturia decreased from 2 times to 1 time per night, he thinks that his first diary was atypical. However, his AUA symptom score only improved from 27 to 18, which is still considered to be a moderately severe symptom score. This points out the importance of not relying on objective criteria alone. Diaries and symptoms scores are very useful, but only when they are put into clinical perspective by talking to the patient.

Objectively, his improvement was manifest by an increase in bladder capacity from 210 to 410 mL. However, his urinary stream is not very different than when he began treatment, and objectively, his uroflow remains quite low and has a long plateau shape, consistent with his documented prostatic urethral obstruction (**Table 2**).

So, what got better? It is doubtful that his obstruction is improved. If anything, his most recent uroflow suggests that it is either worse, or

A

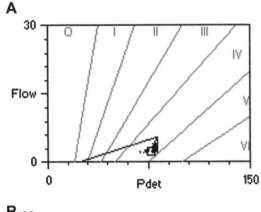

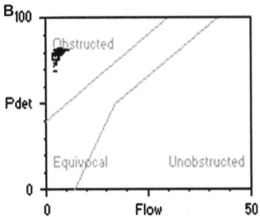

Fig. 3. (*A*) KM. Schafer nomogram showing grade 4 urethral obstruction. (*B*) KM Abrams-Griffiths nomogram showing obstruction.

he has developed impaired detrusor contractility. The only way of finding out is to repeat his video-urodynamic studies (VUDS), but this was not done because from a symptomatic viewpoint he felt so much better. Serial renal and bladder ultra-sounds were done in KM to be sure that his voiding

pattern was not causing bladder or renal compli-cations. His bladder diverticulum appears unchanged and, aside from a benign appearing renal cyst, the kidneys remained normal.

Why did his bladder capacity improve? We don't know, but there were many comments from the panel.

Dr Lerner: It has been suggested, by Cucci I believe, that development of frequency as a func-tion of diminished bladder compliance is a compensatory response of the detrusor to increased outlet resistance that is done to make bladder emptying more energy efficient. It may be simply that α-blockers interrupt this compensa-tory response.

Dr Weiss: I agree with the aforementioned. There may be a "clinic" effect that amounts to placebo benefit from generally being followed in a genitourinary office. Just doing voiding diaries can change drinking and voiding behavior to result in the perception of improvement from treatment received.

Dr Leach: An obvious possibility could be the chronic distension from increasing residuals.

Dr McVary: From a urodynamic perspective, α-adrenergic blockade in patients with urodynami-cally proven obstruction receiving terazosin causes a significant decrease in urethral resis-tance at 26 weeks of therapy compared with none of the patients without obstruction. However, the actual improvement in urodynamic parameters is less impressive than improvement in free urinary flow and symptoms using the international pros-tate symptom score. Further studies are needed to identify reasons for the symptomatic benefit gleaned from α-blockers out of proportion to improvement in urodynamic parameters of pres-sure flow and urethral resistance factors.

Dr Petrou: I don't know that it really matters, since there's no compelling evidence that

Table 2
Data summarizing symptoms of patient in case history 1

Date	Terazosin Dose (mg)	AUA Score	No. of Day Voids	No. of Night Voids	Bladder Capacity	Usual Voided Volume	Qmax	Voided Volume	PVR
11/94	0	27	7	2	210	90–120	4	85	55
2/95	3		10	1	250		7	62	
3/95	4						7	230	83
8/95	4	22	8	0	460	130–165	10	289	
10/96	7	19	10	1	350	130–230	7	304	93
11/97	9		8	0	240	140–230	9	355	19
7/99	5	18	9	1	410	160–200	4	398	149

unrelieved obstruction moves inexorably to worsening symptoms or acute urinary retention. If the symptoms are relieved—that's enough. However, I would have offered the man a transurethral incision of the prostate (TUIP) as a very good alternative. A 1-hour procedure with minimal morbidity would be likely to provide even greater symptomatic improvement and obviate a lifetime of medication.

Dr Weiss: As long as the patient is happy, with no worrisome symptoms such as worsening urgency or development of incontinence and the PVR is not rising, I would continue indefinitely with conservative therapy. The only long-term potential problem I know of from the use of chronic α-blockers is the effect on the eye, especially with respect to the risk of complications from cataract surgery.

Dr Leach: We know that α-blockers may affect bladder function by changing outflow resistance or can possibly have a direct effect on bladder function. A urodynamic study would have been helpful in determining the etiology of the change in capacity.

Dr Kreder: α-Blockers have been shown to increase bladder capacity in one abstract presented at a recent International Continence Society meeting that comes to mind.[1] The investigators used endorectal ultrasound to assess blood flow to the bladder and prostate as well as bladder capacity before and after 5 weeks of tamsulosin. The bladder was filled with NaCl followed by KCl to mimic irritative symptoms. The maximum urodynamic bladder capacity increased by 100 mL for the KCl group treated with tamsulosin. There was no change for the NaCl group. No mechanism was proposed for this effect, other than the observation that blood flow was increased significantly by tamsulosin.[2] This would be consistent with the findings in this case.

CASE 2 (PD). OVERACTIVE BLADDER PREDOMINANT LUTS TREATED WITH SURGERY

Patient: PD is a 56-year-old insurance broker with OAB predominant LUTS.

Urologic history: His chief complaint is urinary frequency, urgency, and nocturia of over 10 years' duration. He voids more often than once an hour during the day and has nocturia about every 1 to 2 hours at night. He has never been incontinent, but "I've been close." He always has hesitancy and a weak stream. He is currently being treated with tamsulosin, 4 mg twice a day and finasteride, 5 mg every day. PSA has ranged from 6.3 to 7 for the last 5 years, and he has had 2 sextant prostate biopsies that have shown benign prostate hyperplasia (BPH). The last biopsy was 6 months ago.

Prior treatment: doxazosin (4 mg every day), terazosin (every day). Each was discontinued because of lightheadedness.

Medical history: mild asthma.

AUA symptom score: 27.

Physical examination: Prostate estimated 15 to 20 g in size, normal consistency, and no nodules.

Laboratory: Total PSA = 3.30 mg/mL.

Free PSA = 0.49 mg/mL (15%).

Urinalysis = normal.

VOID: 7/62/20 **Fig. 4**

Questions for the panel: It's been 6 months since his last biopsy; would you recommend another or more aggressive biopsy? Anything else to aid in the diagnosis of prostate cancer?

Answer:

Dr Weiss: Yes. Our recent study of a large database of men undergoing prostate biopsy concluded that the ideal ratio of prostate volume/core ratio to maximize the diagnosis of prostate cancer is 3 mL/core biopsy.[3] Assuming his prostate is actually 20 mL, a sextant biopsy (and even better, 2 of these sessions) should adequately cover such a gland. His PSA has

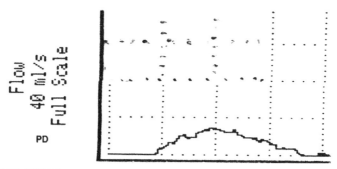

Fig. 4. PD. Uroflow. VOID: 7/62/20.

appropriately come down in response to finasteride, from between 6 and 7 to 3.3. However, the elevated PSA on its own mitigates saturation biopsies, which in this case would be 12 in all.

Dr Petrou: Since the diagnosis of prostate cancer is an issue in view of the history of finasteride and his free PSA total, then I would ask him to undergo a transperineal ultrasound guided templated prostate biopsies. This would also be an ideal way of obtaining a very accurate prostate volume if further therapy is being considered.

Dr Lerner: First, I'd like to make sure that his urinalysis is negative and that his OAB symptoms aren't related to hematuria/bladder cancer. Second, what was the prostate size on TRUS? Is that the 15 to 20 g? Third, has he had any response at all to meds? Did they improve his symptoms, even a little bit? I think this is important to know because it helps us know if this is a BPH/bladder outflow obstruction (BOO) kind of picture versus a high bladder neck. Fourth, did they see inflammation on the biopsies consistent with prostatitis, which could explain his PSA? Lastly, is there a family history of prostate cancer and/or Agent Orange exposure or something that makes us worry about prostate cancer other than the PSA?

Dr Rutman: I would tell him that sextant biopsies are not the standard of care in 2009. Considering he is on finasteride (Proscar) and his PSA is significantly elevated with a palpably small gland, I would recommend a 12-core biopsy if he was interested in being screened for prostate cancer.

Dr Leach: Yes, I would repeat prostate biopsy (6 times each side).

Dr Donnell: In light of his young age, the elevated PSA, the decreased percent free PSA, the reported small prostate size without evidence of inflammation on biopsy, I would repeat a more aggressive biopsy. From this information I would also confirm the prostate size by ultrasound. The diagnosis of prostate cancer would certainly change my approach to his LUTS over the near future.

Question: Assuming that he does not have prostate cancer and he does not want surgery, would you continue to treat him empirically or do you want more studies (urodynamics, cystoscopy)?

Dr Weiss: If his urinalysis and cytology are normal, cystoscopy is optional although I find it useful and would recommend it. The next step before UDS is a voiding diary, preferably several. This will tell us what the functional bladder capacity would be and whether some extraurologic condition such as global polyuria or nocturnal polyuria are contributing to his symptoms. In view of the long-standing nature of his symptoms, urodynamics are indicated as they are in anyone with near-urgency incontinence.

Dr Lerner: It would depend on his response to meds. If he is not responding well to meds, I would encourage a pressure flow study.

Dr Rutman: If he is not interested in surgery and wishes to proceed with medical therapy, I would not perform urodynamics. I would only perform cystoscopy if he had microscopic hematuria.

Dr Donnell: Assuming that he does not have prostate cancer, a urinalysis, cytology, and voiding diary are acceptable. I would then proceed with urodynamics.

Dr Leach: I would do urodynamics and cystoscopy.

Dr Petrou: I would do cystoscopy, urodynamics, and urine cytology.

Question: Assuming that he does not have prostate cancer, and he does not want surgery, how would you treat him now?

Dr Weiss: I would not treat such a patient empirically. He has had quite enough of that for years. Treatment would be tailored to the most specific diagnosis I could derive from analysis of the voiding diary, cystoscopy, and urodynamic study.

Dr Lerner: Urinary urgency always concerns me regarding bladder compensation/decompensation. If he didn't want surgery, I would encourage him to make sure that his bladder wasn't "asking for help." I would consider anticholinergics, but his age suggests that if obstruction were found, a lot of his instability could resolve after treatment.

Dr Rutman: I would add anticholinergics to treat his storage symptoms. Since he also has obstructive symptoms, I would use an α-blocker in addition. If he did not have obstructive symptoms, I would use the anticholinergic alone. I do not believe there is a significant difference between anticholinergic agents as a class, with the caveat that some agents work better in some patients in a completely unpredictable fashion.

Dr Leach: His diagnosis is bladder outlet obstruction and probable detrusor overactivity. With a small prostate (20 g) I would discontinue finasteride and continue tamsulosin, and add an anticholingeric (darifenacin 7.5 mg every bedtime).

Dr Petrou: I'd recommend combined therapy with α-blockers and anticholinergics.

Question: If you recommend anticholinergics, do you think it is necessary to always use α-blockers as well? Do you think there are significant differences among anticholinergics?

Answers:

Dr Petrou: Single-agent initial therapy is acceptable; significant differences are an active point of debate among many of our colleagues, although if the patient does have some postvoid residual present, trospium chloride may be of value in view of its unmetabolized direct effect on the urothelium. Of attractiveness for the contemporary male patient may be the topical gel anticholinergics, in view of the non-pill format and the acceptance of hormone replacement in this fashion.

Dr Weiss: If I'm not sure if a man is obstructed I tend to start an α-blocker as "pretreatment" before institution of anticholinergics. While different patients respond in variable fashion at times to available anticholinergics, we do not have the ability to predict which patients will respond best to which of these. The theoretical differences in receptor affinity among the newer anticholinergics do not translate into major predictable clinical responses. (Perhaps in the elderly one might consider trospium, as it crosses the blood-brain barrier less well than all others owing to its status as a charged amine.) For this reason, and for reasons of economy, assuming there is no history of narrow-angle glaucoma I begin with oxybutynin at a low dose, 2.5 mg twice a day, then have them return in 3 to 4 weeks with a fresh diary for Q, PVR, and questionnaire.

Dr Lerner: No, I do not always think it is necessary to use an α-blocker with an anticholinergic. Yes, there are some differences between drugs, but some patients just do better with one drug over another. I start with oxybutynin, then go to tolterodine, then onwards from there. I tend to avoid the long-acting meds, simply because I don't think they work as well in obstruction-related instability. Neurogenics and age-related instability may do well with long acting, but I have anecdotally found that the peaks of shorter-acting meds are more efficacious.

Dr Leach: I would not give an anticholinergic without the α-blocker in an obstructed man with BPH. I prefer darifenacin due to the lack of "cortical" side effects (memory loss and so forth).

Dr Bushman: I would start anticholinergics along with the α-blocker, establishing the response, and then remove the α-blocker.

Dr Donnell: If I recommend an anticholinergic I refer to the presence or absence of my urodynamics. I will empirically start an α-blocker before an anticholinergic. I do believe that there are differences between the drugs, but for the majority of patients there is little difference in efficacy and a larger concern for side effects.

Question: What is the role for MIST in a patient who says that he doesn't want surgery? Do you consider MIST to be "surgery?" What do you tell the patient?

Dr Weiss: I have been personally disappointed with nonvaporizing treatments that heat the prostate, and do not use or recommend them. They certainly are capable of causing catastrophic complications such as severe bladder neck stenosis. They are inequitably (compared with transurethral resection of the prostate [TURP], TUIP, laser prostatectomy) well compensated by third-party carriers, which in my view is the main reason they persist in urologic practice.

Dr Lerner: I NEVER do MIST, ever.

Dr Rutman: I would discuss all options including Prostiva radiofrequency ablation (RFA) and Microwave, although I am not a huge advocate of these procedures. I would still inform him of the options and refer him if that was a strong consideration. I consider the RFA to be the better option of the two, but I would let him know of all potential outcomes including worsening of his storage symptoms, retention, and lack of efficacy. Since the patient has a small prostate he may be amenable to a TUIP. Otherwise he would be a candidate for any intervention to relieve his obstruction.

Dr Leach: I would not do MIST in a man with OAB symptoms. In my experience, if they get any relief from their OAB symptoms, it is only temporary and they usually get worse before they get better.

Dr Petrou: The larger the volume the less inclination for minimally invasive technique. All surgery including minimally invasive techniques are major surgeries to the person receiving the therapy.

Dr Donnell: MIST therapy can certainly play a role for the patient who does not want surgery and even for that patient who does not want to take pills. I share with my patients that transurethral needle ablation (TUNA) and transurethral microwave therapy (TUMT) are procedures requiring a well-performed regional bloc of the prostate and oral pain medications. While not surgery, I share with them that their time commitment and recovery effort the first day are similar to regular surgery.

Question: How does prostate size influence your treatment recommendations?

Dr Weiss: Men with larger, more glandular prostates may respond better to 5α-reductase inhibitors, especially when the PSA is slightly elevated above normal. I favor KTP laser prostatectomy for small to medium-size prostates and TURP for larger glands. For prostates over 100 mL it is reasonable to consider open prostatectomy, especially in the presence of bladder stones.

Dr Lerner: Size makes a difference between a TUIP versus a more complete trilobar surgery.

Dr Rutman: I would recommend urodynamics to evaluate his bladder function. If he had good bladder function, I would recommend an outlet reductive procedure such as a TUIP or a Green Light HPS Laser prostatectomy.

Dr Leach: Only in that I would not use finasteride with a prostate less than 50 g in size.

Dr Donnell: We do need to be aware of prostate size due to the technical limitations of these particular therapies. An ultrasound would provide information concerning prostate volume, the presence of a median lobe with intravesicle protrusion, which appear to be important parameters associated with increased failure of minimally invasive therapies. Certainly there is a size relationship with TUIP and 5α-reductase inhibitors. There also appears to be a size relationship with Botox, TUNA, and TUMT. Early evidence would support that Botox is possibly more appropriate in the smaller gland as would be TUNA, while TUMT may be better served in that patient with a larger prostate.

Question: If he says that he will follow your advice and do whatever treatment you think will achieve the best outcome, what is your advice?

Dr Weiss: I don't have enough data at this point to recommend a treatment pathway. I want to see the results of the voiding diary, cystoscopy, and urodynamic study.

Dr Lerner and Dr Donnell: I would do UDS and then decide.

Dr Rutman: If we were going to prescribe an antimuscarinic agent, I'd see him back 4 to 6 weeks after instituting therapy. If there was any concern about increasing retention, maybe sooner to check a postvoid residual (2 weeks after starting the antimuscarinic).

Dr Leach: I suggest an α-blocker combined with an anticholinergic agent at this point.

Back to the patient:
Voiding diary:

24-hour voided volume	1,500 mL
Awake hours: # voids	9
Sleep hours: # voids	4
Usual voided volume	120 mL
Functional bladder capacity	240 mL
Nocturnal urinary volume	480 mL
NUV/Total	32%
NBC/Index	3
Nocturia index (NUV/FBC)	2

Cystoscopy: The prostatic urethra was over 6 cm in length and there was a very large intravesical lobe. The bladder was 4+ trabeculated.

Urodynamic study: (8 April, 1999) Tracing is depicted in **Fig. 5**

Fig. 6A, B depict the bladder during filling and voiding.

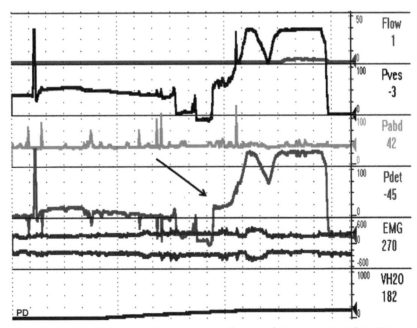

Fig. 5. PD. Urodynamic tracing. The *arrow* denotes an involuntary detrusor contraction. He was aware of the contraction, and by contracting his sphincter, was able to prevent incontinence, but unable to abort the contraction. This is called type 3 OAB. pdet @ Qmax = 139 cm/H$_2$O; Qmax = 4 mL/s.

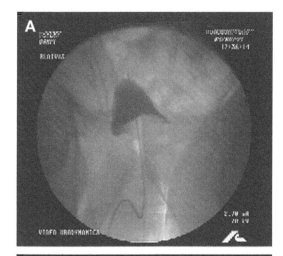

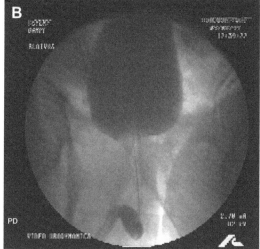

Fig. 6. (*A*) PD. This radiograph was taken with about 50 mL in the bladder. Note the prostate impression on the bladder base. (*B*) PD. This radiograph was taken at Qmax. Note the entire prostatic urethra is markedly narrowed.

Urodynamic diagnosis:

1. Prostatic obstruction
2. Type 3 OAB (detrusor overactivity)

Repeat sextant TRUS prostate biopsy showed nodular BPH without signs of chronic inflammation. The prostate was estimated to be about 80 g in size.

Question: How would you treat this patient? Please describe how you came to your decision.

Dr Weiss: With the large gland and intravesical component, suprapubic prostatectomy is the treatment of choice although many skilled resectionists would feel TURP may be done safely with a similar outcome while avoiding an incision. KTP laser prostatectomy is safe and effective in the hands of those accustomed to performing this procedure on large prostates, and may be the treatment of choice for

men on anticoagulant therapy, even if it means staged procedures would be necessary.

Dr Lerner: I would have done UDS early in this man because of his failure to respond to meds. Then, I would have recommended holmium laser enucleation of the prostate. I had a feeling that his TRUS volume was different than that of his DRE. If BOO is present, then surgery is where I go next. Anticholinergics may be necessary during the postoperative recovery phase, and I use them often.

Dr Rutman: This case played out differently than I expected since the prostate volume was estimated at 15 mL on physical examination. I would have likely offered the patient a Green Light Laser prostatectomy, bipolar TURP, and an open prostatectomy (if the median lobe was gigantic and essentially unresectable transurethrally). I would not recommend a MIST for a patient with a large gland.

Dr Leach: I would also do an open prostatectomy.

Dr Petrou: Single medical therapy followed by multimodal therapy, then followed by tissue ablative therapy if needed.

Dr Donnell: The final outcome of this patient would not warrant a MIST therapy at the time of his presentation for TURP. I would offer him a high-power laser ablation. One would question whether the minimally invasive therapies would have altered his final presentation in either the final presenting symptoms or the time course of the disease. With the HPS laser system the number of open prostatectomies I perform has decreased dramatically.

Back to the patient:

Treatment: Suprapubic prostatectomy was performed without incident. Pathology was nodular BPH (no inflammation).

Follow-up: (4 weeks postop): He said he was voiding with a better stream than he could ever remember, but was disappointed that he still had OAB symptoms and was most bothered by the persistent nocturia.

VOID: 19/207/52 (**Fig. 7**).

Voiding diary:

24-hour voided volume	1,620 mL
Daytime urinary volume	900 mL
Nocturnal urinary volume	720 mL
Awake hours: # voids	8
Sleep hours: # voids	3
Usual voided volume	120 mL
MVV	240 mL
NP index	44%
NBC index	1
Nocturia index (NUV/MVV)	3

The diary showed persistence of nocturnal poly-uria He was started on a low-key behavioral program with particular emphasis on cutting back on fluid intake after his nighttime meal, and made considerable improvement. A bladder diary 6 months postop showed complete resolution of his nocturnal polyuria and OAB symptoms. In addition, his functional bladder capacity increased to 350 mL. He said "I can't believe that I had to wait 5 years for this; I'm cured."

Voiding diary: 6 months postop

24-hour voided volume	1750 mL
Awake hours: # voids	4
Sleep hours: # voids	2
Usual voided volume	300 mL
MVV	350 mL
NUV	600 mL
NP index	33%
NBC index	2
Nocturia index (NUV/FBC)	2

He was unchanged at 1 year follow-up and never returned to the office, but responded to a telephone interview and said that he remains "cured." He declined further prostate cancer screening.

Discussion: PD has had over a decade of unsuccessful "conservative therapy" for BPH. He'd failed almost all of the commercially available α-adrenergic agonists and had at various times been advised to undergo a variety of laser, ultra-sonic, and other thermal procedures intended to accomplish prostatic ablation. His symptoms began when he was in his early forties, and he was thought to be "too young" to have prostatic urethral obstruction.

He consulted us about treatment options. Although his PSA had fallen to 3.3, he was being treated with finasteride and his free PSA was 15%. Repeat sextant biopsy was done to rule out prostate cancer. Prostate ultrasound estimated the size of his prostate at only 80 g, but because of the length of the prostatic urethra (>6 cm) and the large intravesical component, open prostatectomy was elected. At the time none of the current laser surgeries were available.

From our perspective, the choice between TURP, laser prostatic ablation, and open prosta-tectomy is a personal one based primarily on the preference of the surgeon (hopefully he or she is a reasonable judge of his or her surgical skills).

We believe that the choice between a retropubic and suprapubic approach is best made at the time of surgery. If there is sufficient prostatic bulk to accomplish an incision in the anterior prostatic capsule, we prefer a retropubic approach because we believe that it is easier to control bleeding. However, if most of the prostate is intravesical, as it was in this case, a suprapubic approach is technically easier.

For the first month or so his storage symptoms (frequency, urgency, and nocturia) were unabated despite a marked improvement in flow from 7 to 19 mL/s, but his most bothersome symptoms (noctu-ria) was due to a nonurologic condition—nocturnal polyuria—and was effectively treated by behavior modification. By 6 months postop he was totally asymptomatic.

There is, of course, a concern about prostate cancer, given his PSA history, but we respect his decision to decline further screening.

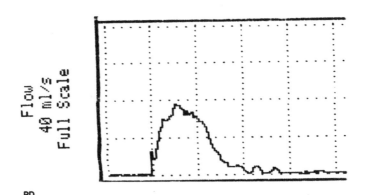

Fig. 7. PD. Uroflow obtained 4 weeks post suprapubic prostatectomy. VOID: 19/207/52.

CASE 3 (AT). OVERACTIVE BLADDER TREATED WITH MEDICATIONS

Patient: AT is a 58-year-old married Greek immigrant who works as a bridge painter (big bridges; high up)!

Date: May 25, 2004

History: His chief complaint was "I pee a lot... I can't see water...I have to go." He voids more often than once an hour for the last 4 to 5 years and has nocturia 1 to 2 times at night. "The urine comes out easy, but not too strong." He has daily urgency but never had urge incontinence.

He has had 4 negative prostate biopsies because of an elevated PSA. The last biopsy was about 6 months ago. Current PSA is 7.9. He also complains of premature ejaculation for the last 3 or 4 months.

He was empirically treated with finasteride and long-acting tolterodine, but found them ineffective and discontinued them.

Current medications: None.

Allergies: None.

Surgery: None.

Family diseases: None.

Social history: He has a 40-year history of smoking 2 packs of cigarettes per day, but does not drink alcohol and does not use drugs.

Physical examination:

Prostate: 2+ in size, normal consistency, no nodules.

Neuro-urologic examination: Normal.

Bladder diary showed 12 voids in 24 hours with a maximum voided volume of 510 mL.

VOID: 35/394/4

He underwent 18-core TRUS-guided prostate biopsy, which was negative for cancer.

Question for the panel: Any further diagnostic tests now? How would you treat him?

Dr Petrou: I would check urine cytology and do cystoscopy. I'd recommend an a-blocker and discuss possible empiric therapy with antibiotics for possible subclinical prostatitis causing voiding dysfunction and sexual dysfunction, as well as an elevated PSA.

Dr Rutman: I'd do urodynamics and cystoscopy. I agree with your assessment. I would also want him to do a full voiding diary including fluid intake to assess his caffeine intake.

Dr Donnell: I also agree with workup so far. I too would ask for a voiding diary with intake/output and urodynamics. With the prominence of the irritative voiding symptoms and his strong tobacco history, I would also perform a cystoscopy.

Dr Weiss: Post prostate massage urine culture to exclude smoldering prostatitis. Urine cytology. If he has sterile pyuria I would obtain urine for acid-fast bacilli. VUDS and cystoscopy. Consider

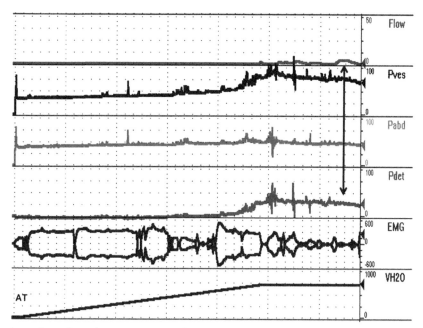

Fig. 8. AT. Urodynamic tracing. There were no involuntary detrusor contractions. A patient with OAB without detrusor overactivity is classified as type 1 OAB. He has a weak detrusor contraction (pdet @ Qmax = 28 cm H_2O) and a weak flow (Qmax = 5 mL/s). The *arrow* points to Qmax.

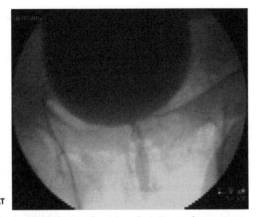

AT

Fig. 9. AT. Radiograph exposed at Qmax shows a narrowed prostatic urethra.

a 4-week course of empiric antibiotics just to make sure we're not dealing with prostatitis while being scheduled for cysto and UDS. If antibiotics cure him, just do the cysto.

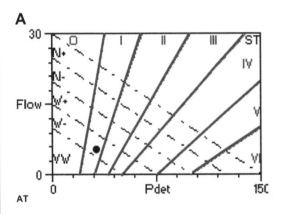

A

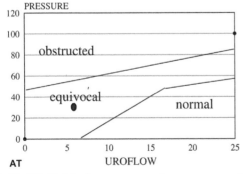

B   Abrams - Griffiths Nomogram

Fig. 10. (A) AT. Schafer nomogram shows a very weak detrusor contraction and a grade 1 urethral obstruction, which is considered equivocal. (B) AT. Abrams-Griffiths nomogram shows equivocal obstruction.

Back to the patient. He underwent cystoscopy and VUDS. Cystoscopy showed a 4-cm prostatic urethra with trilobar enlargement and diffuse 3+ bladder trabeculations (**Figs. 8** and **9**).

Videourodynamic study showed type 1 OAB and definite impaired detrusor contractility, and equivocal urethral obstruction according to P/Q, but his free flow was normal and residual urine was only 4 mL. The impaired detrusor contractility and equivocal urethral obstruction are depicted on the Schafer and Abrams-Griffiths nomograms (**Fig. 10**).

Question for the panel: How do you explain the normal unintubated uroflow and the impaired detrusor contractility and equivocal obstruction?

Dr Petrou: Is his detrusor contraction really that impaired?

Dr Rutman: The contractility equation is pdet @ Qmax + 5 [Qmax]. Therefore if his pressures are low (possibly secondary to a decompensated bladder based on the severe trabeculations on cysto), he will have impaired contractility and this would explain his equivocal BOO. Free flow is a nice initial test, but you need pressure flow to diagnose obstruction.

Dr Weiss: He has urgency without involuntary contractions by definition. Equivocal obstruction occurs when the urethral resistance is variable, and the urethra does not relax during maximum uroflow on the UDS. He does not have impaired detrusor contractility since his free flow is normal. Most likely his external urethra doesn't relax during micturition at least on a consistent basis. This suggests he has sensory urgency and/or pelvic floor dysfunction.

Dr Bushman: By my criteria, I think that a TURP would reduce afterload on the impaired bladder and improve his symptoms.

Question for the panel: Do these urodynamic findings change the way you would treat him?

Dr Petrou: No.

Dr Rutman: Yes, I would warn him that if we take a watchful waiting approach, he may experience detrusor failure and require catheterization. However, I think trying an antimuscarinic agent and behavioral changes is reasonable to assess his symptoms. If there is significant improvement, I would carefully monitor his PVR over time.

Dr Donnell: The patient has already trialed one antimuscarinic without success. If he does not have elevated PVR on follow-up and other antimuscarinics are not effective, it is possible that in the future Botox may be an attractive agent for such a patient. The agent is investigational at present, but the symptom complex is attractive to the theoretical properties of this agent. Further, the patient is quite young and such a minimally invasive procedure would be less likely to impact future therapies if he required treatment for prostate cancer.

Dr Weiss: Since he voids at highly variable volumes, has normal bladder capacity and no evidence of fixed obstruction based on the excellent free flow, the diagnosis is acquired voiding dysfunction, which is best treated with behavior modification with or without biofeedback.

Question for the panel: Are you concerned about the impaired detrusor contractility vis-a-vis using anticholinergics?

Dr Petrou: Not overly.

Dr Rutman and Dr Donnell: As long as his residuals are low, I would not be afraid to use a trial of antimuscarinics.

Dr Weiss: No. Close follow-up will exclude development of urinary retention.

Question for the panel: How do you think he would respond to ablative prostate surgery?

Dr Petrou: Potentially very well.

Dr Rutman: I would think he would do well if he has some bladder function.

Dr Donnell: Agree, if there is adequate detrusor contraction, he should do well.

Dr Weiss: Poorly.

Back to the patient. He was started on tolterodine LA, 4 mg at bedtime.

Question for the panel. Does the impaired detrusor contractility alter when you would see him again?

Dr Petrou: I would lean toward seeing him sooner as opposed to later.

Dr Bushman: I would see him in 1 month.

Dr Rutman: I would see him 1 or 2 weeks later to check his PVR, or sooner if he has any difficulty voiding.

Dr Donnell: With impaired contractility a PVR is usually checked in the next 1 to 2 weeks.

Dr Weiss: Yes: Within 2 weeks of initiating anticholinergics if in fact that was his therapy (which is not my choice, please see earlier discussion).

Back to the patient:
June 15, 2004: He was seen again 3 days after starting the tolterodine to be sure he was voiding normally.

VOID: 18/173/25 (**Fig. 11**), but he did not notice any difference in symptoms.

Question for the panel: How long do you treat with medication before changing the dose, adding or switching meds?

Dr Petrou: Arbitrarily, 6 weeks.

Dr Bushman: Two weeks.

Dr Rutman: I would give him at least 4 weeks.

Dr Donnell: Three to 4 weeks.

Dr Weiss: I give anticholinergics if that is an option 2 to 3 weeks before changing dose or switching medications. There may be a central mechanism by which these medications work; it takes that long to stabilize brain levels of any medication that crosses the blood-brain barrier.

Back to the patient:
July 20, 2004: He was seen again 5 weeks later. He says he is much better, "I go much less times in the bathroom."

Voiding diary:
24-hour volume = 1350 mL; 6 voids; MVV = 360 mL.
VOID: 12/109/6.
October 28, 2004: "Doing much better than before; since I started the pills, beautiful."
VOID: 16/139/0. Diary 24-hour volume = 1575 mL with 8 voids, nocturnal volume = 255 mL with 1 void, FBC = 240.

Diary date: February 2, 2005

Total 24-hour volume	1860
Total daytime volume	1380
Total nighttime volume	480
Daytime # voids	8
Nighttime # voids	1
Largest voided volume	480
Smallest voided volume	120

VOID: 21/160/0.
He continued to do well. PSA rose to 8.6 and on examination the prostate is 3+ slightly irregular and slightly firm, but not hard.

He underwent TRUS biopsy and was found to have left lateral Gleason 3 + 3 = 6 adenocarcinoma of the prostate, involving 1 of 4 tissue cores, less than 5% of the total tissue examined.

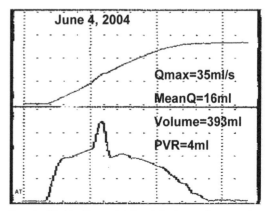

Fig. 11. AT. Uroflow obtained 3 days after starting tolterodine. VOID: 18/173/25.

Question for the panel: Do you think there is any relationship between prostate cancer and his symptoms?

Dr Rutman: No, not with low volume, low grade disease.

Dr Weiss: No

Dr Bushman: No.

Dr Donnell: No.

Question for the panel: How does this affect your recommendations for prostate cancer treatment?

Dr Petrou: I would recommend a prostatectomy over radiotherapy options or focal therapy in view of his baseline voiding dysfunction.

Dr Rutman: He is 58. If he desires treatment for his cancer, I would be hesitant to advise radiation for his cancer, due to his LUTS. I would likely recommend a radical prostatectomy.

Dr Weiss: I would treat him with radical prostatectomy. If he indeed has impaired detrusor contractility, urethral resistance will be decreased with the operation which if anything will facilitate emptying. Radiation therapy will increase outlet resistance ultimately and be associated with increased risk for exacerbation of his symptoms.

Dr Donnell: It doesn't.

Discussion: AT presented with what appeared to be refractory OAB. Cystoscopy looked like typical BPH with obstruction and severe bladder trabeculations, but VUDS confirmed neither detrusor overactivity nor prostatic obstruction. The only abnormality was impaired detrusor contractility, but his weakened bladder was sufficient to afford a normal Q; his flow was impaired only when his urethra was intubated. Why does he have a normal Q without the catheter, but appears obstructed with it? Part of the answer is apparent in the pressure flow tracing. The flow is interrupted and there is sporadic electromyographic (EMG) activity, suggesting that he is contracting and relaxing his sphincter, interrupting the stream. This is assuredly a (nonpathologic) response to the catheter. But that is not the whole answer. His pdetmax is only about 35 cm H_2O, so by any account his bladder is weak. It is likely that the added resistance offered by the catheter taking up part of the cross-sectional area of the urethra is just enough to cause the low flow.

What caused the impaired detrusor contractility? That, we don't know. I doubt that it is due to prolonged untreated bladder outlet obstruction because without the catheter his uroflow was normal, so even if there is obstruction, it must be very mild. There are no neurologic findings to suggest a neurologic bladder. Perhaps it is the consequence of long-standing untreated detrusor overactivity, but that is pure conjecture.

What about the propriety of using anticholinergics in the presence of impaired detrusor contractility, especially in this patient who doesn't even have detrusor overactivity on urodynamic study? Medicine is still, at least part, art, and myself and the panel respondents all thought it appropriate to empirically treat him with anticholinergics. And they worked! But we all proceeded with the same caveat—follow the patient and the PVRs closely. My usual practice in men with impaired contractility or prostatic obstruction in whom I start anticholinergics is to have them take the pill for the first time in the evening and come into the office the next morning for flow and residual urine. That might be overkill, but it works for me.

CASE 4 (SJ). PROGRESSION TO RENAL FAILURE WHILE ON "EFFECTIVE" MEDICAL TREATMENT OF LUTS

Patient: SJ is a 64-year-old cable TV executive.

Urologic history:

Age 55 (1994): Complained of a 1-year history of urinary frequency, urgency, and hesitancy. He voided about 9 times during the day and had nocturia 2 times per night. His maximum voided volume was 140 mL, but he did not find the symptoms very bothersome and did not elect any treatment. Prostate was 2+ in size and benign feeling. VOID: 9/160/77; urinalysis normal; creatinine = 1.2 mg/dL, PSA 1.9. Intravenous pyelography (IVP) was normal, but there was a large prostatic impression on the bladder base.

Question to panel:

Dr Blaivas: I do not practice "cost-effective medicine." I give the patient the choice as to how much of a diagnostic evaluation to pursue. When patients have symptoms, but decline treatment, I recommend upper tract imaging because if there is hydronephrosis, I urge treatment. Of course now, we'd get ultrasonography (USG), not IVP. What are your thoughts about this?

Dr Donnell: In the absence of bothersome symptoms I would obtain a PVR and hold off further investigation.

Dr Lerner: I would get a PVR and if it was low, I wouldn't go any further.

Dr Bushman: I evaluate and treat symptoms only. If he had a PVR that was more than 250 mL I would get an ultrasonogram to rule out hydro. Otherwise, I'd let him be.

Dr Rutman: I agree with you. If his symptoms were not bothersome, I would hold off on any investigation.

Dr Weiss: With no bother, normal urinalysis, modest PVR. and normal renal function, I would not feel compelled to go further from a diagnostic standpoint.

Question for panel: He has a low flow and a maximum voided volume of only 140 mL. Would you recommend treatment even though he'd rather not? If so, what/how would you follow him and how often?

Dr Lerner: If he didn't want treatment, I would follow his PVR and watch for worsening of urge symptoms.

Dr Rutman: I would not recommend treatment, unless he was bothered. I would however warn him that we do not know the natural history of his voiding dysfunction. and he may develop bladder decompensation and even renal failure. I think it is important to explain this to patients so they do not come back in 2 years with an acontractile detrusor.

Dr Weiss: I agree.

Age 56 (1995): His symptoms worsened. He developed urinary frequency, urgency, more difficulty initiating micturition, and the stream was weaker. VOID: 8/126/75. He agreed to treatment.

Panel: What would you recommend?

Dr Lerner: I would start with terazosin.

Dr Rutman and Dr Donnell: I would typically start with an α-blocker (tamsulosin or uroxatral).

Dr Weiss: I would hold treatment until he had repeat diary plus cystoscopy (I want to make sure that the new onset of urgency is not owing to the development of bladder cancer); one may forego the latter if repeat urinalysis and cytology are negative.

Back to the patient: He started 2 mg terazosin at bedtime. After 1 month he felt very much improved. "I no longer have any urinary symptoms." A voiding diary revealed that he voided 11 times in 24 hours for a total of 900 mL. Most voids were between 30 and 90 mL; maximum voided volume was 150 mL. Renal ultrasound normal. Terazosin was increased to 4 mg every bedtime.

Age 56 (1996): He continued to feel very well on 4 mg terazosin. "When I am busy I can go 6 hours without voiding." VOID: 5/125/115. He clinically remained about the same for several years, but routine renal ultrasound showed subtle, bilateral pyelocaliectasis. Serum creatinine was 1.5. He left for an extended business trip and was advised to return for evaluation.

Age 64 (1999): That was quite an extended business trip! He did not come back for 3 years and then was seen on an urgent basis because of a 1-month history of enuresis. Aside from the enuresis, he said his bladder symptoms were unchanged. VOID: 6/69/265. Renal ultrasound showed bilateral hydronephrosis and serum

creatinine was 2.5. He was advised that he needed urgent treatment and agreed to TURP pending the results of VUDS and cystoscopy.

Past medical history: unremarkable, no neurologic deficits.

AUA symptom score: 20.

Physical examination: Prostate 35 to 45 g; smooth, symmetric, and benign feeling.

Neuro-urologic examination: Normal.

Cystoscopy: There was trilobar prostatic enlargement encroaching the lumen throughout. Estimated prostatic length was 2.5 cm. The bladder was 4+ trabeculated, and there were multiple cellules and small diverticula. The ureteral orifices were normal.

Voiding diary:

24-hour voided volume	2,885 mL
Awake hours: # voids	15
Sleep hours: # voids	5
Usual voided volume	175 mL
MVV	300 mL
Nocturnal urinary volume	1,185 mL
NP index	41%
NBC index	2
Nocturia index	3.95

VUDS: Fig. 12.
Radiograph obtained @ Qmax: Fig. 13.
Urodynamic diagnosis:

1. Prostatic urethral obstruction
2. Low bladder compliance
3. Multiple small bladder diverticula

Treatment: TURP.

One week postoperatively he was voiding about every hour with a very strong stream, stronger than he can ever remember. VOID: 9/96/0. Creatinine = 1.7. Pathology showed BPH. At 1 year he was voiding every 5 to 7 hours during the day and did not have nocturia. VOID: 11/113/9. The stream remained "very strong." Creatinine fell to 1.5. He was followed for 6 more years and then, incredibly enough, did not return for follow-up and declined prostate cancer screening. Last VOID: 12/347/36.

Discussion: This case demonstrates the potential fallibility of relying on symptoms alone and the importance of close follow-up in patients undergoing conservative therapies. At a time when he thought he was doing well and had a PVR of only 115 mL, he already had pyelocaliectasis on renal USG, but despite our advice, he did not return for follow-up. According to the AUA guidelines,

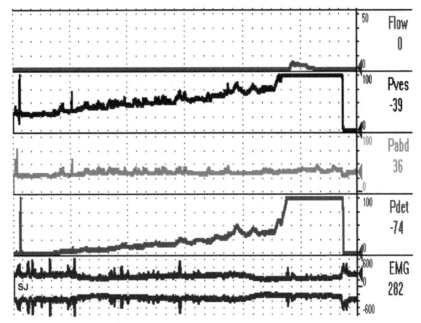

Fig. 12. SJ. Urodynamic tracing. Note the steep increase in detrusor pressure during bladder filling. Bladder capacity 500 mL; pdet @ bladder capacity = 50 cm H$_2$O; bladder compliance = 10 mL/cm H$_2$O. The pdet tracing was clipped by the software. pdet @ Qmax = 113 cm H$_2$O; Qmax = 7 mL/s.

renal USG was not indicated at this time because his creatinine was normal; nevertheless the USG alerted us that further evaluation and treatment were necessary, but the patient declined.

This "conservative therapy" for BPH led to temporary (4 years) amelioration of LUTS while the underlying condition worsened and led to silent renal failure. Fortunately, he developed enuresis and this was a sufficient warning to

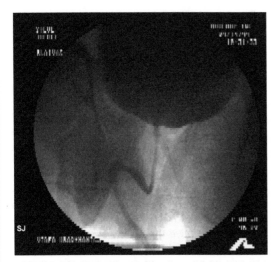

Fig. 13. SJ. Radiograph obtained at Qmax depicting a trabeculated bladder and narrowed prostatic urethra.

prompt full evaluation including blood urea nitrogen (BUN) and creatinine, renal ultrasound, VUDS, and cystoscopy. We have previously documented that the acute onset of adult enuresis is a harbinger of underlying prostatic obstruction.[4] A summary of these findings is presented in **Table 3**.

Of note, until the onset of enuresis he never found his symptoms bothersome at all, even though 6 months before the development of enuresis his residual urine had risen to about 250 mL, renal ultrasound showed very mild pyelocaliectasis, and his creatinine had risen to 1.5, and was already 2.0 when the enuresis began and 2.5 by the time the TURP was done 1 month later. The urodynamic study showed 2 significant risk factors for the development of hydronephrosis: low bladder compliance and severe prostatic obstruction (pdetmax = 131 cm H$_2$O). He underwent TURP. His creatinine normalized within several days and PVR was nil. Repeat ultrasound showed complete resolution of the hydronephrosis. Although repeat UDS have not been performed, in other men with similar findings we have documented the reversibility of low bladder compliance after successful treatment by TURP.

The real (and unanswered) question is how to determine which men with LUTS are at risk for renal and/or bladder damage, when to intervene, and how to treat. The AUA guidelines on BPH recommend that upper tract imaging should not

Table 3
Clinical summary of SJ

Date	VOID	Renal USG	Creatinine (mg/dL)
1994	9/160/77	Wnl	1.2
1995	8/150/	Wnl	1.2
1996	11/78/48	Wnl	1.1
1997	8/58/72	Wnl	1.2
1998		Slight hydronephrosis	1.5
1999	6/69/265	Bil hydronephrosis	2.5
TURP (10/99)			
2002	11/113/9	Wnl	1.5
2003	11/315/31	Wnl	1.5
2005	12/347/36	Wnl	1.5

be performed in men with BPH unless the serum creatinine is 2.5 mg/dL or higher. They seem to suggest that you should not screen for reversible forms of renal failure until the patient already has renal failure (which may or may not be reversible by the time it is discovered). I strongly oppose that position. If this man (and many others like him) undergo VUDS much earlier on in the course of their disease, we will likely be able to determine who is at risk and who requires earlier intervention. Further, by understanding the underlying pathophysiologies, it is likely that we will develop new, less invasive, and simpler therapies that are specifically designed for particular abnormalities uncovered by the diagnostic evaluation.

Until these questions are answered, I recommend that men with LUTS and low flows or residual urine be screened yearly with renal and bladder ultrasound, and measurement of serum BUN and creatinine. It may not be "cost effective," but it is good medicine!

Question to the panel: Any comments about the discussion?

Dr Lerner: If his PVR was rising at each visit, I would have encouraged him to go on to UDS. I agree that medications can help but also "hide" worsening bladder function, but in general, something changes, like the PVR or the continued presence of urge. I often have to really elicit this history from the patient, but with specific questioning, continued urge—or worsening urge—prompts me to move forward. I likely would have put him on anticholinergics and clean intermittent catheterization (CIC) to improve his compliance before surgery, I have to say. I am sure this is just a preference, but I like to get the bladder looking better before I head on to surgery.

Dr Rutman: I agree wholeheartedly with your discussion. I think a Q and PVR, and symptomatic assessment (ie, AUA symptom score) is enough. If there is a significant residual (>150 mL) than I would do a renal bladder USG and creatinine monitoring.

Dr Weiss: Agreed. When I meet a man for the first time who presents with urinary retention I ask "how long have you been wetting the bed?"; the response will determine the length of time that the limits of bladder compliance have been continuously met, corresponding to the duration of time the kidneys have been suffering the effects of high intrarenal pressure. The longer that duration, the less reversible will be his secondary renal insufficiency. If he has been dry at night, so much the better though of course renal insufficiency may still be an issue.

Dr Bushman: We know what the incidence of retention is in patients followed longitudinally, but we don't know what percentage are "silent retention"—the kind that produces renal insufficiency. Without that number, I don't know that we can decide the cost-effectiveness of following patients. While PVR is highly flawed, it is cheap. It is rare for patients to develop hydro with a modest PVR. So I use PVR to determine in whom an upper tract study is indicated.

Dr Donnell: Minimally invasive therapies may have played a role earlier in this patient's treatment course if the patient had pursued additional therapies beyond medical therapy. Our current guidelines depend on absolute and relative indicators. While not perfect, they have brought improvements to our care of the patient with LUTS. Once the medical therapy appeared to fail one would question the ability to use a minimally invasive therapy. Whether minimally invasive therapies would prevent the complications of progression is unknown. Certainly one needs to ask whether partial therapies are better than no therapy at all in the patient who presents with a similar scenario.

However, his initial presentation with such a large component of irritative symptoms would be theoretically attractive to the use of Botox. Obviously this is an investigative technique and will require additional information to establish its role in the care of the patient with LUTS.

CASE 5 (MC). YOUNG MAN PRESENTING WITH RENAL FAILURE

Patient: MC is a 31-year-old married Portuguese swimming pool installer.

History: Two years ago he presented to his primary care doctor with the sudden onset of pedal edema, and was found to have a creatinine of 7.8. He denied any voiding symptoms at all, but ultrasound revealed bilateral grade 3 hydronephrosis and a bladder volume of about 800 mL. He underwent multichannel urodynamics and cystoscopy was said to have an "areflexic bladder" with a capacity of 600 mL. He was treated with intermittent self-catheterization 4 to 5 times a day, and could not void at all. His creatinine fell to 2.2, and after a few months he began to void on his own. The intermittent catheterization was reduced to twice a day, but he had catheterized volumes as high as 2500 mL.

He sought 2 other opinions from urologists and underwent repeat urodynamics and cystoscopy, and was told that "there is no blockage" and that he should continue intermittent catheterization, but he discontinued it and sought another opinion.

AUA symptom score: 7.

Physical examination: Prostate 1+, smooth, symmetric, and benign feeling.

Urinalysis: normal.

Neuro-urologic examination: Normal (anal sphincter tone and control, perianal sensation, bulbocavernosus reflex).

VOID: 4/112/825.

Questions for the panel: Any further evaluation? Different treatment? Empiric prostate surgery? MIST?

Dr Rutman: I would obtain the urodynamics report to see up to what volumes they filled his bladder. A voiding diary and diary of catheter volumes would be helpful as well.

Dr Weiss: The patient has high catheter volumes (2500 mL as part of a twice-a-day catheterization schedule) suggesting the possibility that he has global polyuria. Thus, a 24-hour catheter/void diary done over the course of 7 days will determine whether polyuria is a clinical diagnosis, which could then be investigated further with overnight water deprivation studies.

Dr Donnell: The patient is very young with what appears to be complications from long-standing impaired lower urinary tract function. He is not a candidate for any of the MIST therapies. I agree that a voiding diary would help identify intake and output. I would also recommend a watch with a preset timer to improve his catheterizing schedule and reduce bladder volumes.

Back to the patient:

Further evaluation included a bladder diary and VUDS. He declined cystoscopy because recent cystoscopy (his third) was said to be normal.

Voiding diary:

24-hour voided volume	1560 mL
Usual voided volume	90–120 mL
MVV	210 mL
Awake hours: # voids	8
Sleep hours: # voids	2

Videourodynamic study: Fig. 14.

At a bladder volume of about 1200 mL he felt comfortably full and when asked to void, he had a detrusor contraction of about 20 cm H_2O, but could not void.

Question for the panel: Anything more to do?

Dr Rutman: I would continue to fill him since he has a large capacity bladder as long as he was not in pain.

Dr Weiss: In view of the catheterized volumes in excess of 2 L, it behooves the urodynamicist to proceed to fill the bladder toward its viscoelastic limits to see if a detrusor contraction will occur at filling volumes closer to the patient's actual bladder capacity.

Back to the patient: Bladder filling was continued and finally, at a bladder volume of about 1400 mL he had a sustained detrusor contraction that reached 100 cm H_2O (**Figs. 15–18**).

Question for panel: Diagnosis? Further workup? Treatment?

Dr Weiss: The lack of contrast below the bladder neck associated with a pdet = 100 cm H_2O indicates he has bladder neck obstruction. Because contrast did not enter the prostatic urethra, it's impossible to say if the patient also has pelvic floor dysfunction from a urodynamic standpoint.

Back to the patient:

Our diagnosis was primary bladder neck obstruction and he was scheduled for transurethral incision or resection of the prostate. Spinal anesthesia was administered and at cystoscopy there was a tight meatal stenosis that would not admit passage of a 17F cystoscope. The meatus was dilated to 28F, but was very tight, and the scope was gripped by the stricture. A 24

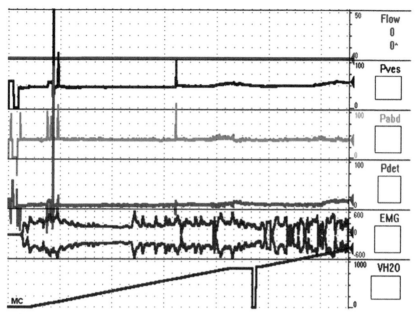

Fig. 14. MC. Urodynamic tracing. At a bladder volume of 1100 mL, he was asked to void and had a voluntary detrusor contraction to 20 cm H_2O, but could not void.

resectoscope would not pass. An incision was made at the 6 o'clock position from meatus about 2 cm proximal through the entire thickness of the distal urethra, cutting through the strictured area. The resectoscope was then passed without difficulty. The remainder of the urethra was normal.

There was mild trilobar enlargement with a prominent elevation and circumferential narrowing of the vesical neck. Prostatic length was approximately 3 cm. The bladder wall was 3+ trabeculated.

Question for the panel: Would you continue with the prostate surgery or wait and see how he

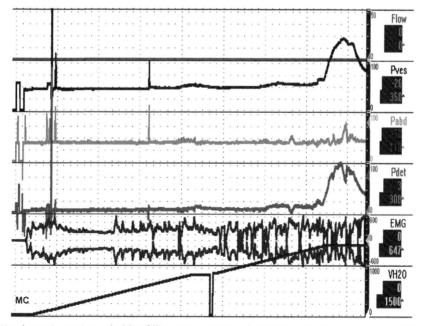

Fig. 15. MC. Urodynamic tracing. Bladder filling was continued and at a bladder volume of 1400 mL, he had a voluntary detrusor contraction to 100 cm H_2O, but no contrast was seen in any part of the urethra.

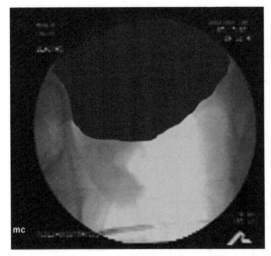

Fig. 16. MC. Radiograph obtained during attempt to void shows no contrast in the urethra and a trabeculated bladder.

does? If you elect the former, do you think it makes a difference whether you do TURP, TUIP, or laser surgery?

Dr Rutman: Considering his VUDS showed a narrowed prostatic urethra and he had 2 other supposedly normal cystoscopies, I do not believe the meatal narrowing was a source for his symptoms. I would have proceeded with a outlet procedure. I think as long as his bladder neck is opened a TURP or Green Light Laser is reasonable.

Dr Donnell: I too would continue with the TUIP given the urodynamics findings. I think that the patient could be treated with a TUIP, a Green Light Laser, or the Bipolar device.

Dr Weiss: At his young age, it would be preferable to perform TUIP, as this operation affords a maximum chance for antegrade ejaculation while effecting a decrease in urethral resistance adequate to assure complete emptying.

Dr Petrou: I would elect to treat in view of age and renal insufficiency. Secondary to the history of the self-catheterization, there may be some compression of the prostate tissue deemphasizing the obstructive component of same. For that reason, I would proceed with TURP as opposed to TUIP. Laser therapy is an option but in challenging cases I would lean toward traditional therapies to lessen the variables in the equation of therapy. A secondary question, for the meatal stricture, was the incision made with an Otis urethrotome or with an incision?

Dr Blaivas: An incision with a #15 blade.

Dr Petrou: Does this warrant follow-up for in one of the radiographic images, I believe there may be columnization of contrast to the fossa navicularis. Our pediatric colleagues will vouch for the ability of meatal stenosis to cause upstream hydronephrosis in select cases.

Back to the patient:

He underwent uncomplicated TURP and the pathology showed nodular hyperplasia. One week postoperatively he was voiding 4 to 6 times

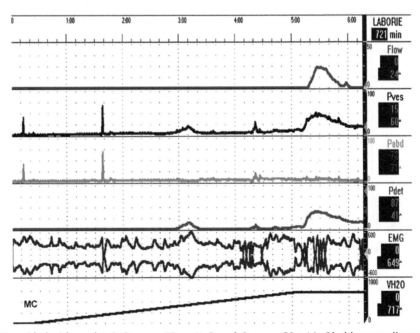

Fig. 17. MC. He voided with a pdet @ Q_{max} = 45 cm H_2O and Q_{max} = 20 mL/s. Bladder compliance was normal.

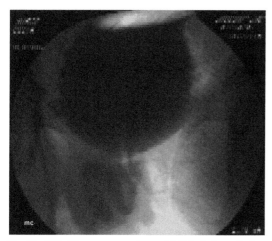

Fig. 18. MC. There was a large TURP defect during filling that is not pictured here. The voiding cystourethrogram showed a wide open urethra, but the anterior urethra seemed a bit wider than usual.

per day. VOID: 24/335/34. Four months later he was completely asymptomatic, voiding 4 to 6 times per 24 hours. VOID: 34/420/0. His creatinine, though, did not fall any further and remained stable at 2.2. The hydronephrosis was unchanged on ultrasound. Noncontrast computed tomography (CT) scan was done, which showed bilateral hydronephrosis with mildly dilated ureter down to the ureterovesical junction (UVJ).

Question for the panel: Any further diagnostic evaluation/further treatment?

Dr Rutman: I would have repeated VUDS as well.

Dr Weiss: The bilateral hydronephrosis is probably chronic and will not yield further to measures to influence vesicourethral function. It's possible that the bladder wall involving the intramural ureters is locally stiff and of low compliance, due to his long-standing obstruction.

Dr Donnell: I agree that the hydronephrosis is probably chronic, but I would repeat the urodynamics given we have not identified a definitive etiology for his initial presentation.

He underwent repeat VUDS. There was a large TURP defect during filling that is not pictured here. He voided with a pdet @ Qmax = 45 cm H_2O and Qmax = 20 mL/s. Bladder compliance was normal. The voiding cystourethrogram showed a wide open urethra, but the anterior urethra seemed a bit wider than usual.

Question for the panel: Why did his hydronephrosis not improve? Any further treatment?

Dr Rutman: I would make sure he does timed voiding to not allow his bladder to become overly stretched. I would likely just monitor his symptoms. The hydro is likely from chronic distension,

although you would expect some improvement with his outlet reductive procedure.

Dr Weiss: A diuretic renogram may determine if the ureters remain obstructed. Placement of bilateral ureteral stents with follow-up renal function testing will be a straightforward way to tell if there is an element of reversible renal dysfunction.

Dr Donnell: I agree.

Dr Petrou: At this point a Lasix renogram may be of help identify the point of obstruction at the UVJ, prostate, or fossa navicularis. Before a bilateral ureteroneocystostomy is performed, bilateral stenting should be considered for an acceptable time frame to assure the obstruction is at the level of the UVJ.

Back to the patient: We discussed the possibility of bilateral ureteroneocystostomy but neither the patient, his wife, nor his doctor was very enthusiastic about doing that. He has remained asymptomatic for the duration of his follow-up (6 years postop). At his last visit (3 months ago) his creatinine and renal USG were unchanged. VOID: 39/940/34.

Comment: MC likely had a remedial cause of renal failure from his initial presentation—primary bladder neck obstruction.[5] Unfortunately, his prior urologists failed to fill his bladder sufficiently to produce a detrusor contraction. Most urodynamic units use prefilled chambers containing 600 to 1000 mL of infusant, and many urodynamicists are reluctant to fill the bladder much more than that. MC, though, had recorded residual urines of 2500 mL and, in our judgment, it is critically important to fill the bladder to capacity (whatever that is) because some patients can only generate a voluntary detrusor contraction at capacity.[6] Had this been done, MC may have undergone surgery before his renal failure became irreversible.

CASE 6 (MH). PROSTATIC OBSTRUCTION AND MEDIUM-SIZED BLADDER DIVERTICULUM

Patient: MH is a 61-year-old Turkish man with symptoms of urinary frequency and urgency every 1.5 hours, nocturia × 2, decreased stream; AUASS = 16.

Laboratory: UA and culture negative; PSA = 2.1; creatinine 1.2.

Prostate: 25 g, smooth, benign feeling.

Neuro-urologic examination: normal.

Prior treatment: α-Blockers, anticholinergics.

VOID: 7/113/150.

Cystoscopy revealed trilobar prostatic enlargement, prostatic urethra 4 cm in length, narrow mouth bladder diverticulum, 1+ bladder trabeculations.

Question for the panel: Would anyone proceed without urodynamics?

Dr Weiss: No.

Dr Rutman: No.

Dr Donnell: No.

Dr Petrou: No, I feel complete evaluation would be very helpful.

Dr Kreder and Dr Powell: Because of the severe urgency and frequency I'd want to see if the patient demonstrated detrusor overactivity.

Dr Bushman: If the diverticulum were tiny, I would not do urodynamics. If I thought paradoxic filling was an issue, then I would.

Question for the panel: Are you selective or do you do VUDS for all men that undergo urodynamics?

Dr Kreder and Dr Powell: We do video on everyone, men and women, and in this case it would have picked up the diverticulum if cystoscopy were not performed. One might ask "when would you NOT want more information?"

Dr Weiss: We are selective.

Dr Rutman: Anyone for whom I am planning surgery gets VUDS.

Dr Petrou: Routinely I perform them on most patients.

Dr Bushman: Selective.

Dr Donnell: We are selective. VUDS shows severe prostatic obstruction and a bladder diverticulum that fills as the patient voids.

Back to the patient:

VUDS (**Fig. 19**) shows severe prostatic obstruction. The voiding cystourethrogram (**Fig. 20**) shows that as he voids the bladder diverticulum fills, and that most of the PVR is contained by the diverticulum.

Question for the panel: How would you treat him? If you think the diverticulum requires surgery, do you do that first, synchronously with the prostate or afterwards? How do you decide the order?

Dr Weiss: I would definitely treat the prostate first, as it is my contention that high-pressure voiding is the genesis of the diverticulum. This bladder has plenty of power to empty. I would do a TURP. We hope that when urethral resistance is reduced by surgery, it empties more into the commode than into the diverticulum. Follow-up will tell, based on post-TURP measurement of sequential PVRs. If the diverticulum doesn't empty despite adequately reduced urethral resistance, diverticulectomy may be done if his symptoms warrant it. If the diverticular orifice is too narrow it may not empty well, regardless of how low the urethral resistance becomes post-TURP. However, if the patient is asymptomatic, the diverticulum may be treated expectantly. There is a higher likelihood of cancer developing in the diverticulum, and this should be followed endoscopically.

Dr Rutman: I would do the outlet first, Green Light Laser or Bipolar TURP. I'd monitor symptoms afterwards and observe the diverticulum. If the prostate was larger and I was planning on doing a suprapubic prostatectomy, I would do them simultaneously. Whether to do diverticulectomy depends on the size of the diverticulum.

Dr Donnell: I agree.

Dr Petrou: I have found that delayed fluoroscopic images with contrast will help determine how well the diverticulum empties and whether the residual is from the diverticulum, bladder, or a combination of same. This will help guide the need to address the diverticulum. After full discussion with the patient, I will usually address the outlet obstruction first endoscopically with a classic TURP. This will either be done on a synchronous basis at one operative setting or metachronous, depending on the patient's preference for relative efficiency or desire for a minimally invasive approach. While initially preferring an extraperitoneal approach for the diverticulectomy, we have recently found that robotic assisted laparoscopic diverticulectomy offers some potential advantages with good clinical applicability.

Dr Kreder and Dr Powell: We address the bladder outlet first, because if this is not done we feel the diverticulum will eventually recur. Recurrent infection, presence of tumor on cystoscopy, or suspicious cytology (which we do on all diverticula regardless of size), elevated postvoid residual, narrow neck diverticulum, stone in the diverticulum, and ipsilateral hydronephrosis are all indications to operate on the diverticulum in our opinion. Young age is another relative indication. We will start with TURP or α-blockers and recheck uroflow and possibly repeat pressure flow studies. After that we address the diverticulum. It is reasonable to do TURP or open prostatectomy at the same time as the diverticulectomy. If the diverticulum is less than 100 mL volume and the prostate is less than 60 g by TRUS, we will do simultaneous TURP and rollerball the diverticulum, which has been shown to contract over time afterwards.[7,8] If it is a large prostate, we perform suprapubic prostatectomy or simple retropubic prostatectomy in conjunction with open diverticulectomy. If the diverticulum is near the ureteric orifice we don't hesitate to place 5F pediatric feeding tubes to identify the ureters intraoperatively. All diverticula should be sent for pathologic examination.

Back to the patient: He underwent TURP. Pathology was benign. His symptoms completely resolved. VOID: 17/325/86. He was followed for 4

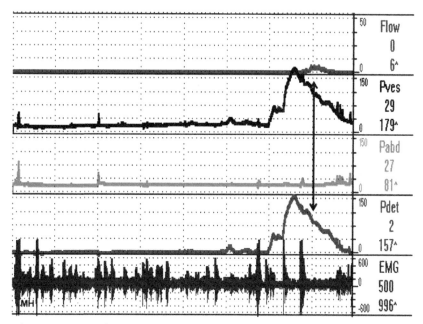

Fig. 19. MH. Urodynamic tracing. There is a voluntary detrusor contraction. pdet @ $Qmax$ = 75 cm H_2O; $Qmax$ = 6 mL/s, indicating Schafer grade 4 urethral obstruction.

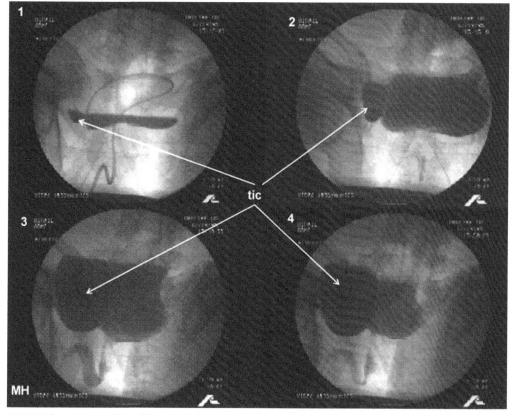

Fig. 20. MH. The cystogram (**1** and **2**) and voiding cystourethrogram (**3** and **4**) show that as he voids the bladder diverticulum fills, and that most of the PVR is contained by the diverticulum. Note the narrowed prostatic urethra.

more years and remained unchanged. Renal and bladder USG were stable and the tic remained about the same size. Yearly follow-up continued for another 5 years via mail, and his status was unchanged. He never required further treatment during that period of time.

CASE 7 (GG). LARGE BLADDER DIVERTICULUM

Patient: GG is a 59-year-old man referred for evaluation of large postvoid residual urine volume.

History: One year ago he underwent uneventful percutaneous placement of coronary artery stents and was treated with clopidogrel (Plavix). He subsequently developed gross hematuria and clot retention. He underwent emergency cystoscopy that showed no cause for the hematuria. The prostate was small, but bladder capacity was very large. Abdominal and pelvic CT scan were normal except for slight fullness of the collecting system and an enormous, thin-walled bladder. He was treated with an indwelling catheter for several weeks. After removal of the catheter, he voided without difficulty, but was found to have postvoid residual urine volumes of about 4500 mL.

For as long as he could remember he voided infrequently, in large amounts, every 10 hours or so, but denied any other urologic symptoms and never had a urinary tract infection or stones.

When apprised of his current condition, his 96-year-old mother told him that when he was a child, she was worried about how infrequently he voided and used to remind him to void more frequently.

After removal of the catheter he voided about every 4 hours. The strength of his stream was, and remained very variable, usually on the weak side, but sometimes very strong. He had been treated with terazosin and then tamsulosin (Flomax) because his family doctor thought he had an enlarged prostate.

Medical history: Unremarkable.

Prior surgery: Percutaneous coronary stent.

Physical examination: Prostate: 2+ in size, normal consistency, no nodules.

Neuro-urologic examination: Normal.

Motor and sensory examination in the lower extremities was normal.

Cystoscopy: The prostatic urethra was about 3 cm in length and had minimal prostatic enlargement. The ureteral orifices were normal. The bladder was 4+ trabeculated and appeared to have a huge bladder diverticulum.

VOID: 14/560/4800 (the uroflow had a bell-shaped curve).

Videourodynamic study is seen in **Fig. 21** and a radiograph obtained at maximum uroflow is seen in **Fig. 22**.

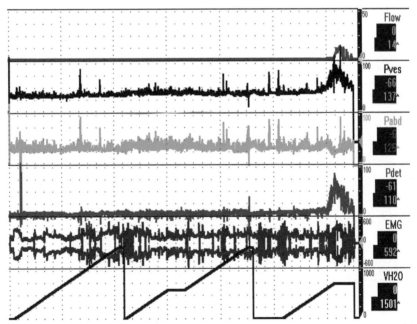

Fig. 21. GG. Urodynamic tracing. The first urge occurred at 4200 mL with a detrusor pressure of 5 cm H_2O and a severe urge occurred at 4880 mL, with a detrusor pressure of 6 cm H_2O. During bladder filling there were no spontaneous involuntary detrusor contractions. Bladder capacity was 5013 mL, at which time he had a voluntary detrusor contraction. Qmax = 14 mL, pdet @ Qmax = 48 cm H_2O, pdetmax = 49 cm H_2O, Voided volume = 730 mL, Postvoid residual = 4177 mL.

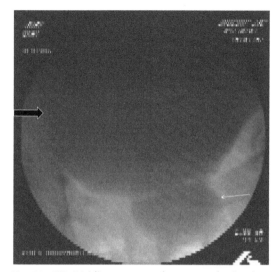

Fig. 22. GG. Voiding cystourethrogram obtained at maximum uroflow. What appears to be a dilated posterior urethra (*small arrow*) is actually the large bladder diverticulum posterior to the prostate, and what appears to be a large bladder diverticulum above the bladder (*large arrow*) is actually the large bladder.

Discussion: He has an enormous bladder capacity (over 5 L) and a postvoid residual of about 4 L. There are only 2 possible causes of incomplete bladder emptying—impaired detrusor contractility or urethral obstruction—and, at present, the only means of distinguishing between the 2 is synchronous detrusor pressure uroflow studies. At a bladder volume of over 5 L, he voided with a sustained detrusor contraction. pdetmax = 88 cm H_2O; pdet @ Qmax = 48 cm H_2O with a Qmax = 16 mL/s. When plotted on the Schafer nomogram (**Fig. 23**), these values are equivocal urethral obstruction and slightly weak detrusor contraction strength. Therefore, neither condition

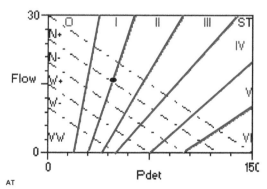

AT

Fig. 23. GG. Schafer nomogram shows equivocal urethral obstruction and a slightly weak bladder.

is really severe enough to account for his enormous bladder capacity and residual urine.

Question for the panel: Any idea what caused this?

Dr Lerner: This is a Hinman bladder, in my opinion. I am actually shocked he was capable of generating the detrusor contraction he had at 5 L.

Dr Weiss: He has voiding dysfunction since childhood. Therefore he is likely afflicted with the dysfunctional voiding syndrome characterized by failure to relax the external urethral sphincter during voluntary micturition. It's possible he has a "blown out" end stage of Hinman syndrome, the "nonneurogenic neurogenic bladder." Another possibility is Williams syndrome, a forme-fruste of prune belly syndrome only involving the bladder. Posterior urethral valves constitute a congenital obstructive process, but these should be evident endoscopically and, in any event, he is not demonstrated to have urethral obstruction by UDS.

Dr Rutman: I agree.

So why doesn't he empty? He doesn't empty because, even though his bladder contracts strongly enough, it does not contract long enough.

Dr Lerner: ...Or early enough. He doesn't get a signal to void until his bladder is really full. This is what concerns me the most. If he was signaled to void sooner, then maybe the length of the contraction would not be as important.

To void to completion at a normal Qave, his bladder would need to contract for over 8 minutes; during the urodynamic study he voided over 700 mL in 73 seconds which, although normal, is insufficient to empty. In this sense, then, his bladder is impaired, but we don't know why.

Dr Rutman: I agree with these statements.

Back to the patient:

Treatment is indicated if there are complications such as hydronephrosis, stones, infection, or significant symptoms. He has none of these and has likely had this condition since birth. Accordingly, treatment is elective. Of course there is a concern that the bladder might decompensate to the point where he could no longer void at all. His bladder was emptied at the conclusion of the UDS and he did not void for 3 days, after which he resumed his usual voiding habits. Somehow, that convinced him that he should consider treatment.

Question for the panel: Does he need treatment?

Dr Rutman: I would treat him if he wants to have a chance to void spontaneously in the future.

Question for the panel: How would you treat him?

Dr Lerner: Reduction cystoplasty with CIC afterwards is his only option, in my opinion, for potential intervention. If his capacity was reduced, and he maintained his detrusor contraction, he could be "trained" to keep his volumes under 500 mL. And with time, he may very well void on his own.

Dr Weiss: I would suggest a trial of CIC on a three-times-a day basis. This will protect his upper tracts and possibly improve his detrusor contractility. Reduction cystoplasty may improve emptying efficiency, as the issue is the lack of detrusor power required to deal with a very large volume. Reduction cystoplasty will greatly reduce this volume and presumably result in a better matchup of detrusor contractility and bladder volume.

Dr Rutman: I would put him on catheterization around the clock to keep his void plus residual to 500 mL or less and repeat UDS 4 to 6 months later to evaluate his bladder function.

Back to the patient: Cholinergic agonists such as bethanechol could be tried, but we have never found these to be efficacious. There seemed to be little alternative to reduction cystoplasty, but this procedure is rarely reported. It has been used in some children with "decompensated bladders" due to posterior urethral valves or megacystis, but over the long term, this procedure has proved ineffective. In our unpublished experience, though, reduction cystoplasty has been effective in a small group of highly selected patients such as this who, despite very large bladder capacity, have normal detrusor contractility. If urethral obstruction is present it is treated at the same time.

He elected to undergo reduction cystoplasty. At the time of surgery, it was apparent that there were innumerable bladder diverticula but there was no single large one to account for his massive bladder capacity. There were 2 large diverticula that extended behind the prostatic urethra and accounted for the appearance of a normal bladder and large bladder diverticulum on the voiding cystourethrogram (see **Fig. 22**). These 2 diverticula were excised transvesically, as was a large portion of the bladder. The vesical neck was palpably tight and would not admit even the tip of a small finger. It felt like hypertrophied muscle. A 5 & 7 o'clock prostatotomy and bladder neck Y-V plasty was done because the prostate was too small for open prostatectomy. He did very well postoperatively and at 6-month follow-up said "I'm doing great...I can sleep nights...it all comes out...a marvelous thing." He voids about every 4 hours during the day and does not have nocturia. He reports his stream is very strong. VOID: 30/284/119. Unfortunately, he has not returned for further follow-up, but by telephone said he was unchanged at 1 year. The etiology of his condition was never determined.

CASE 8 (DB). DECOMPENSATED LARGE CAPACITY BLADDER

Patient: DB is a 59-year-old married professional bridge player with type 1 diabetes who has been on sterile intermittent catheterization (SIC) for about 2 years.

History: He saw a urologist 2 years ago because of an asymptomatic kidney stone and was started on intermittent self-catheterization because of large residual urine and a large capacity, areflexic bladder, but he denied any symptoms. He had a severe febrile kidney infection about a year later, and underwent lithotripsy and basket extraction of a ureteral stone. Ever since, he complained of recurrent lower UTIs characterized by urinary frequency, urgency, and positive urine cultures.

He had been catheterizing erratically, varying from once a day to 4 times a day, and voiding between times. PVRs have been as high as 1400 mL and voided volumes as large as 220 mL.

Medical history: He has well-controlled type 1 diabetes mellitus and an extensive neurologic history. He has had symptomatic herniated discs that have resulted in numbness, tingling, and weakness that have responded well to the surgeries listed below. At the present time he has no neurologic symptoms.

Prior surgery:

Discectomy & fusion C 3-4	1990
Discectomy & fusion C 4-5	1994
Discectomy & fusion C 2, 3,	2001
Lithotripsy & basket extraction of stone	2008

Physical examination: Prostate: 2+ in size, normal consistency, no nodules.

Neuro-urologic examination: Anal tone and control: normal. Bulbocavernosus reflex: normal. Perianal sensation: normal.

Deep tendon reflexes were 2+ at the knees, but ankle jerks were absent.

Motor examination in the lower extremities was normal.

Laboratory: Urinalysis had 5 to 10 white blood cells per high-power field; culture had more than 100,000 cfu/mL *Klebsiella pneumoniae*; PSA = 2.7; creatinine 1.3.

13 January, 2009: Cystoscopy showed moderate trilobar prostatic enlargement and the prostatic urethra was about 3 cm in length. The

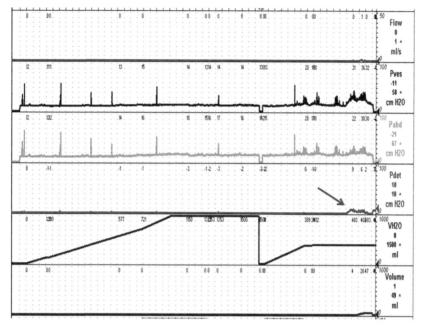

Fig. 24. DB. Urodynamic tracing. impaired detrusor contractility: Qmax = 1.4 mL/s, pdet @ Qmax = 5.2 cm H_2O, pdetmax = 9 cm H_2O; Voided volume = 40 mL, Postvoid residual = 1860 mL. The detrusor contraction is marked by the 100,000 cfu/mL. Not the barely visualized uroflow.

ureteral orifices were not seen because of modest intravesical protrusion. The bladder was capacious and at least 2 L. I could not see well enough because of the large bladder size to rule out a bladder diverticulum. There were multiple hard bladder stones, the largest of which was about 2 cm in size.

Videourodynamic study:

Urodynamic tracing (Fig. 24) showed impaired detrusor contractility:

Radiograph is shown in **Fig. 25**A, B.

Renal and bladder USG showed normal upper tracts and a large bladder with multiple stones,

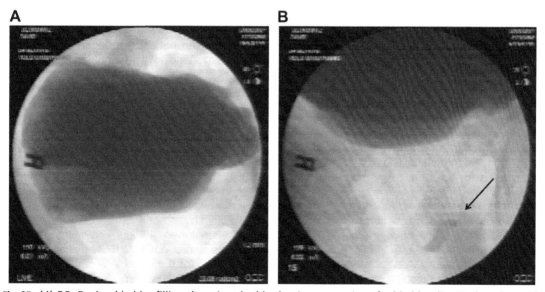

Fig. 25. (*A*) DB. During bladder filling there is a double density, suggestive of a bladder diverticulum, but with further filling (too large to capture on a single film) there were no signs of diverticulum. (*B*) DB. During voiding, there is faint visualization of the anterior urethra (*arrow*), but the prostatic urethra is not seen at all.

the largest of which was about 2 cm. There were no signs of bladder diverticulum.

Questions for the panel: What do think caused this large capacity bladder with impaired contractility? Diabetic cystopathy? Any role for the cervical disks?

Dr Weiss: Diabetic cystopathy may explain this man's condition though end-stage detrusor due to chronic outlet obstruction secondary to BPH or long-standing pelvic floor dysfunction are possibilities. The EMG tracing is not provided but the lack of involuntary contractions excludes detrusor external sphincter dyssynergia (DESD) unless the bladder has become flaccid for other reasons. If that were the case, the consequences of DESD are no longer an issue as his lower tract is like that of an augmented bladder.

Dr Rutman: Likely a combination of both.

Dr Lerner: I think this is hard to say. I am sure it is multifactorial with some component of back surgery and his diabetes and his lack of compliance. When he was found to have a large PVR (which I think is likely from him diabetes), he needed to be compliant, but wasn't, so he volitionally worsened his symptoms. The other thing to consider is medication. I am guessing that if he has had back issues, he is on chronic pain medications, which may have been affecting his bladder sensation leading to decreased voiding frequency, sort of like a medicated Hinman bladder, and further exacerbating his condition.

Dr Donnell: I agree, it is likely to be multifactorial with his history of surgery, diabetes, pain medications, and possibly behavior.

Dr Kreder and Dr Powell: I think the BPH and high-pressure voiding caused the diverticulum, and in combination with diabetic cystopathy caused bladder decompensation and impaired contractility. I would expect the cervical discs to most likely cause detrusor instability. There is no EMG on his urodynamic study so I can't comment on overactive or dyssenergic sphincter.

Dr Petrou: Very difficult to pinpoint and one that would be open for an extensive academic discussion; it may be multifactorial in nature.

Question for the panel: Any more diagnostic studies? How do you exclude a bladder diverticulum in men with huge bladder capacity?

Dr Weiss: I make a great effort to visualize the internal bladder architecture in these patients with large bladders and particulate matter obscuring endoscopic vision. I repeatedly aspirate "dirty" urine and replace it with fresh irrigant until I can see in which case I would expect to identify easily whether a diverticulum is present or not.

Dr Rutman: It is difficult, but I would try and fill him up on cystoscopy until he was close to his capacity or uncomfortable.

Dr Lerner: Fill him to capacity and see what you find at fluoroscopy. You can also do a rigid cystoscopy, which is better than a flexible, as we know.

Dr Petrou: I would be inclined to obtain a non-contrast CT scan of the abdomen and pelvis to determine status of his urolithiasis and to help identify a bladder diverticulum. If needed, a pelvic CT scan after bladder instillation of contrast would help with diverticulum position.

Dr Kreder and Dr Powell: CT scan especially if cystoscopy, which was done already, was felt to be suboptimal.

Question for the panel: How would you treat him?

Dr Weiss: If the stones broke up adequately using the Holmium laser or electrohydraulic lithotripsy apparatus I would attempt to clear the stones endoscopically. It is usually difficult to see well enough after such a lengthy lithotripsy procedure to do a concurrent TURP or TUIP (the prostate was described as short in length so should be amenable to one or the other); the latter may be staged at a separate time. I don't like doing suprapubic prostatectomy on small glands. However, if TRUS demonstrated the prostate volume to be over 50 mL, a concomitant open vesicolithotomy and suprapubic prostatectomy may be done. The decision as to whether to do a diverticulectomy at the time of surgery would depend on the results of my repeat endoscopy as described earlier.

Dr Kreder and Dr Powell: I would do a transurethral laser lithotripsy of this bladder stone, followed by TUIP or TURP at the same time.

Back to the patient: He underwent reduction cystoplasty, removal of the stones, and excision of an unusual type of bladder diverticulum and suprapubic prostatectomy. Despite the appearance (double density) seen on the radiograph, I did not think that he had a bladder diverticulum. At the time of surgery, though, in addition to the stones and a capacious bladder he was found to have a depression behind the trigone, which I believe is an unusual type of bladder diverticulum that I have seen in patients like this. This was excised transvesically and the detrusor muscle reapproximated. Pathology showed only BPH. Postoperatively, he voided about every 4 hours with a strong stream. 2 months postop VOID: 12/166/49.

Question for the panel: Any comments?

Dr Donnell: This is a very nice outcome. He was managed with intermittent self-catheterization (ISC) for 2 years, and one has to question whether the patient would have recovered sufficiently to warrant earlier urodynamic evaluation and possibly completed therapy sooner if he was compliant with his ISC program.

Dr Lerner: Before I considered a reduction cystoplasty, I would have gotten him to be more compliant on doing intermittent catheterization. I would have considered an outlet reduction procedure, and would certainly have treated the stones, but would have told him that he may not void any better, but it could make catheterizing better. I admit that reduction cystoplasty is not something I do very often.

Dr Weiss: I suggest placement of stents intraoperatively as the intramural ureters are at risk for injury with operation on any nearby diverticulae.

Dr Rutman: Very interesting. I have never done a reduction cystoplasty. It makes sense. Are you the only person who has ever done this?

Dr Petrou: Very fascinating case, I completely concur with the open procedure, especially performing a suprapubic prostatectomy. And is transrectal volume determination needed preoperatively since he has the other conditions that need addressing, or should it be considered if a prostatotomy would suffice?

Dr Kreder and Dr Powell: I think that is a good result. It is possible that he did not need the reduction cystoplasty.

Dr Blaivas: Reduction cystoplasties have been reported sporadically in the past, but were never really accepted because of 2 problems—lack of efficacy and overzealous resection resulting in small capacity bladder. In my unpublished experience in about 15 such patients (out of over 15,000 patients who underwent UDS), the long term outcome has been good with only about 20% requiring SIC. All of the successful patients had either a voluntary detrusor contraction (coming at a very large bladder capacity).

I agree that a classic suprapubic prostatectomy is difficult when the prostate is small, but I use a different technique for these—I circumscribe the bladder neck and use Metzenbaum scissors for the dissection rather than my finger, and do a "Y-V" plasty of the bladder neck.

CASE 9 (SO). EMPIRIC TREATMENT OF URINARY RETENTION IN A MAN WITH LOW BLADDER COMPLIANCE

I added this case after the panel had concluded because I think it makes another important point about empiric treatment of LUTS, especially patients in urinary retention.

Patient: SO is a 77-year-old retired home builder.

History: (8 June, 2004) He has been on intermittent catheterization ever since a transurethral "stretching of the urethra...first they said was a stricture...he cut it and it bled a lot...at the same time he cut a little of the prostate out...he said the bladder was all stretched." Before the surgery he thought he voided normally, but had cystoscopy because of microhematuria. Subsequently he was found to have very large PVRs. He currently self catheterizes every 4 to 5 hours. He was treated with bethanechol; never on α-blockers. He was told to stop catheterizing and see how he did, but he developed too much difficulty voiding and resumed. He is sometimes is able to void a small amount now.

Medications: None.

Prostate: small, flat, firm in size.

Neuro-urologic examination: Normal.

He was empirically started on doxazosin 0.4 mg. After 1 month he noted no change in symptoms and the dose was doubled, but after another month, he was clinically unchanged.

8 September, 2004—Cystoscopy: The prostatic urethra was about 3 cm in length and showed signs of prior TURP, but there was a moderate amount of remaining prostatic tissue in the distal half of the prostatic urethra. The ureteral orifices were normal. The bladder was 4+ trabeculated with multiple cellules.

VUDS is seen in **Figs. 26** and **27**. It shows low bladder compliance, but no detrusor contraction. Voiding by straining shows a flow too low to activate the flowmeter and a narrowed prostatic urethra.

He underwent KTP laser ablation of the prostate on 27 September, 2004 without incident.

6 October, 2004: He is very pleased, says he is voiding better than he can ever remember. Residual urine was negligible at home and he discontinued intermittent catheterization. Void: 4/94/373; second void 6 hours later void = 14 mL, VV = 582 mL, PVR = 271 mL. He said, though, that he has been voiding much better at home than either of these flows show.

9 November, 2004: Voiding diary showed a total 24-hour volume of 1830 mL with 5 voids. MVV = 480 mL; smallest = 270 mL. VOID: 17/419/129.

12 January, 2005: "I'm doing very, very well, except when I come here...the flow test makes me nervous...I usually urinate great...this one is not good." VD = Total volume = 2340 mL with 7 voids, Nocturnal volume = 390 mL with 1 void, MVV = 240 mL. VOID: 3/142/353; He came back 5 hours later and voided again. VOID: 14/603/21.

He was followed at yearly intervals and when last seen (23 September, 2008) he said he is

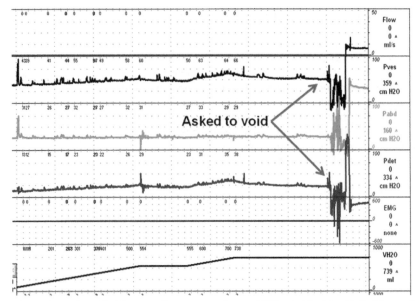

Fig. 26. SO. Urodynamic tracing. Bladder compliance at a volume of 750 mL-20 mL/cm H_2O. When asked to void he strained and voided out the urodynamic catheter. There was no detrusor contraction.

completely asymptomatic. A voiding diary showed a 24-hour volume of 1830 mL with 6 voids; MVV = 390; VOID: 13/643/9.

Discussion: Remember back to SJ? He had low bladder compliance and severe prostatic obstruction documented by pressure flow studies. SO was not so fortunate. He had low bladder compliance and urinary retention, but did not have a detrusor contraction during the urodynamic study and would be thought, by most, to have an

areflexic or acontractile detrusor. Such a patient is often denied the opportunity of outlet reducing surgery because his obstruction has not been "proven."

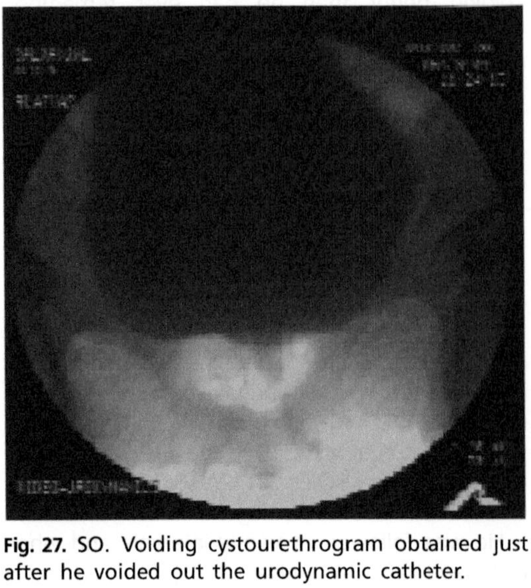

Years ago, as a young academic, I brought a urodynamic tracing with me to the annual meeting of the AUA. It was similar to SO—low bladder compliance and urinary retention, but no detrusor contraction. I had treated him with SIC, but he was not satisfied and wanted something more. The BPH/urodynamic pundits at the time all gave the same advice—"just TURP him; he'll do fine." And so I did and so he was, and I acquired an important lesson. The science of medicine can take you just so far. There are things that we just don't yet understand, but experience is still a good teacher—that's what empirical medicine (as opposed to evidence-based medicine) is all about. I think there is still room for both.

Does that mean that you should offer ablative prostatic surgery to all men with urinary retention and low bladder compliance who do not have detrusor contractions? No! Therein lies the importance of VUDS. Obviously, if the prostatic urethra is wide open during bladder filling or attempts to void, prostatic surgery has no place and may cause sphincteric incontinence. These findings (an open bladder neck and acontractile, low compliance bladder) are characteristic of thoracolumbar neurologic disorders and peripheral sympathetic and parasympathetic decentralization after radical

Fig. 27. SO. Voiding cystourethrogram obtained just after he voided out the urodynamic catheter.

pelvic surgery.[8] In the case of SO, there was a TURP defect during filling, but his was due to prior prostatic surgery.

REFERENCES

1. Strasser H, Pinggera GM, Hohlbrugger G, et al. Alpha-blockers increase vesical and prostatic blood flow and bladder capacity. Heidelberg, Germany: International Continence Society; 2002. abstract #455.
2. Pinggera GM, Mitterberger M, Pallvein L, et al. Alpha-blockers improve chronic ischaemia of the lower urinary tract in patients with lower urinary tract symptoms. BJU Int 2008;101(3):319–24.
3. Sfakianos JP, Weiss JP, Dovirak O, et al. The significance of prostate volume to biopsy core sample ratio on cancer detection rates. J Urol 2009; 181(4):710.
4. Sakamoto K, Blaivas JG. Adult onset nocturnal enuresis. J Urol 2001;165:1914–7.
5. Blaivas JG. Urodynamic diagnosis of primary bladder neck obstruction. World J Urol 1984;2:191.
6. Purohit RS, Blaivas JG, Saleem KL, et al. The pathophysiology of large capacity bladder. J Urol 2008; 179(3):1006–11.
7. Clayman RV, Shahin S, Reddy P, et al. Transurethral treatment of bladder diverticula. Alternative to open diverticulectomy. Urology 1984;23(6): 573–7.
8. Barbalias GA, Blaivas JG. Neurourologic implications of the pathologically open bladder neck. J Urol 1983; 129:780–3.

Index

Note: Page numbers of article titles are in **boldface** type.

Urol Clin N Am 36 (2009) 571–575
doi:10.1016/S0094-0143(09)00089-5

urologic.theclinics.com

United States Postal Service

Statement of Ownership, Management, and Circulation
(All Periodicals Publications Except Requestor Publications)

1. Publication Title	2. Publication Number	3. Filing Date
Urologic Clinics of North America	0 0 0 - 7 1 1	9/15/09

4. Issue Frequency	5. Number of Issues Published Annually	6. Annual Subscription Price
Feb, May, Aug, Nov	4	$269.00

7. Complete Mailing Address of Known Office of Publication (Not printer) (Street, city, county, state, and ZIP+4®)

Elsevier Inc.
360 Park Avenue South
New York, NY 10010-1710

Contact Person
Stephen Bushing
Telephone (Include area code)
215-239-3688

8. Complete Mailing Address of Headquarters or General Business Office of Publisher (Not printer)

Elsevier Inc., 360 Park Avenue South, New York, NY 10010-1710

9. Full Names and Complete Mailing Addresses of Publisher, Editor, and Managing Editor (Do not leave blank)

Publisher (Name and complete mailing address)

John Schrefer, Elsevier, Inc., 1600 John F. Kennedy Blvd. Suite 1800, Philadelphia, PA 19103-2899

Editor (Name and complete mailing address)

Kerry Holland, Elsevier, Inc., 1600 John F. Kennedy Blvd. Suite 1800, Philadelphia, PA 19103-2899

Managing Editor (Name and complete mailing address)

Catherine Bewick, Elsevier, Inc., 1600 John F. Kennedy Blvd. Suite 1800, Philadelphia, PA 19103-2899

10. Owner (Do not leave blank. If the publication is owned by a corporation, give the name and address of the corporation immediately followed by the names and addresses of all stockholders owning or holding 1 percent or more of the total amount of stock. If not owned by a corporation, give the names and addresses of the individual owners. If owned by a partnership or other unincorporated firm, give its name and address as well as those of each individual owner. If the publication is published by a nonprofit organization, give its name and address.)

Full Name	Complete Mailing Address
Wholly owned subsidiary of	4520 East-West Highway
Reed/Elsevier, US holdings	Bethesda, MD 20814

11. Known Bondholders, Mortgagees, and Other Security Holders Owning or Holding 1 Percent or More of Total Amount of Bonds, Mortgages, or Other Securities. If none, check box ☐

Full Name	Complete Mailing Address
N/A	

12. Tax Status (For completion by nonprofit organizations authorized to mail at nonprofit rates) (Check one)
The purpose, function, and nonprofit status of this organization and the exempt status for federal income tax purposes:
☐ Has Not Changed During Preceding 12 Months
☐ Has Changed During Preceding 12 Months (Publisher must submit explanation of change with this statement)

PS Form 3526, September 2007 (Page 1 of 3 (Instructions Page 3)) PSN 7530-01-000-9931 PRIVACY NOTICE: See our Privacy policy in www.usps.com

---

13. Publication Title	14. Issue Date for Circulation Data Below
Urologic Clinics of North America	August 2009

15. Extent and Nature of Circulation			Average No. Copies Each Issue During Preceding 12 Months	No. Copies of Single Issue Published Nearest to Filing Date
a. Total Number of Copies (Net press run)			3475	3200
b. Paid Circulation (By Mail and Outside the Mail)	(1)	Mailed Outside-County Paid Subscriptions Stated on PS Form 3541. (Include paid distribution above nominal rate, advertiser's proof copies, and exchange copies)	1313	1217
	(2)	Mailed In-County Paid Subscriptions Stated on PS Form 3541 (Include paid distribution above nominal rate, advertiser's proof copies, and exchange copies)		
	(3)	Paid Distribution Outside the Mails Including Sales Through Dealers and Carriers, Street Vendors, Counter Sales, and Other Paid Distribution Outside USPS®	1106	1057
	(4)	Paid Distribution by Other Classes Mailed Through the USPS (e.g. First-Class Mail®)		
c. Total Paid Distribution (Sum of 15b (1), (2), (3), and (4))		►	2419	2274
d. Free or Nominal Rate Distribution (By Mail and Outside the Mail)	(1)	Free or Nominal Rate Outside-County Copies Included on PS Form 3541	112	102
	(2)	Free or Nominal Rate In-County Copies Included on PS Form 3541		
	(3)	Free or Nominal Rate Copies Mailed at Other Classes Through the USPS (e.g. First-Class Mail)		
	(4)	Free or Nominal Rate Distribution Outside the Mail (Carriers or other means)		
e. Total Free or Nominal Rate Distribution (Sum of 15d (1), (2), (3) and (4))		►	112	102
f. Total Distribution (Sum of 15c and 15e)		►	2531	2376
g. Copies not Distributed (See instructions to publishers #4 (page #3))		►	944	824
h. Total (Sum of 15f and g)		►	3475	3200
i. Percent Paid (15c divided by 15f times 100)			95.57%	95.71%

16. Publication of Statement of Ownership
If the publication is a general publication, publication of this statement is required. Will be printed
in the November 2009 issue of this publication. ☐ Publication not required

17. Signature and Title of Editor, Publisher, Business Manager, or Owner

Stephen R. Bushing – Subscription Services Coordinator
Date September 15, 2009

I certify that all information furnished on this form is true and complete. I understand that anyone who furnishes false or misleading information on this form or who omits material or information requested on the form may be subject to criminal sanctions (including fines and imprisonment) and/or civil sanctions (including civil penalties).

PS Form 3526, September 2007 (Page 2 of 3)

Moving?

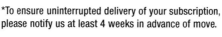